Push your Career Publish your Thesis

Science should be accessible to everybody. Share the knowledge, the ideas, and the passion about your research. Give your part of the infinite amount of scientific research possibilities a finite frame.

Publish your examination paper, diploma thesis, bachelor thesis, master thesis, dissertation, or habilitation treatises in form of a book.

A finite frame by infinite science.

Infinite Science
Publishing

A University Press imprint of
Infinite Science GmbH
MFC 1 | Technikzentrum Lübeck
BioMedTec Wissenschaftscampus
Maria-Goeppert-Straße 1
23562 Lübeck
book@infinite-science.de
www.infinite-science.de

Infinite Science
Publishing

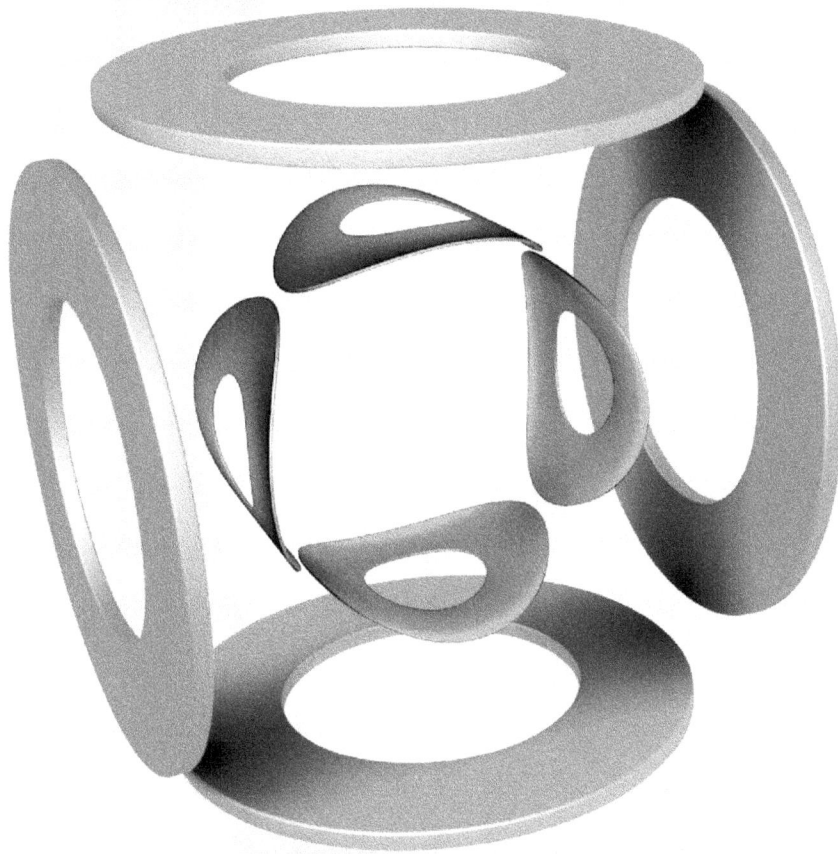

8th International Workshop on

Magnetic Particle Imaging
IWMPI 2018

March 22–24, 2018 | Hamburg, Germany

Book of Abstracts

T. Knopp and T. M. Buzug (Eds.)

© 2018 Infinite Science Publishing
         University Press and
         Academic Printing

Imprint of Infinite Science GmbH,
MFC 1 | BioMedTec Wissenschaftscampus
Maria-Goeppert-Straße 1
23562 Lübeck, Germany

Cover Design and Illustration: Uli Schmidts, metonym
Editorial: Universität zu Lübeck

Publisher: Infinite Science GmbH, Lübeck, www.infinite-science.de
Printed in Germany, BoD, Norderstedt

ISBN Paperback: 978-3-945954-48-5

Bibliografische Information der Deutschen Nationalbibliothek:
Die Deutsche Nationalbibliothek verzeichnet diese Publikation in der Deutschen Nationalbibliografie; detaillierte bibliografische Daten sind im Internet über http://dnb.d nb.de abrufbar.

Scientific Commitees

Workshop Chairs

Tobias Knopp	University Medical Center Hamburg-Eppendorf (UKE)	Germany
Thorsten M. Buzug	University of Lübeck	Germany

Program Committee

Gerhard Adam	University Medical Center Hamburg-Eppendorf (UKE)	Germany
Christoph Alexiou	University Medical Center Erlangen	Germany
Meltem Asilturk Akdeniz	University, Antalya	Turkey
Jörg Barkhausen	UKSH Lübeck	Germany
Volker Behr	University of Würzburg	Germany
Ayhan Bingolbali	Yildiz Technical University, Istanbul	Turkey
Jeff Bulte	John Hopkins University, Baltimore	USA
Thorsten M. Buzug	University of Lübeck	Germany
Steven M. Conolly	University of California, Berkeley	USA
Nurcan Dogan	Gebze Institute of Technology, Kocaeli	Turkey
Silvio Dutz	Technical University of Ilmenau	Germany
Matthew Ferguson	LodeSpin Labs, Seattle	USA
Dominique Finas	Evangelisches Krankenhaus Bielefeld	Germany
Patrick W. Goodwill	University of California, Berkeley	USA
Mark Griswold	Case Western Reserve University, Cleveland	USA
Urs Häfeli	University of British Columbia, Vancouver	Canada
Jens Haueisen	Technical University of Ilmenau	Germany
Michael Heidenreich	Bruker BioSpin MRI GmbH, Ettlingen	Germany
Ulrich Heinen	Pforzheim University of Applied Sciences	Germany
Yasutoshi Ishihara	Meiji University, Tokyo	Japan
Peter Jakob	University of Würzburg	Germany
Fabian Kiesling	UKA Aachen	Germany
Tobias Knopp	University Medical Center Hamburg-Eppendorf (UKE)	Germany
Kannan Krishnan	University of Washington, Seattle	USA
Wenzhong Liu	Huazhong University of Science and Technology	China
Frank Ludwig	Technical University of Braunschweig	Germany
Mauro Magnani	University of Urbino	Italy
Kenya Murase	Osaka University	Japan
Jan Niehaus	CAN Center für Applied Nanotechnology, Hamburg	Germany
Stefan Odenbach	Technical University of Dresden	Germany
Quentin Pankhurst	University College London	UK
Ulrich Pison	Charité Universitätsmedizin Mitte, Berlin	Germany
Anna Cristina Samia	Case Western Reserve University, Cleveland	USA
Emine Ulku Saritas	Bilkent University, Bilkent/Ankara	Turkey
Meinhard Schilling	Technical University of Braunschweig	Germany
Jörg Schnorr	Charité Universitätsmedizin Mitte, Berlin	Germany
Ludek Sefc	Charles University, Prague	Czech Republik
Michael Taupitz	Charité Universitätsmedizin, Berlin	Germany
Bennie ten Haken	University of Twente, Enschede	Germany
Alexey Tonyushkin	University of Massachusetts, Boston	USA
Lutz Trahms	PTB Physikalisch-Technische Bundesanstalt, Berlin	Germany
John B. Weaver	Dartmouth-Hitchcock Medical Center, Lebanon	USA
Oliver Weber	Philips Hamburg	Germany
Antoine Weis	University of Fribourg	Switzerland
Jürgen Weizenecker	University of Applied Sciences, Karlsruhe	Germany
Frank Wiekhorst	PTB Physikalisch-Technische Bundesanstalt, Berlin	Germany
Barbara Wollenberg	University Medical Center Schleswig-Holstein, Lübeck	Germany

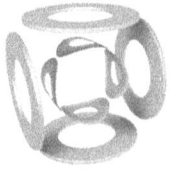

International Workshop on
Magnetic Particle Imaging
IWMPI

Technical Commitees

Organization

Infinite Science is in charge of marketing, registration and publication of IWMPI. Infinite Science provides the platforms iwmpi.org and the open access journal IJMPI https://journal.iwmpi.org.

Registration and Administration

Kanina Neideck, General Manager, Infinite Science GmbH
E-mail: neideck@infinite-science.de

Infinite Science GmbH
BioMedTec Wissenschaftscampus
Maria-Goeppert-Str. 1, 23562 Lübeck, Germany
Email: info@iwmpi.org

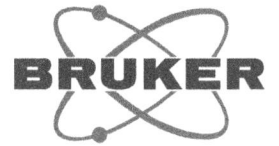

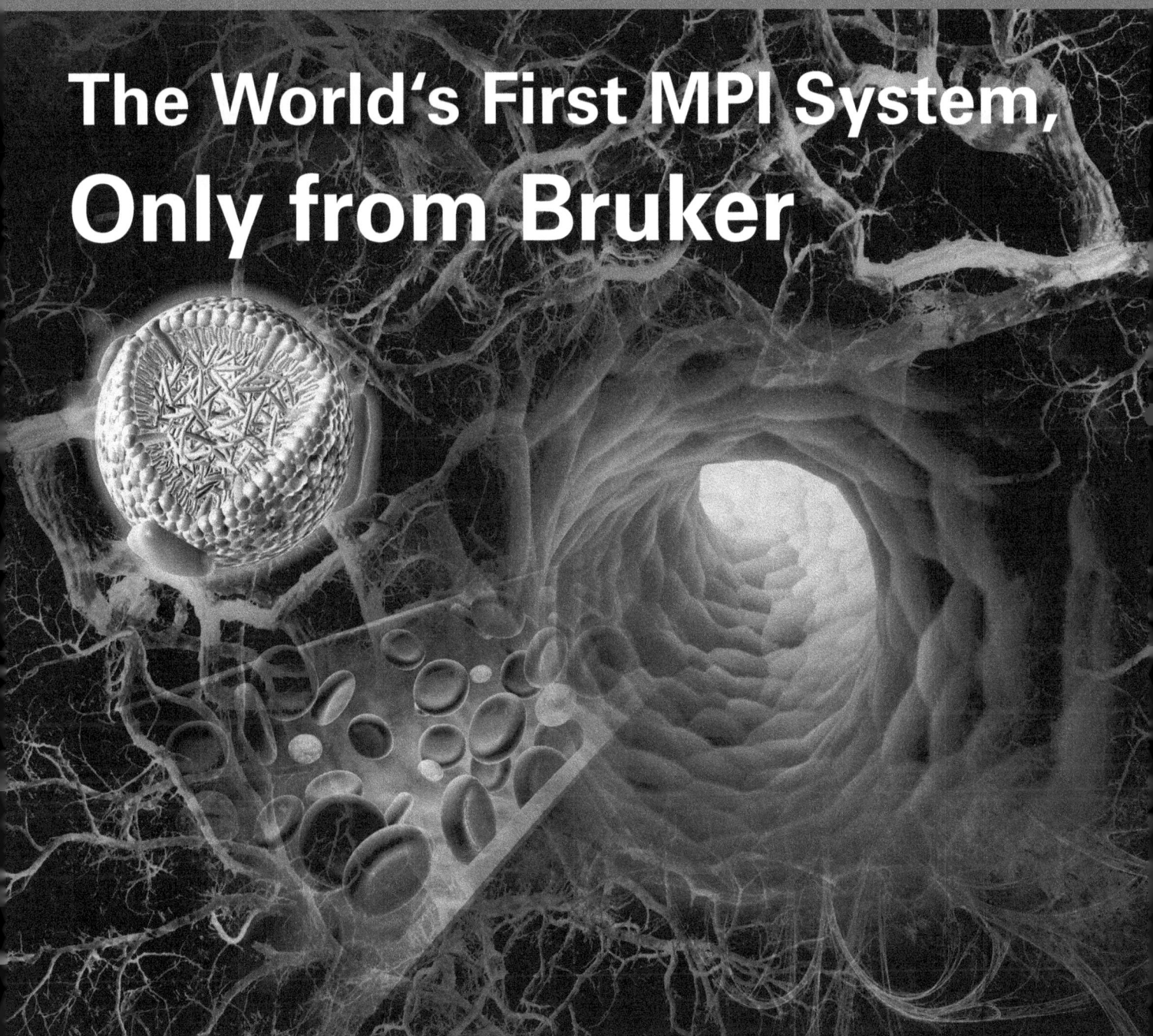

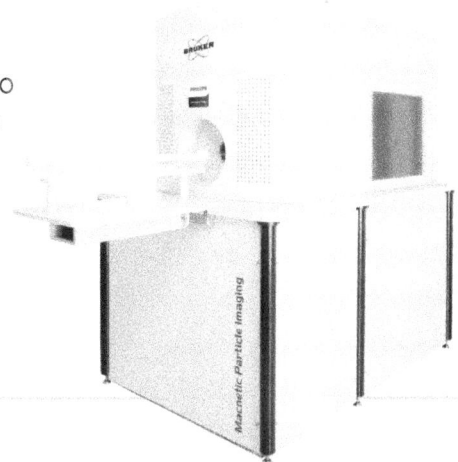

Titles on Magnetic Particle Imaging by Infinite Science Publishing

Bildgebungs-konzepte für das Magnetic Particle Imaging
Mandy Ahlborg
EUR 79,90
Hardcover, 156 S.

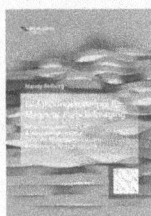

Magnetic Particle Imaging mit einer asymmetrischen Spulentopologie
Ksenija Gräfe
EUR 79,90
Hardcover, 162 S.

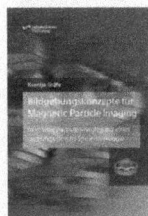

Echtzeitbildgebung mittels Magnetic Particle Imaging
Klaas Bente
EUR 79,90
Hardcover, 172 S.

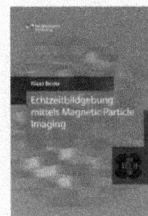

Behandlung von Imperfektionen bei Magnetic Particle Imaging
Alexander Weber
EUR 89,90
Hardcover, 196 S.

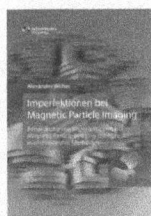

Neuartige Bildge-bungskonzepte mit einer feldfeien Linie
Matthias Weber
EUR 89,90
Hardcover, 194 S.

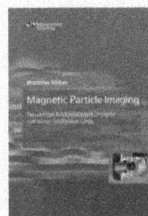

Strategien zur ef-fizienten Nutzung und Erweiterung des Messfeldes
Christian Kaethner
EUR 89,90
Hardcover, 224 S.

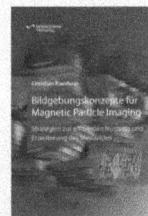

Scannertopologien und Optimierung von Feldsequen-zen für Magnetic Particle Imaging
Timo F. Sattel
EUR 89,90
Hardcover, 184 S.

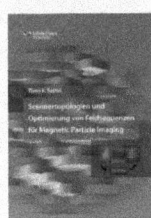

Biokompatible superpara-magnetische Nanopartikel
David Heinke
EUR 59,90
Paperback, 142 S.

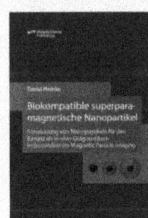

Lernen spärlicher Repräsentationen für die verbesserte MPI-Rekonstruktion
Patrik Bedei
EUR 39,90
Paperback, 76 S.

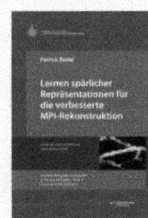

Infinite Science Publishing

www.publishing.infinite-science.de

Infinite Science GmbH
MFC 1 | BioMedTec Wissenschaftscampus
Maria-Goeppert-Str. 1, 23562 Lübeck
book@infinite-science.de

micromod **Partikeltechnologie GmbH**

For more than **20 years** micromod has been the reliable supplier of particle-based system components for *in vitro* diagnostics, high-throughput screening, magnetic bio-separation, cell labeling as well as a partner in R&D of novel components for diagnosis (MPI, MRI) and cancer therapy (hyperthermia). A modern quality management according to EN ISO 13485:2012/AC:2012 ensures a high quality standard in the development and production of **micro- and nanoparticles**.

synomag® - our new Nanoflower-shaped Magnetic Nanoparticles with Excellent Properties

➡ as tracer for Magnetic Particle Imaging (MPI)

➡ as contrast agent for Magnetic Resonance Imaging (MRI)

➡ for hyperthermia applications

➡ as tool for biosensor and lab-on-chip applications

Magnetic Particle Spectra:

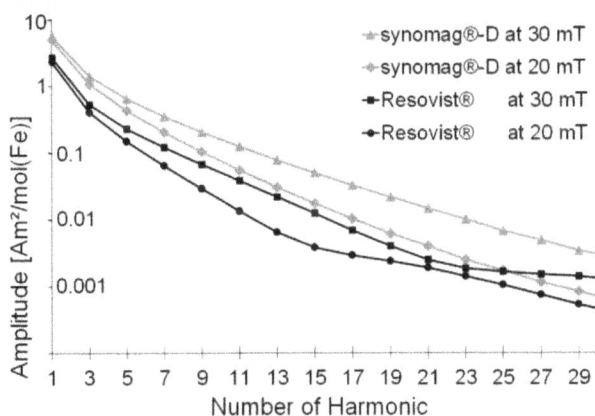

Magnetic Particle Spectra (MPS) of 50 nm synomag®-D particles at 20 and 30 mT, amplitude of odd harmonics scaled to the amount of iron compared to Resovist®
(C. Grüttner *et al. Proceedings of IWMPI 2018*)

TEM images of synomag®-D:

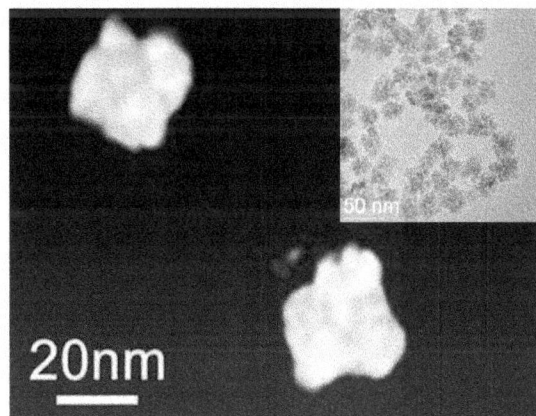

TEM tomography image of synomag®-D with a closer look at two particles viewed parallel to the electron beam direction
(L.J. Zeng, Chalmers University of Technology, Göteborg)

- **The amplitude A3 of the 3rd harmonic in the MPS spectrum of synomag® Is more than twice as high as that of Resovist®.**

- **synomag®-D have a very high intrinsic loss power (ILP) of about 7 nHm²/kgFe** (P. Bender et al. J. Phys. Chem. C, 2017, DOI: 10.1021/acs.jpcc.7b11255)

(12) INTERNATIONAL APPLICATION PUBLISHED UNDER THE PATENT COOPERATION TREATY (PCT)

(19) World Intellectual Property Organization
International Bureau

(43) International Publication Date
4 January 2007 (04.01.2007)

PCT

(10) International Publication Number
WO 2007/000350 A1

(51) International Patent Classification:
A61K 49/18 (2006.01)

(21) International Application Number:
PCT/EP2006/006319

(22) International Filing Date: 29 June 2006 (29.06.2006)

(25) Filing Language: English

(26) Publication Language: English

(30) Priority Data:
05014059.9   29 June 2005 (29.06.2005)   EP

(71) Applicant (*for all designated States except US*): SCHERING AG [DE/DE]; Müllerstrasse 170-178, 13342 Berlin (DE).

(71) Applicant (*for all designated States except DE, US*): KONINKLIJKE PHILIPS ELECTRONICS N.V. [NL/NL]; Groenewoudseweg 1, NL-5621 BA Eindhoven (NL).

(71) Applicant (*for DE only*): PHILIPS INTELLECTUAL PROPERTY & STANDARDS GMBH [DE/DE]; Steindamm 94, 20099 Hamburg (DE).

(72) Inventors; and
(75) Inventors/Applicants (*for US only*): BRIEL, Andreas [DE/DE]; Garnestrasse 10, 10245 Berlin (DE). GLEICH, Bernhard [DE/DE]; Rübenhofstrasse 41, 22335 Hamburg (DE). WEIZENECKER, Jürgen [DE/DE]; Reekamp 39, 22415 Hamburg (DE). ROHRER, Martin [DE/DE]; Victoriastrasse 13, 12203 Berlin (DE). WEINMANN, Hanns-Joachim [DE/DE]; Westhofener Weg

23, 14129 Berlin (DE). PIETSCH, Hubertus [DE/DE]; Ingwäonenweg 147, 13127 Berlin (DE). LAWACZECK, Rüdiger [DE/DE]; Bevschlagstrasse 8c, 13503 Berlin

(74)

(81)

(84)

GM, KE, LS, MW, MZ, NA, SD, SL, SZ, TZ, UG, ZM, ZW), Eurasian (AM, AZ, BY, KG, KZ, MD, RU, TJ, TM), European (AT, BE, BG, CH, CY, CZ, DE, DK, EE, ES, FI, FR, GB, GR, HU, IE, IS, IT, LT, LU, LV, MC, NL, PL, PT, RO, SE, SI, SK, TR), OAPI (BF, BJ, CF, CG, CI, CM, GA, GN, GQ, GW, ML, MR, NE, SN, TD, TG).

Published:
—   *with international search report*

For two-letter codes and other abbreviations, refer to the "Guidance Notes on Codes and Abbreviations" appearing at the beginning of each regular issue of the PCT Gazette.

(54) Title: COMPOSITIONS CONTAINING MAGNETIC IRON OXIDE PARTICLES, AND USE OF SAID COMPOSITIONS IN MAGNETIC PARTICLE IMAGING

(57) Abstract: The present invention relates to complexes which contain magnetic iron oxide particles in a pharmaceutically acceptable shell, said particles having a diameter of 20 nm to 1 μm with an overall particle diameter/core diameter ratio of less than 6, and ... ... complexes in magnetic particle imaging (MPI). Particular preference is given to the use of these compositions in ... ... of the heart and cranial components, in the diagnosis of arteriosclerosis, infa...

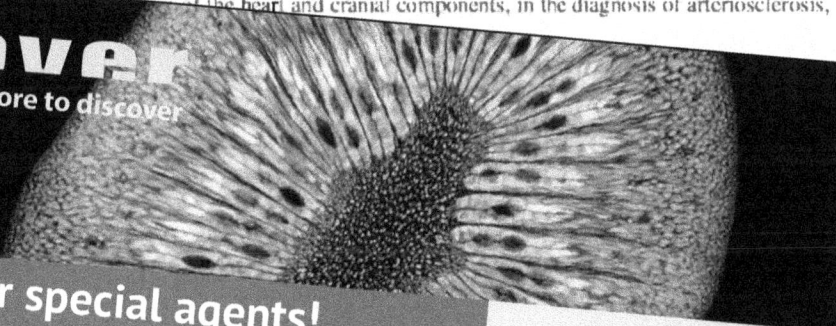

WO 2007/000350 A1

Unser Qualitätsmaßstab ganz oben

Höchste Qualität in allen Bereichen: Produktion, Service, Fortbildungen.

Auf Bayer Radiologie können Sie sich verlassen.

radiologie.bayer.de

L.DE.MKT.DI.04.2017.0836

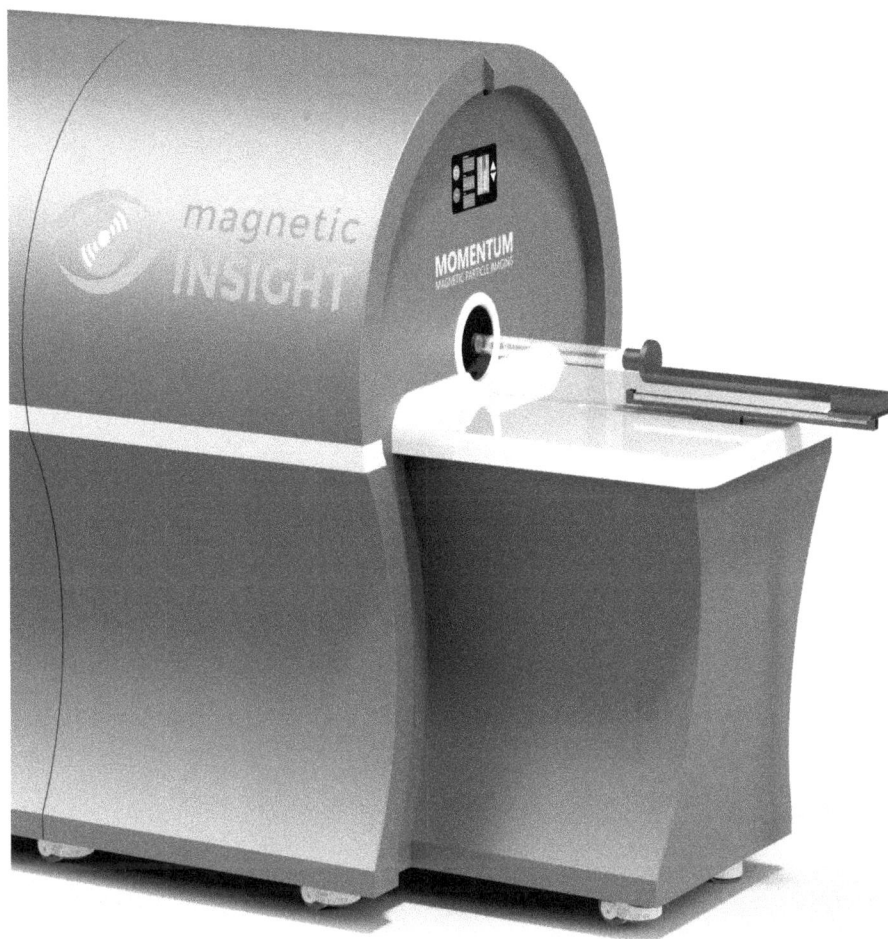

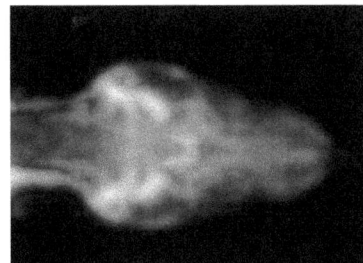

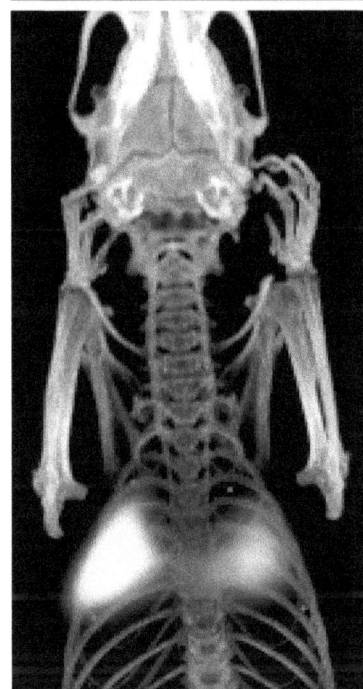

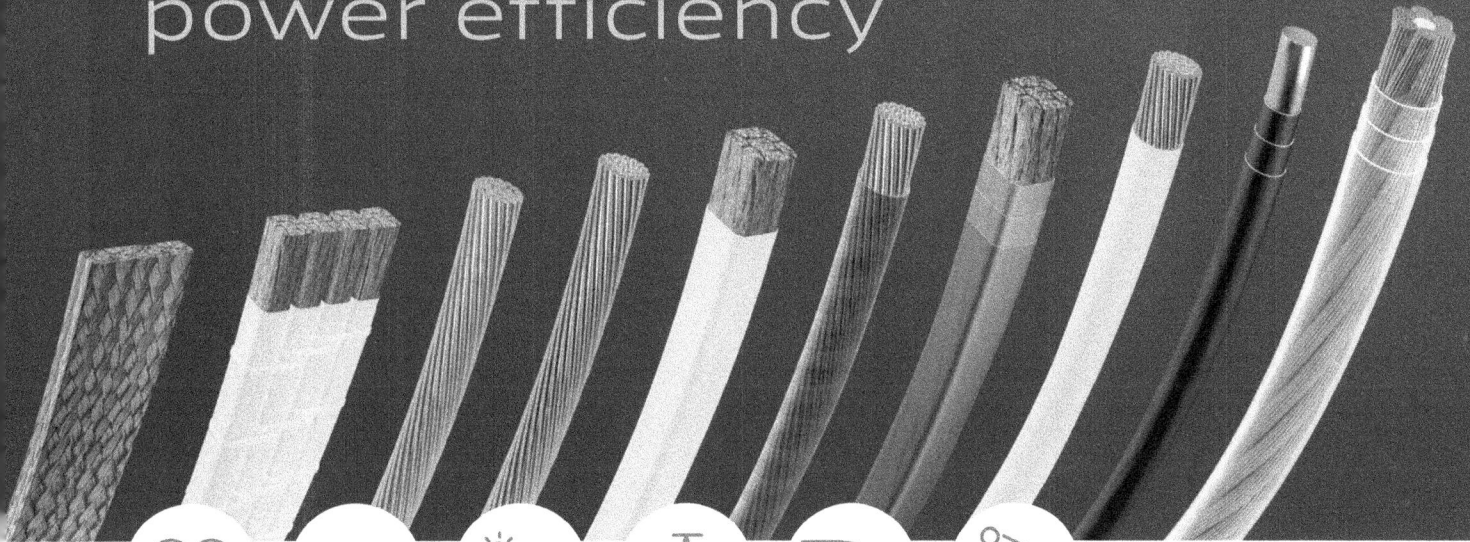

mps

pd
pure devices

Magnetic Particle Spectrometer

mps unit
magnetic particle spectroscopy

drive

Characterization of

contrast agents
magnetic particles
MPI tracers
ferrofluides

Specifications

drive field: 0 - 30 mT
frequency: 20 kHz
bandwidth: 2.5 MHZ
test tubes: 6 mm

easy to set up

easy to operate

pd
pure devices

Pure Devices GmbH
Eisenbahnstr. 53
97084 Würzburg
GERMANY

www.pure-devices.com
info@pure-devices.com
Tel.: +49 (0) 931 71053590
Fax: +49 (0) 931 71053595

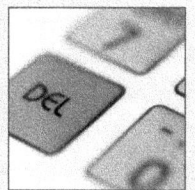

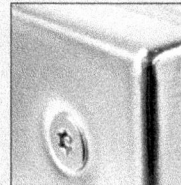

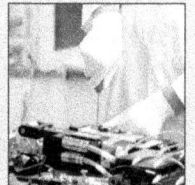

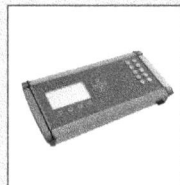

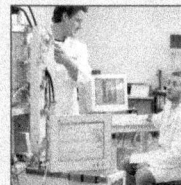

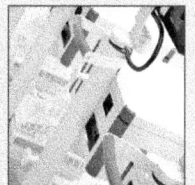

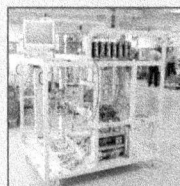

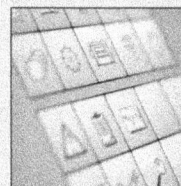

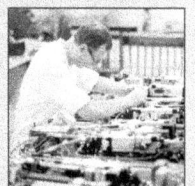

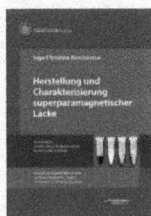

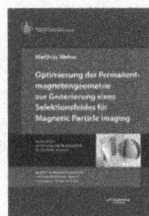

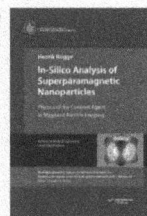

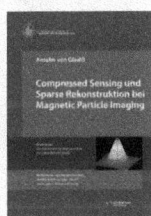

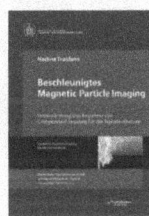

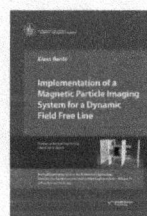

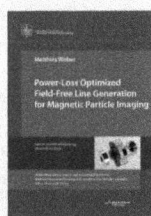

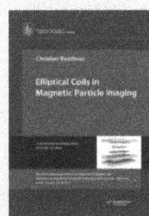

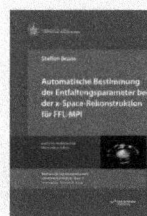

Book of Abstracts 2018

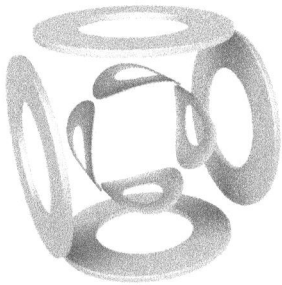

International Workshop on
Magnetic Particle Imaging
IWMPI

Preface and Acknowledgements

Dear Colleagues,

we are very pleased to host the 8th International Workshop on Magnetic Particle Imaging in Hamburg and would like to thank Ludek Sefc, Charles University and his team for the outstanding meeting IWMPI2017 in exciting Prague. We are proud to announce contributions of participants from 10 countries presenting 45 talks and 47 posters. This year's keynote speech is given by Lawrence L. Wald, Professor of Radiology, Harvard Medical School on 'Assessing MPI as a Functional Brain Imaging Modality'.

Since the first workshop in 2010, the International Workshop on MPI (IWMPI) has been the premier forum for researchers working in the MPI field. The workshop aims at covering the status and recent developments of both the instrumentation and the tracer material, as they are equally important in designing a well performing MPI system. The main topics presented at the workshop include hardware developments, image reconstruction and systems theory, nanoparticle physics and theory, nanoparticle synthesis, spectroscopy, patient safety, and medical/research applications of MPI.

We encourage you and your colleagues to contribute your research and results to IWMPI, where you will have an opportunity to interact and collaborate with the greater MPI community, and to take steps in advancing the field of MPI. The workshop will provide a great opportunity to present your research results, as well as to learn more about the technical aspects and clinical potential of MPI.

In 2015, the International Journal on Magnetic Particle Imaging (IJMPI) has been launched as a future format for publishing high quality research articles on MPI (journal.iwmpi. org). The scope of the IJMPI ranges from imaging sequences and reconstruction over scanner instrumentation as well as particle synthesis and particle physics to pre-clinical and potential future clinical applications. Journal articles will be published online with open access under a Creative Commons License. In order to share ideas and experiences with a focused audience, we encourage submission of research papers to the new journal. IJMPI will publish research articles that can be submitted at any time.

As chairs of the workshop we would like to thank the members of the program committee for their exceptional service for the MPI community: G. Adam, University Medical Center Hamburg-Eppendorf (UKE); C. Alexiou, University Medical Center Erlangen; M. Asilturk, Akdeniz University, Antalya; J. Barkhausen, UKSH Lübeck; V. Behr, University of Würzburg; A. Bingolbali, Yildiz Technical University, Istanbul; J. Bulte, John Hopkins University, Baltimore; T. M. Buzug, University of Lübeck; S. M. Conolly, University of California, Berkeley; N. Dogan, Gebze Institute of Technology, Kocaeli; S. Dutz, Technical University of Ilmenau; M. Ferguson, LodeSpin Labs, Seattle; D. Finas, Evangelisches Krankenhaus Bielefeld; P. W. Goodwill, University of California, Berkeley; M. Griswold, Case Western Reserve University, Cleveland; U. Häfeli, University of British Columbia, Vancouver; J. Haueisen, Technical University of Ilmenau; M. Heidenreich, Bruker BioSpin, Ettlingen; U. Heinen, Pforzheim University of Applied Sciences; Y. Ishihara, Meiji University, Tokyo; P. Jakob, University of Würzburg; F. Kiesslinh, UKA Aachen; T. Knopp, University Medical Center Hamburg-Eppendorf; K. Krishnan, University of Washington, Seattle; Liu Wnezong, Huazhong University of Science and Technology; F. Ludwig, Technical University of Braunschweig; M. Magnani, University of Urbino; Kenya Murase, Osaka University; J. Niehaus, CAN Center for Applied Nanotechnology, Hamburg; S. Odenbach, Technical University of Dresden; Quentin Pankhurst, University College London; U. Pison, Charité, Berlin; A. C. Samia, Case Western Reserve University, Cleveland; E. U. Saritas, Bilkent University, Bilkent/ Ankara; M. Schilling, Technical University of Braunschweig; J. Schnorr, Charité, Berlin; Ludek Sefc, Charles University, Prague; Michael Taupitz, Charité Universitätsmedizin, Berlin; B. ten Haken, University of Twente, Enschede; Alexey Tonyushkin, University of Massachusetts, Boston; L. Trahms, PTB, Berlin; J. B. Weaver, Dartmouth-Hitchcock Medical Center, Lebanon; Oliver Weber, Philips Hamburg; Antoine Weis, University of Fribourg; J. Weizenecker, University of Applied Sciences, Karlsruhe; F. Wiekhorst, PTB, Berlin; B. Wollenberg, UKSH Lübeck.

Most importantly, we would like to thank our partners for their support and cooperation: Bruker BioSpin, magnetic INSIGHT, nanoPET Pharma, Micromod, Bayer Vital, PMB of IOP, Pure Devices, PACK LitzWire, Lacon Group, Schwartau and we would also like to extend our gratitude to the marketing alliance with the World Molecular Imaging Society (WMIS), the German Scociety of Biomedical Engineering (DGBMT), and the Germany Life-Science North Cluster (LSN). Special thanks go to the members of the local organization teams at UKE Hamburg and Infinite Science for their outstanding efforts and work.

We wish all of us an inspiring workshop.

Tobias Knopp, Thorsten M. Buzug
Hamburg, March 2018

Partner of IWMPI 2018

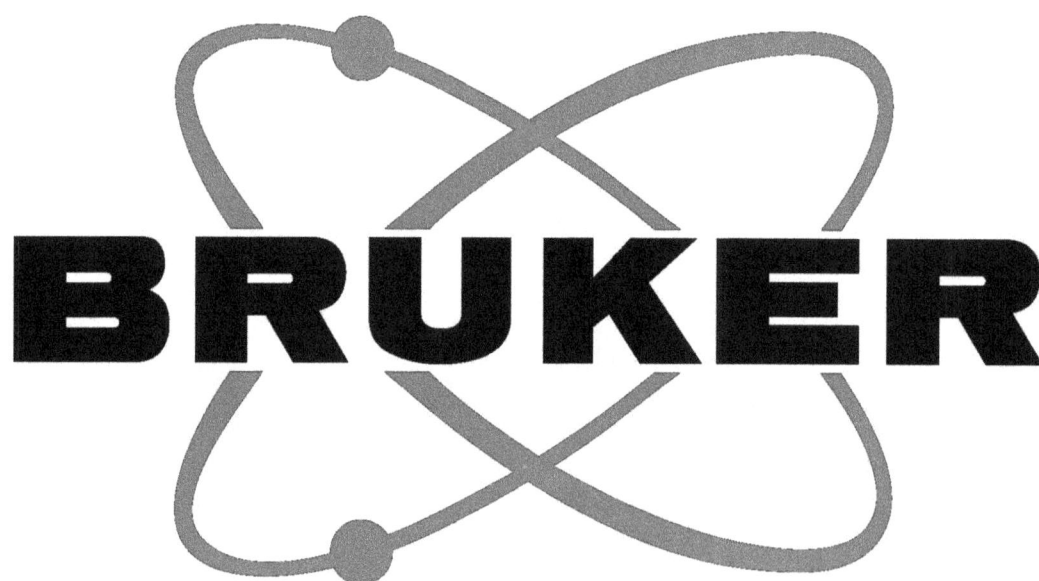

Marketing Alliance IWMPI 2018

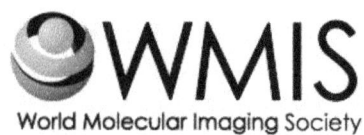

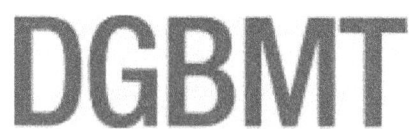

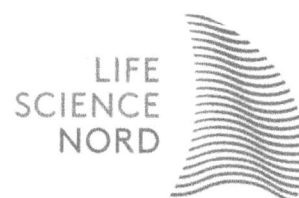

Sponsors and Exhibitors of IWMPI 2018

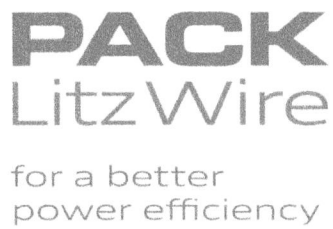

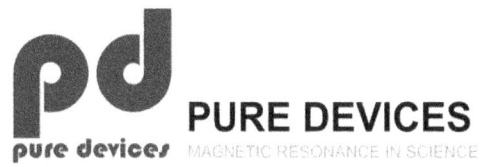

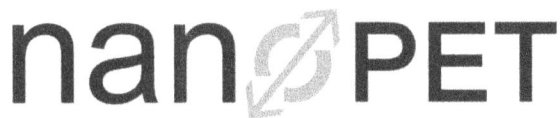

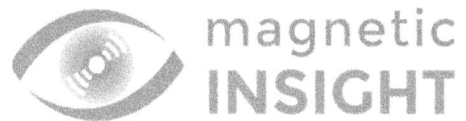

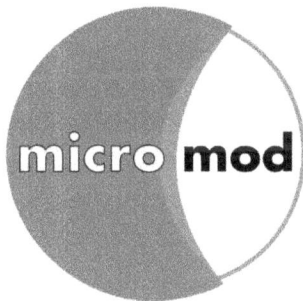

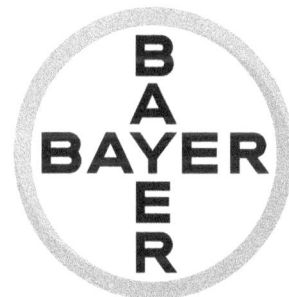

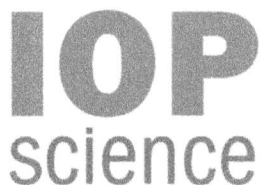

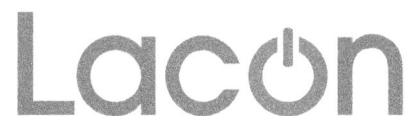

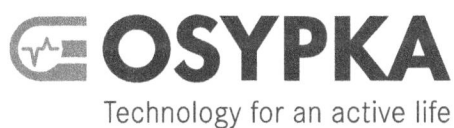

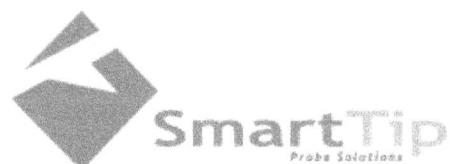

PACK LitzWire
for a better
power efficiency

pd pure devices **PURE DEVICES** MAGNETIC RESONANCE IN SCIENCE

nanoPET

magnetic INSIGHT

micro mod

BAYER

IOP science

Lacon

OSYPKA
Technology for an active life

SmartTip
Probe Solutions

Table of Contents

Session 11 - Applications III

Session 12 - Survey on Applications

Session 13 - Instrumentation IV

Keynote by Lawrence L. Wald

Keynote: Assessing MPI as a Functional Brain Imaging Modality

Lawrence L. Wald [a,b,c,*], Cooley Clarissa [a,b], Erica Mason [a,c], Eli Mattingly [a], Mathias Davids [d]

[a] A.A. Martinos Center, Dept. of Radiology, Massachusetts General Hospital, Bosotn, USA
[b] Harvard Medical School, Boston, MA, USA
[c] Harvard-MIT Health Sciences & Technology, Cambridge, MA, USA
[d] Comp. Assist. Clinical Medicine, Medical Faculty Mannheim, Heidelberg University, Heidelberg, Germany
[*] Corresponding author, email: wald@nmr.mgh.harvard.edu

I. Introduction

Functional brain imaging has played an important role in recent advances in human neuroscience, allowing traditional psychology experiments to be carried out during non-invasive imaging sensitive to the metabolic or hemodynamic effects of brain activation. This has allowed human neuroscience to move from indirect measurements such as subject responses and reaction times to direct interrogation of the brain regions and circuits used in a task. The application of functional brain imaging has become so central to human neuroscience that most major psychology/neuroscience departments at US universities now operate an fMRI facility.

While fMRI is valued for its ability to noninvasively map the hemodynamic response to brain activation, its sensitivity is relatively low. Studies typically require repeated trials and are averaged across multiple subjects to achieve statistical significance. The consequence of low CNR extends beyond the inconvenience of averaging and missing subtle effects. It prevents fMRI from impacting clinical medicine where decisions must be made for an individual, not a group average. The ability to make statements about a brain circuit's function or dysfunction in individuals could provide means of phenotyping spectrum diseases such as the major mental illnesses; a potential breakthrough for diagnosis and treatment.

II. Material and Methods

MPI [1] offers an attractive and potentially very sensitive compliment to fMRI. We propose using a similar hemodynamic contrast mechanism; the local Cerebral Blood Volume changes during activation.[3] Since injected SPIONs do not cross the blood-brain barrier, the direct measure of SPION concentration provided by MPI is a measure of local CBV and CBV changes (~20% during brain activation) will be directly effected in a time-series of MPI images. Such CBV measures are currently the most sensitive way to perform fMRI. We validated the sensitivity of MPI detection to CBV changes by applying controlled periods of O_2/CO_2 inhalation in a rat while monitoring the MPI signal. These hypoxic and hyperoxic challenge are known to modulate global brain CBV about 25% and showed promising CNR compared to fMRI. We also observed physiological fluctuations in the rodent resting CBV levels similar to those seen in fMRI. This raises the possibility that brain regions displaying correlated hemodynamic MPI resting state signals could be used to establish functional connectivity networks in an analogous way to resting-state fMRI.

III. Results

Together, this has motivated us to continue to develop fMPI. We are constructing FFL [2] imagers further targeting rodent fMPI and a larger scanner for primate fMPI including humans. Since Peripheral Nerve Stimulation (PNS) is an important concern for human MPI, we have focused on advancing our understanding and ability to predict this effect. Our model consists of a comprehensive body model for EM simulations, a detailed atlas of human nerve fiber geometry and properties, and a numerical model describing nerve responses to the induced electrical fields. We show that this model can correctly estimate the observed experimental PNS thresholds in MPI solenoids[4] and MRI gradient coils[5]. Perhaps more importantly it shows the location and etiology of the stimulation and allows the testing of mitigation strategies.

ACKNOWLEDGEMENTS
Funding from the National Institutes of Health under award number U01EB025121.

REFERENCES
[1] B. Gleich and J. Weizenecker. Tomographic imaging using the nonlinear response of magnetic particles. *Nature*, 435(7046):1217-1217, 2005. doi: 10.1038/nature03808.
[2] J. Weizenecher, B. Gleich, Borgert J. Magnetic Particle Imaging using a field free line. J Phys Appl Phys. 2008;41:105009.
[3] E. Mason, C.Z. Cooley, S.F. Cauley, M.A. Griswold, S.M. Conolly, L.L. Wald. Design analysis of an MPI human functional brain scanner. J Magn Part Imaging. 2017;3(1), doi: 10.18416/ijmpi.2017.1703008
[4] M. Davids, B. Guerin, M. Malzacher, L.R. Shad, and L.L. Wald. Predicting Magnetostimulation Thresholds in the Peripheral

Nervous System using Realistic Body Models. *Scientific Reposts*, 7(1):5316, 2017. doi: 10.1038/s41598-017-05493-9.

[5] M. Davids, B. Guerin, V. Klein, L.R. Shad, and L.L. Wald.. *Prediction of Peripheral Nerve Stimulation Thresholds of MRI Gradient Coils*. Proc. of the ISMRM, Paris France, June 2018.

Lawrence L. Wald, Ph.D., is currently a Professor of Radiology at Harvard Medical School, Affiliated Faculty of the Harvard-MIT Division Health Sciences Technology and Sara & Charles Fabrikant Research Scholar at the Massachusetts General Hospital. He received a BA in Physics at Rice University, and a Ph.D. in Physics from the University of California at Berkeley in 1992 under the direction of Prof. E.L. Hahn with a thesis related to optical detection of NMR. He obtained further (postdoctoral) training in Physics at Berkeley and then in Radiology and MRI at the University of California at San Francisco (UCSF). He began his academic career as an Instructor at the Harvard Medical School and since 1998 has been at the Massachusetts General Hospital Dept. of Radiology A.A. Martinos Center for Biomedical Imaging. His recent work focuses on improving methods for functional brain imaging. He has worked on the benefits and challenges of highly parallel MRI and its application to faster image encoding and parallel excitation and ultra-high field MRI (7 Tesla) methodology, and also improved method for studying the Human Connectome and portable MRI technology. Recent work has included studying the feasibility of functional brain imaging with Magnetic Particle Imaging (MPI) using Cerebral Blood Volume (CBV) contrast and analysis of the instrumentation needed for fMPI of humans. This has also led to extending understanding of Peripheral Nerve Stimulation (PNS) in human MPI and MRI using electromagnetic body models with full nerve atlases and a detailed neuro-dynamic model to predict magneto-stimulation thresholds. Dr. Wald is a Fellow of the International Society of Magnetic Resonance (ISMRM) and the College of Fellows of the American Institute for Medical and Biologial Engineering (AIMBE). He will serve as President of the ISMRM in 2019.

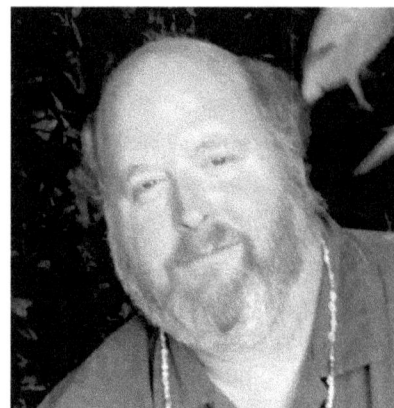

Session 01 - Talks

Tracer Synthesis and Characterization I

Synthesis and Characterization of $Zn_{0.1}Co_{0.9}Fe_2O_4$

Nurcan Doğan [a,*], Meltem Asiltürk [b], Faik Mikailzade [a], Ayhan Bingölbali [c], Zerin Yeşil Acar [d]

[a]Department of Physics, Gebze Technical University, Kocaeli, Turkey
[b]Department of Materials Science &Engineering, Akdeniz University, Antalya 07058, Turkey
[c]Department of Bioengineering, Yıldız Technical University, Istanbul 34220, Turkey
[d]Department of Chemistry, Akdeniz University, Antalya, Turkey
[*] Corresponding author, email: nurcandogan80@gmail.com

I. Introduction

Iron oxides with spinel structures have been emerged as one of the important magnetic materials since they exhibited high electrical resistance, low eddy current losses, high frequency applicability, greater heat resistance and higher corrosion resistance. Therefore, it can be used in enormous technological applications. It is well known that specific properties of it depend on preparing methods, chemical ingredients, cation distributions. In this study, $Zn_{0.1}Co_{0.9}Fe_2O_4$ was prepared by using hydrothermal method that divalent and trivalent metal salts of nickel, cobalt and manganese were used. This synthesis method was performed in two steps: At first, the particle was precipitated at alkaline condition by using reflux method. Secondarily, the mixture was then transferred to teflon-lined stainless steel autoclave. X-ray powder diffractometry (XRD), scanning electron microscopy (SEM), and energy-dispersive X-ray spectroscopy (EDX) and physical property measurement system (PPMS) were used to characterize the structural, morphological and magnetic properties of the sample.

II. Results and Discussions

II.I. Crystal structure and microstructure

The XRD patterns of Co-Zn doped on Fe_2O_4 nanoparticle is shown in Fig. 1. The diffraction peaks have demonstrated the presence of secondary structural phase.

Additionally, the size and morphology of the synthesized nanoparticles were characterized by SEM and EDS. The SEM graphs of the samples is shown in Fig. 2. According to the SEM micrographs of Co-Zn doped on Fe_2O_4 nanopowders. Chemical structure of $Zn_{0.1}Co_{0.9}Fe_2O_4$ system obtained and we can this results according EDS atomic percentage.

The particle size of $Zn_{0.1}Co_{0.9}Fe_2O_4$ particle ranked in the range of 50-100 nm.

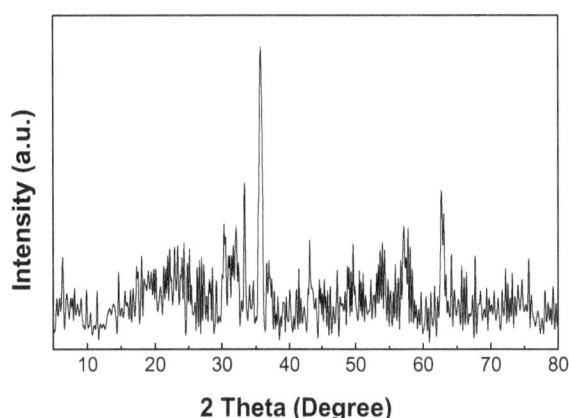

Figure 1: The XRD patterns of as-synthesized samples of $Zn_{0.1}Co_{0.9}Fe_2O_4$.

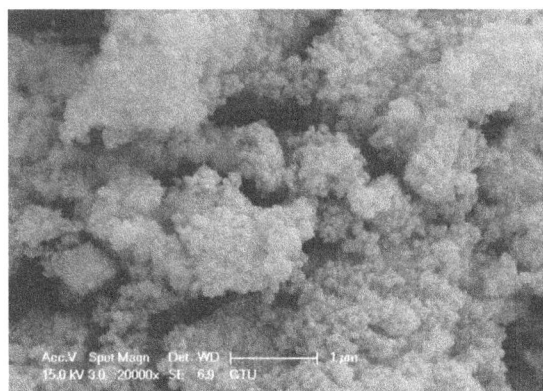

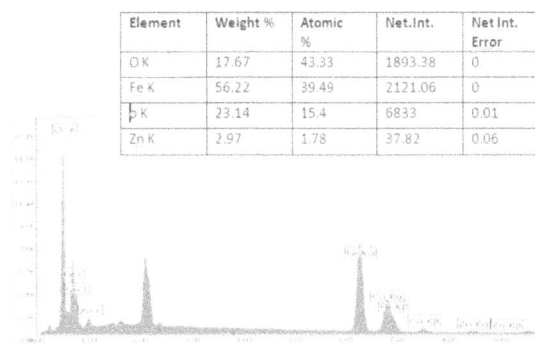

Element	Weight %	Atomic %	Net.Int.	Net Int. Error
O K	17.67	43.33	1893.38	0
Fe K	56.22	39.49	2121.06	0
p K	23.14	15.4	6833	0.01
Zn K	2.97	1.78	37.82	0.06

Figure 2. SEM and EDS patterns of $Zn_{0.1}Co_{0.9}Fe_2O_4$.

II.II. Magnetic Characterizations

To investigate the influence of Co-Zn doped Fe_2O_4 nanoparticle on the magnetic behavior of the $Zn_{0.1}Co_{0.9}Fe_2O_4$ system, the magnetic field dependences of the magnetization of all sample was measured at room temperature. The result is shown in Fig. 3. It has been obtained that the sample is ferromagnetic at room temperature. As it is seen from the figure, *M(H)* curve of the sample clearly show narrow hysteresis loop, presumably due to remanent magnetization (M_r). The value of remanent magnetization is found 18.3 emu/g and coercivity field of the sample is 550 Oe. The saturation magnetization value of the samples (Ms) is value of its was 58.03 emu/g.

ACKNOWLEDGEMENTS

The present work was supported by the TUBITAK (Project number:115E776 and 115E777).

REFERENCES

[1] B. Gleich and J. Weizenecker. Tomographic imaging using the nonlinear response of magnetic particles. *Nature*, 435(7046):1217-1217, 2005. doi: 10.1038/nature03808.

[2] T. Knopp and T. M. Buzug. *Magnetic Particle Imaging: An Introduction to Imaging Principles and Scanner Instrumentation.* Springer, Berlin/Heidelberg, 2012. doi: 10.1007/978-3-642-04199-0.

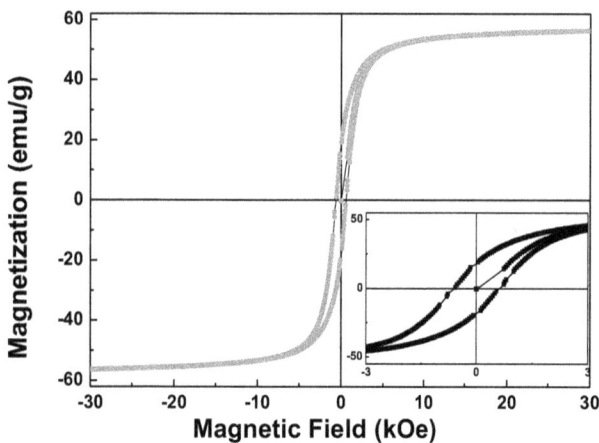

Figure 3: *M(H)dependences of $Zn_{0.1}Co_{0.9}Fe_2O_4$ sample measured at room temperature.*

III. Conclusions

Thus, the structural investigations of magnetic $Zn_{0.1}Co_{0.9}Fe_2O_4$ particle were performed. The peaks of X-ray diffraction patterns of the samples were indexed which confirms that the prepared nanoparticles are in hexagonal structure. This result well agrees with literature. The morphology of the prepared samples was identified by using scanning electron microscopy technique. MPS experiments will be conducted until workshop date. The toxicity investigations of the $Zn_{0.1}Co_{0.9}Fe_2O_4$ particle were observed that it was not toxic. The cytotoxicity assays of the sample will be presented in the poster. The room temperature studies of the magnetic properties of $Co_{0.1}Cu_xZn_{0.9-x}O$ particles revealed ferromagnetic behavior.

Response of Suspensions of Microfabricated Magnetic Discs to Time Varying Fields

Per A. Löthman[a,b], Tijmen Hageman[a,b], Jordi Hendrix [b], Hans Keizer [b], Henk van Wolferen [b], Kees Ma [c], Melissa van de Loosdrecht [b], Bennie ten Haken [b], Thijs Bolhuis [b], Leon Abelmann [a,b*]

[a] KIST Europe, Saarbrücken, Germany
[b] University of Twente, Enschede, The Netherlands
[b] MicroCreate, Enschede, The Netherlands
[*] Corresponding author, email: l.abelmann@kist-europe.de

I. Introduction

At IWMPI 2017 we introduced suspensions of micro-fabricated magnetic discs of 2 and 3 µm diameter as alternatives for colloidal suspensions, and showed their response in magnetic particle spectroscopy at 20 kHz [1]. In this contribution we investigated the magnetic stability of these suspensions at longer time scales, and introduce the first sub-micron discs. In contrast suspensions of superparamagnetic particles, the micro-fabricated discs that we produced up to now have a non-zero remanence. Therefore, magnetostatic interaction between discs is a point of concern. If this interaction is strong, agglomerates will form that might change the magnetic response of the suspension.

II. Material and Methods

The 2 µm diameter discs were prepared from Au(14nm)/NiFe(12nm)/Au(14nm) thin films deposited on a negative photoresist as sacrificial layer by contact mask lithography and ion beam etching [1]. The lithography technique for the 200 nm diameter discs was laser interference lithography. This technique allows for full-wafer exposure within a minute. The transmission of light through a suspension was analyzed by means of a LED-photodiode detection system with two orthogonal coils cells to provide a field in the order of one mT (Fig. 1).

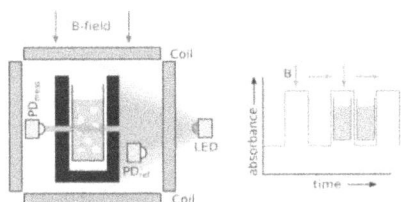

Figure 1: *The transmission of light through a suspension of magnetic discs is analyzed as function of the applied field.*

Vibrating sample magnetometry was performed in a Veeco VSM-10 vector coil system on 50 µL of a suspension of 345 discs/nL. The total measurement time for a loop is one to two hours. The magnetic susceptibility was measured by a homebuilt superpara-magnetic particle analyzer at a drive field of 1.3 mT at 2.5 kHz [2].

III. Results

There is a remarkable difference in the slow magnetic response of the discs when they are still on the production wafer (black curve in Fig. 2) and when in suspension (red curve). A second step at about 5 mT can be observed. This step is not visible in the susceptibility measurement at 2.5 kHz (Fig. 3). In that measurement a peak develops around 1 mT for drive frequencies above 10 kHz. Strangely, this peak does not coincide with the coercivity of the VSM loop.

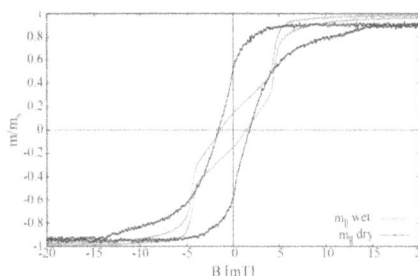

Figure 2: *Magnetic hysteresis loop measured by VSM of a Au/NiFe/Au discs of 2 µm diameter in suspension (red curve) and in dry state (black curve).*

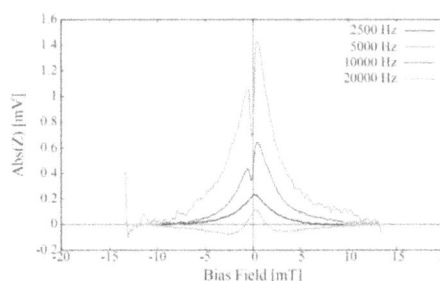

Figure 3: *Magnetic susceptibility of the suspension as a function of bias field for different frequencies.*

We suspect that the low frequency anomaly has an origin in particle chain formation. To further investigate the low frequency behavior, we observed the light transmitted through a suspension of the discs. Fig. 4 shows the normalized absorbance g as a function of applied field angle θ. When the magnetic field is aligned parallel to the light beam ($\theta=0$) the transmission of light is maximal. When the field is tilted perpendicular to the light direction, the discs block the light and the signal on the photodiode decreases.

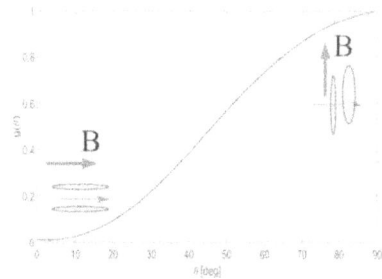

Figure 4: *Normalized absorbance of a suspension of Au/NiFe/Au discs of 2 μm diameter as a function of the applied field angle.*

We rotated the field from parallel to perpendicular every 10 s. After 7 hours, the signal dropped by a factor of two, which can be explained by sedimentation. At the same time however the time constant increases, and the pattern becomes erratic (Fig. 5). We believe this is a clear sign of disc interaction, which could also be the origin of the strange behavior in the VSM loop. We cannot exclude that disc interaction occurs immediately after creating the suspensions, or on a time scale much smaller than we can access with our instrument. Further investigation into this phenomenon of these discs with high remanence is required.

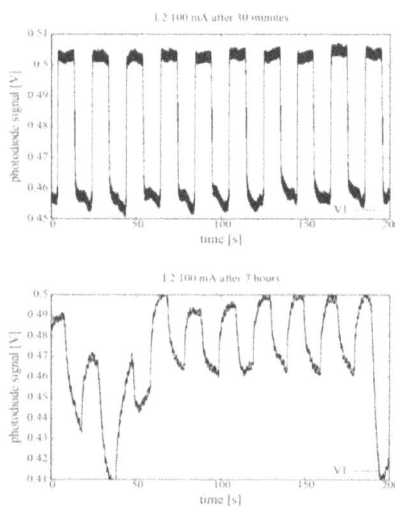

Figure 5: *The response of the suspension to the magnetic field changes dramatically over time. After 30 min (top) the response is fast. After 7 hours (below), the response is much slower and erratic.*

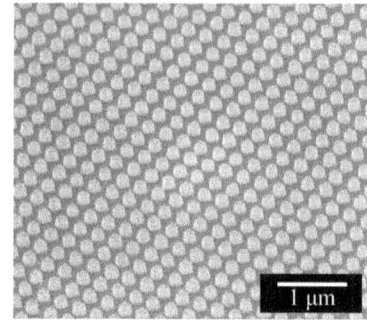

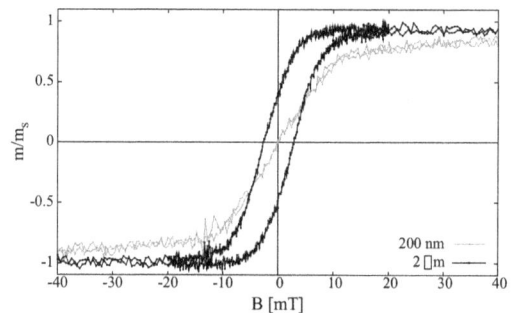

Figure 6: *Top: SEM image of magnetic Au/NiFe/Au discs of 200 nm diameter, prepared by laser interference lithography. The photoresist is still on top of the discs. Bottom: VSM loops. As compared to discs with 2 μm diameter, the hysteresis has entirely disappeared (discs on wafer).*

Next to the anomalous behavior in liquid, at the conference we will present our first results on magnetic disc of only 200 nm in diameter, prepared by laser interference lithography. Fig. 6 shows the patterned Au/NiFe/Au elements when they are still on the production wafer. The VSM loop shows that at this small size, the hysteresis entirely disappears and the discs turn non-remanent.

IV. Conclusions

Microfabricated magnetic discs show a remarkably different magnetic response when they are in suspension, compared to when they are still on the production wafer. At very low frequencies, the magnetic hysteresis loop features a distinct step at 5 mT. This step is not visible in low frequency susceptibility measurements, where at frequencies above 10 kHz a step develops at 1 mT. After several hours in suspension, rotation experiments hint at formation of bigger structures. This behavior in liquids is interesting from a physical point of view, and will have implications for application of these discs in magnetic particle detection and imaging.

REFERENCES

[1] Löthman, P. A., Janson, T. G., Klein, Y. P., Blaudszun, A-R., Ledwig, M., & Abelmann, L. (2017). Microfabrication and Magnetic Particle Spectrometry of Magnetic Discs. International Journal on Magnetic Particle Imaging (IJMPI), 3(2), [1707001]

[2] Van de Loosdrecht, M. M., Waanders, S., Wildeboer, R. R., Krooshoop, H. J. G., & ten Haken, B. (2017). Differential magnetometry to detect sentinel lymph nodes in laparoscopic procedures. IWMPI 2017, Prague.

Evaluation of Magnetic Particle Imaging Using Blood-Pooling Magnetic Nanoparticles

Yuki Matsugi [a], Satoshi Ota [b,*], Takeru Nakamura [a], Ryoji Takeda [c], Yasushi Takemura [c], Ichiro Kato [d], Satoshi Nohara [d], Teruyoshi Sasayama [a], Takashi Yoshida [a], and Keiji Enpuku [a]

[a] Department of Electrical Engineering, Kyushu University, Fukuoka, Japan
[b] Department of Electrical and Electronic Engineering, Shizuoka University, Hamamatsu, Japan
[c] Department of Electrical and Computer Engineering, Yokohama National University, Yokohama, Japan
[d] The Nagoya Research Laboratory, Meito Sangyo Co. Ltd., Kiyosu, Japan
* Corresponding author, email: ota.s@shizuoka.ac.jp

I. Introduction

With respect to the magnetic nanoparticles (MNPs) for magnetic particle imaging (MPI), the high harmonic signal promotes the reconstructed image [1]. The harmonic signal is influenced by the core diameter, structure, and state of MNPs [2]. In this study, the intensity and the half bandwidth of the MPI signal of MNPs were measured. The dependence of the MPI signal on the core diameter and the structure of MNPs was discussed.

II. Material and Methods

Measurements were performed using water-based maghemite nanoparticles (CMEADM-004 (Sample I), CMEADM-023 (Sample II), CMEADM-033 (Sample III), and CMEADM-033-02 (Sample IV). These nanoparticles were supplied by Meito Sangyo Co. Ltd., Kiyosu, Japan. These MNPs were coated by carboxymethyl-diethylaminoethyl dextran, and their core and hydro-dynamic diameters are listed in Table 1. Carboxymethyl-diethylaminoethyl dextran-coated iron oxide nanoparticles are negatively charged and are used as a blood-pooling contrast agent [3].

We prepared the set of permanent magnets, a drive coil, and a pick-up coil to measure the MPI signal of the prepared MNPs for 2D MPI. The third harmonic

Table 1 The core diameter d_c and hydrodynamic diameter d_h of the measured MNPs.

Sample #: measured MNP	d_C [nm]	d_H [nm]
I: CMEADM-004	4	38
II: CMEADM-023	8	83
III: CMEADM-033	5–6	54
IV: CMEADM-033-02	6	64

magnetization was measured as the MPI signal. The gradient field to select the field of view (FOV) was applied by the permanent magnets, whose gradient was 1 T/m and 2 T/m for x-axis and y-axis, respectively. The intensity and the frequency of the applied AC field was 3.5 mT and 3 kHz, respectively.

III. Results and Discussion

Figure 1 shows the 2D images of the measured MNPs. Figure 2 shows the MPI signal intensities of measured MNPs. Table 2 shows the maximal intensity and the half bandwidth of the MPI signal in the measured MNPs normalized by those in Sample I. The maximal intensities of the MPI signals were proportional to the third harmonic intensities shown in Fig. 3. The third harmonic intensity of Sample II was higher than that of Sample I and Sample III because the core diameter of Sample II is larger than that of Sample I and Sample III [2]. The measured MNPs are composed of the particles divided into three types of the structures such as the single-core, multi-core, and chain. In particular, the multi-core structure promotes the magnetization and third harmonic signal because of the large size of the effective core [4]. The third harmonic

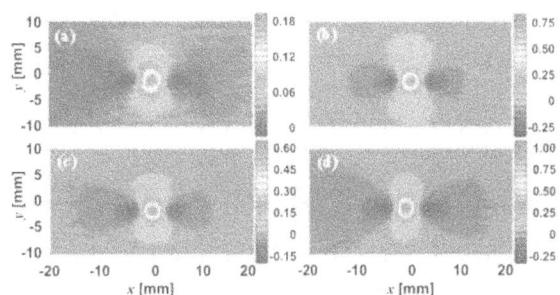

Figure 1 2D MPI images of the (a) I:CMEADM-004, (b) II:CMEADM-023, (c) III:CMEADM-033, and (d) IV:CMEADM-033-02. The intensity and frequency of the applied AC field was 3.5 mT and 3 kHz, respectively. The gradient was 1 T/m and 2 T/m for x-axis and y-axis in the gradient field, respectively.

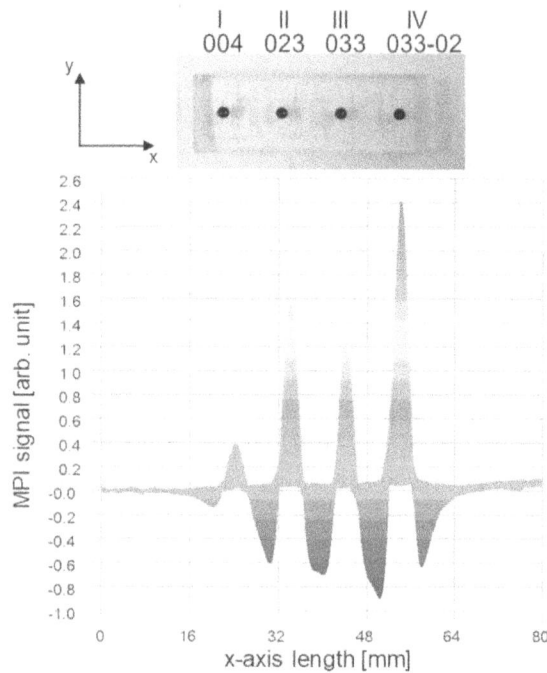

Figure 2 *The MPI signals of the measured MNPs. The intensity and frequency of the applied AC field was 3.5 mT and 3 kHz, respectively. The gradient was 1 T/m and 2 T/m for x-axis and y-axis in the gradient field, respectively.*

Table 2 *The maximal intensity and half bandwidth of the MPI signal in the measured MNPs shown in Fig. 2, which are normalized by those in CMEADM-004.*

Sample #: measured MNP	Maximal intensity	Half bandwidth
I: CMEADM-004	1	1
II: CMEADM-023	3.9	0.86
III: CMEADM-033	3.1	0.81
IV: CMEADM-033-02	6.1	0.76

intensity of Sample IV was higher than that of Sample II whereas the core diameter of Sample IV is smaller than that of Sample II. It is indicated that the distribution of the multi-core particles in Sample IV are narrower than that in Sample II. Actually, Sample IV was prepared by collecting the MNPs with larger magnetization by magnetic separation from Sample III [2].

The third harmonic magnetization normalized by the fundamental magnetization M_3/M_1 is shown in Fig. 3. For the estimation of M_3/M_1, the AC magnetization signal was measured at 10 mT and 10 kHz of the intensity and the frequency in the applied field, respectively. The half bandwidth of the MPI signal estimated from Fig. 2 is depended on the M_3/M_1, which indicates the non-linear response of the magnetization to the applied field. Sample IV shows the highest M_3/M_1 and the smallest half bandwidth in the measured MNPs. In particular, M_3/M_1 of

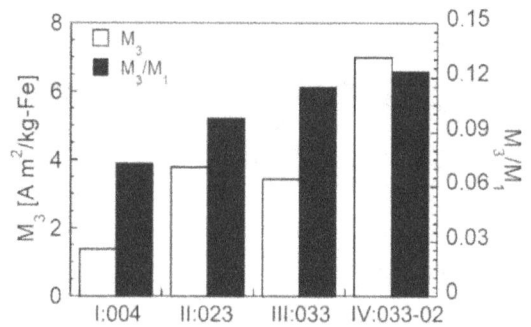

Figure 3 *The third harmonic magnetization M_3 and M_3 normalized by the fundamental magnetization M_1. The intensity and frequency of the applied AC field was 10 mT and 10 kHz, respectively.*

Sample III was higher than that of Sample II. The half bandwidth of Sample III was smaller than that of Sample II, although the maximal intensity of the MPI signal of Sample III was lower than that of Sample II. It suggests that the difference in the structures of Sample II and Sample III influences their maximal intensity and the half bandwidth of the MPI signal.

IV. Conclusions

The MPI images of the blood-pooling MNPs were observed. The maximal intensity of the MPI signal agreed with the third harmonic intensity. In addition, the half bandwidth was depended on M_3/M_1, which indicates the non-linear response of the magnetization to the applied field.

ACKNOWLEDGEMENTS
This work was partially supported by the JSPS KAKENHI Grant Numbers: 15H05764, 17H03275, and 17K14693.

REFERENCES
[1] B. Gleich and J. Weizenecker. Tomographic imaging using the nonlinear response of magnetic particles. *Nature*, **435**, 1217, 2005. doi: 10.1038/nature03808.
[2] S. Ota, R. Takeda, T. Yamada, I. Kato, S. Nohara, and Y. Takemura. Effect of particle size and structure on harmonic intensity of blood-pooling multi-core magnetic nanoparticles for magnetic particle imaging. *Int. J. Magn. Part. Imaging*, **3**, 1703003, 2017. doi: 10.18416/ijmpi.2017.1703003.
[3] N. Nitta, K. Tsuchiya, A. Sonoda, S. Ota, N. Ushio, M. Takahashi, K. Murata, and S. Nohara. Negatively charged superparamagnetic iron oxide nanoparticles: a new blood-pooling magnetic resonance contrast agent. *Jpn. J. Radiol*, **30**, 832, 2012. doi: 10.1007/s11604-012-0133-0.
[4] T. Yoshida, N. B. Othma n, and K. Enpuku. Characterization of magnetically fractionated magnetic nanoparticles for magnetic particle imaging. *J. Appl. Phys.*, **114**, 173908, 2013. doi:10.1063/1.4829484.

Magnetic Fractionation of Resovist® Nanoparticles for Magnetic Particle Imaging

Takashi Yoshida [a,*], Yuki Matsugi [a], Takuru Nakamura [a], Oji Higashi [a], and Keiji Enpuku [a]

[a] Department of Electrical Engineering, Kyushu University, Fukuoka, Japan
* Corresponding author, email: t_yoshi@ees.kyushu-u.ac.jp

I. Introduction

Magnetic particle imaging (MPI) is a new modality for the imaging of the spatial distribution of magnetic nanoparticles (MNPs), especially for in-vivo diagnostics [1]. A commercially available MNP, called Resovist® (FUJIFILM RI Pharma), is one of the candidates for an MPI tracer, since it has already been safely used inside the human body as a contrast agent in magnetic resonance imaging (MRI). However, it was shown that some portion of the MNPs in a Resovist® sample do not contribute to the harmonic signals [2]. Therefore, if we can extract particles responsible for the rich harmonic signals from the original sample, we can expect much improvement in the performance of MPI. To this end, magnetic fractionation of original MNPs will be useful [3], [4]. In this study, we performed magnetic fractionation and characterized the fractionated Resovist® MNPs for MPI application.

II. Material and Methods

II.I. Magnetic fractionation and samples

Magnetic fractionation was performed by using a separation column and a dc magnetic field. The separation column (MS column, Miltenyi Biotec), is filled with soft magnetic iron spheres to increase a magnetic field gradient inside the column. An electromagnet (Model 3470, GMW), was used to generate the dc magnetic field. By performing a single fractionation, an original MNPs sample is divided into two fractions. Here, the fraction from the original MNPs that was captured in the separation column is called positive fraction. While, the fraction that was not captured in the separation column is called negative fraction. To investigate the properties of harmonic magnetization from fractionated Resovist® MNPs, we prepared four fractionated samples (S1-4) by changing the strength of the dc magnetic field $\mu_0 H_{dc}$. Each fractionated sample is the positive fraction from original Resovist® MNPs.

II.II. Static *M-H* curve

Static *M-H* curves of the fractionated samples suspended in water were measured using homemade vibrating

sample magnetometer (VSM). By using a Langevin function L, the static *M-H* curve is given by

$$M(H) = \frac{1}{V_T} \int_0^\infty n(m) mL\left(\frac{\mu_0 mH}{k_B T}\right) dm . \quad (1)$$

Here, V_T is the total volume of MNPs, $n(m)$ is the number of MNPs with a magnetic moment m, k_B is the Boltzmann constant, and T is the absolute temperature. By comparing the measured static *M-H* curve and eq. (1), we can estimate the magnetic moment distribution in the sample [5]. For the estimation, we used non-negative least square (NNLS) method [5].

II.III. DLS

For dynamic light scattering (DLS) measurements, a commercially available particle size analyzer (Zetasizer Nano ZS, Malvern Instruments), was used. Using the software equipped with the DLS setup, Z-average particle size and polydispersity index (PDI) value were obtained.

II.IV. ACS

Frequency dependent ac susceptibilities (ACS) of the fractionated samples suspended in water were measured using homemade ACS setup. The amplitude of the ac excitation field was set to 100 μT, i.e., ACS measurements were performed in linear magnetization regime. It is well recognized that the imaginary part of the ACS in the linear magnetization regime becomes maximum value when the Brownian relaxation time τ_B satisfies the following equation.

$$2\pi f \tau_B = 2\pi f \frac{\pi \eta d_H^3}{2 k_B T} = 1 . \quad (2)$$

Here, η is the viscosity of surrounding medium. As shown in eq. (2), we can obtain the typical hydrodynamic size of the MNPs sample from the frequency at which imaginary part of the ACS becomes maximum value.

II.V. MPS

Harmonic magnetizations of the fractionated samples suspended in water were measured using homemade magnetic particle spectroscopy (MPS). The amplitude and frequency of the ac excitation field were set to 20 mT and 20 kHz, respectively.

Table 1: Parameters of fractionated Resovist® MNPs.

	S1	S2	S3	S4	Original Resovist®
Strength of dc fractionation field $\mu_0 H_{dc}$ (T)	0.67	0.34	0.17	0.07	–
Typical value of magnetic moment ($\times 10^{-18}$ Am^2)	2.8	4.0	6.3	11.2	2.5
Z-average hydrodynamic size (nm)	63.3	67.8	77.7	101.6	62.5
PDI	0.218	0.193	0.172	0.127	0.207
Typical hydrodynamic size obtained from ACS (nm)	63.2	67.2	84.6	98.7	63.6
Amplitude of third harmonic magnetization (a.u.)	1.37	2.24	2.20	1.82	1

III. Results and Discussion

Estimated magnetic moment distributions for all samples are shown in Fig. 1. As can be seen, the value of magnetic moment becomes large with decreasing the strength of the dc magnetic field for fractionation H_{dc}. This indicates that magnetic moment of the MNPs sample can be controlled by adjusting the dc magnetic field for fractionation. The typical values of magnetic moment for all samples are listed in Table 1.

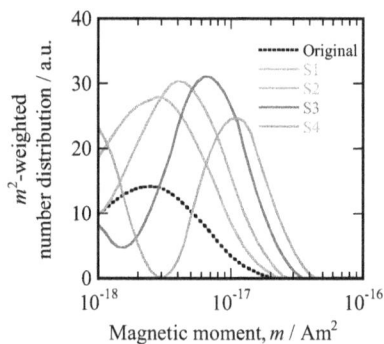

Figure 1: Estimated magnetic moment distribution

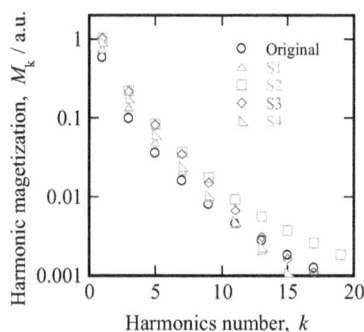

Figure 2: Amplitude of the harmonic magnetization spectrum when an ac excitation field with amplitude $\mu_0 H_{ac}$ = 20 mT and frequency f = 20 kHz was applied.

Hydrodynamic sizes obtained from DLS and ACS measurements are listed in Table 1. As can be seen, Z-average size obtained from DLS measurement and typical hydrodynamic size obtained from ACS measurement nicely fit for all fractionated samples. We also found that hydrodynamic size becomes large and PDI value becomes small with decreasing the strength of the dc magnetic field

for fractionation. As listed in Table 1, hydrodynamic size ranges approximately 60 nm to 100 nm.

Fig. 2 shows the spectral amplitudes of the harmonic magnetization measured by MPS setup. As can be seen, S2 shows the largest harmonic spectrum. As listed in Table I, the amplitude of the 3rd harmonic magnetization of S2 showed the 2.24-hold increase compared to that of original Resovist® sample. As shown in Table 1, the MNPs with magnetic moment value around $4 \times 10^{-18} \sim 6 \times 10^{-18}$ Am^2 is suitable for the enhancement of MPI signals.

IV Conclusions

In this study, we performed magnetic fractionation and characterized the fractionated Resovist® MNPs for MPI. We showed that the harmonic magnetization signals from MNPs, which are used for the detection of MNPs in MPI, can be enhanced by magnetically selecting appropriate MNPs with magnetic moment value around $4 \times 10^{-18} \sim 6 \times 10^{-18}$ Am^2.

ACKNOWLEDGEMENTS

This work was supported by the JSPS KAKENHI 15H05764 and 16K14277.

REFERENCES

[1] B. Gleich and J. Weizenecker. Tomographic imaging using the nonlinear response of magnetic particles. *Nature*, 435(7046):1214-1217, 2005. doi: 10.1038/nature03808.

[2] T. Yoshida, K. Enpuku, F. Ludwig, J. Dieckhoff, T. Wawrzik, A. Lak, and M. Schilling. Characterization of Resovist® Nanoparticles for Magnetic Particle Imaging. *Springer Proc. Phys.*, 140:3-7, 2012. doi: 10.1007/978-3-642-24133-8_1.

[3] T. Yoshida, N. B. Othman, and K. Enpuku. Characterization of magnetically fractionated magnetic nanoparticles for magnetic particle imaging. *J. Appl. Phys.*, 114: 173908, 2013. doi: 10.1063/1.4829484.

[4] N. Löwa, P. Knappe, F. Wiekhorst, D. Eberbeck, A. F. Thünemann, and L. Trahms. Hydrodynamic and magnetic fractionation of superparamagnetic nanoparticles for magnetic particle imaging. *J. Magn. Magn. Mater.*, 380:266–270, 2015. doi: 10.1016/j.jmmm.2014.08.057.

[5] J. van Rijssel, B. W.M. Kuipers, B. H. Erné. Non-regularized inversion method from light scattering applied to ferrofluid magnetization curves for magnetic size distribution analysis. *J. Magn. Magn. Mater.*, 353:110–115, 2014. doi: 10.1016/j.jmmm.2013.10.025.

Session 02 - Posters

Tracer Synthesis and Characterization II

synomag® *Nanoflower* Particles: A new Tracer for MPI, Physical Characterization and Initial *in vitro* Toxicity Studies

Cordula Grüttner[a], Anja Kowalski[a], Florian Fidler[b], Maria Steinke[c], Fritz Westphal[a], Henrik Teller[a*]

[a] *micromod Partikeltechnologie GmbH, Rostock, Germany*
[b] *Fraunhofer-Entwicklungszentrum Röntgentechnik EZRT ein Bereich des Fraunhofer-Instituts für Integrierte Schaltungen IIS, Würzburg, Germany*
[c] *Universitätsklinikum Würzburg - Lehrstuhl Tissue Engineering und Regenerative Medizin, Würzburg, Germany; Fraunhofer-Institut für Silicatforschung ISC, Würzburg, Germany*
* Corresponding author, email: henrik.teller@micromod.de

I. Introduction

Magnetic particle imaging (MPI) provides three-dimensional imaging of magnetic nanoparticle (MNP) tracers with high spatial and temporal resolution[1]. The MPI signal intensity critically depends on the individual non-linear response of the used tracer material as well as the achievable resolution. In terms of resolution, a narrow size distribution and an optimized core diameter were found to be preferable. Since clinical approved tracer materials are still rare, new imaging agents comprising superior magnetic properties along with good bio-compatibility and no systemic toxicity need to be developed. Herein, we report on a new magnetic iron oxide nanoparticle type as tracer for MPI with a unique nano-flower structure. The potential impact of synomag®-particles in regenerative medicine, e.g. homing and track-ing of human mesenchymal stem cells (hMSCs), has been evaluated in cell uptake and initial *in-vitro* toxicity studies.

II. Material and Methods

The new synomag®-particles are multi-core particles featuring a nanosized dendritic (nanoflower) substructure of iron oxide crystallites with an excellent biocompatibility. The particles are synthesized by a polyol method including thermal decomposition of suitable iron precursors[2]. Final coating with dextran provides monodisperse synomag®-D particles with a hydrodynamic diameter of 50 nm and a very narrow size distribution[3]. These particles have been analyzed in a magnetic particle spectrometer (MPS system, Pure Devices, Germany) and compared to the gold standard Resovist®.

MNPs with amino groups on the dextran surface and a moderate positive zeta potential have shown an efficient uptake in hMSCs [4]. To analyze cell-particle interaction *in vitro*, hMSCs were incubated with plain (nearly neutral) and amino functionalized synomag®-D particles with a moderate positive zeta potential for 20 h. Then, trypan blue exclusion test and Prussian blue staining were performed. Non-labeled hMSCs served as controls.

III. Results

III.I. Physico-chemical characterization

The TEM image visualizes the nanoflower structure of the new synomag®-D particles with a mean core size of 22 nm (Figure 1).

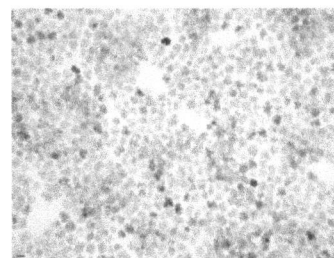

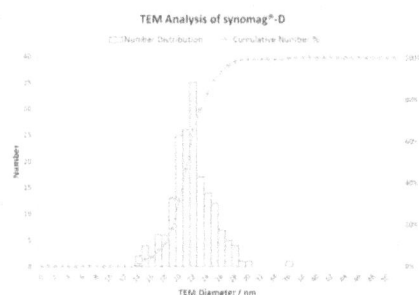

Figure 1: Top: TEM image of 50 nm synomag®-D particles with plain surface, bottom: TEM analysis.

The hydrodynamic diameter and the narrow size distribution of synomag®-D particles are highly reproducible (Figure 2).

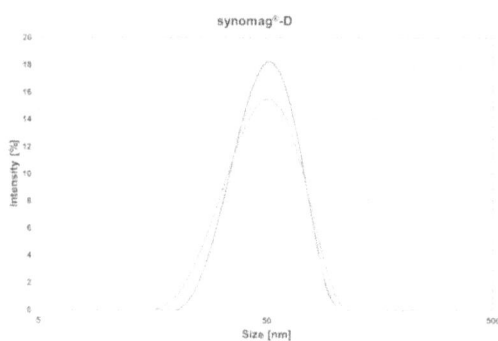

Figure 2: Size distribution of synomag®-D particles (three different batches) measured by dynamic light scattering.

The MPS spectra of synomag®-D particles are shown in figure 3 in comparison to Resovist® as reference. Excitation field strength was 20 and 30mT at a frequency of 20 kHz, averaging was set to 20 times. In addition, the linear phase suggests a monodisperse particle suspension, as predicted from the manufacturing process. Figure 4 plots the resulting magnetization curve of the synomag®-D particles compared to Resovist®.

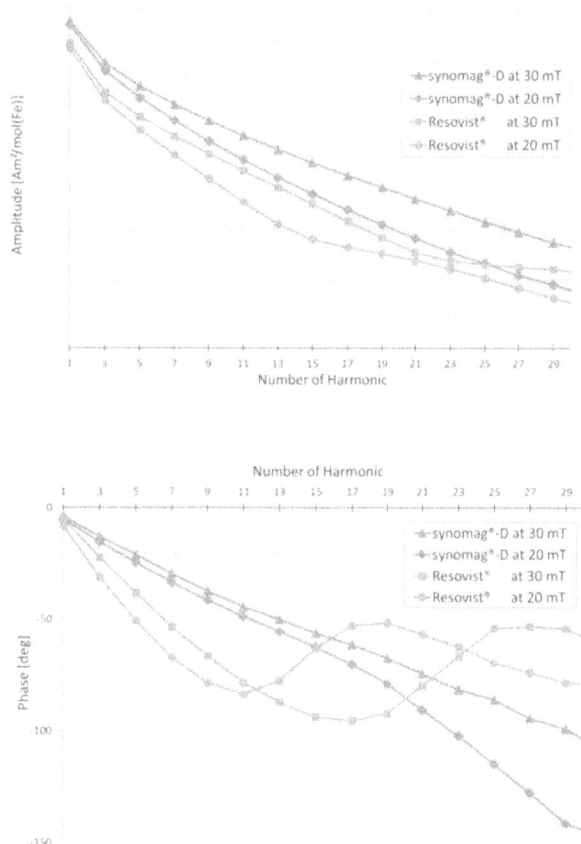

Figure 3: Top: MPS Spectra of 50 nm synomag®-D particles at 20 and 30 mT, amplitude of odd harmonics scaled to the amount of iron (mol Fe) compared to Resovist®; bottom: Phase of odd harmonics.

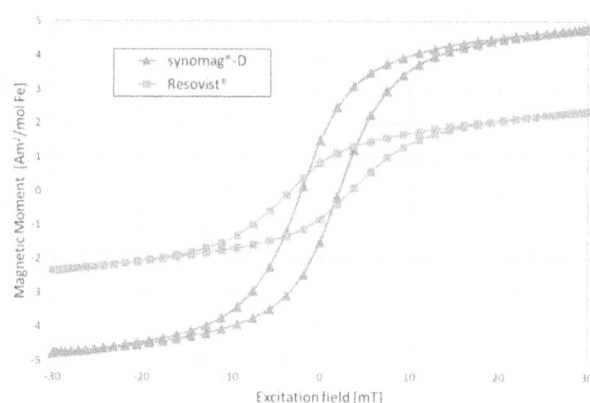

Figure 4: Magnetization curve of synomag®-D particles compared to Resovist®.

III.II. *In vitro* toxicity studies in hMSC

After 20 h of incubation with plain and amino functionalized synomag®-D particles, more than 98% of hMSCs were viable. There was no difference to non-labeled cells. In cytological samples, clear Prussian blue-positive cells were identified with an increasing signal intensity that was dependent on the labeling concentration $(200 < 500 < 1000$ mg ml^{-1} Fe). Moreover, the Prussian blue signal intensity of plain synomag®-D particles was higher compared to corresponding amino functionalized particles.

IV. Discussion

The synomag®-D nanoflower particles lead to increased signal strength per iron compared to Resovist®. Comparison between different batches and coatings does not affect the achievable signal significantly. Our preliminary *in vitro* data indicate that both plain and amino functionalized synomag®-D are not cytotoxic and allow a good cell-particle-interaction. Subsequent tests need to be done, e.g. to analyze the subcellular localization of the particles and to determine the particles' biocompatibility in more detail.

V. Conclusions

synomag® nanoflower particles with a biocompatible dextran coating exhibit a great potential as tracer material for MPI, combining less substance demand with improved signal strength. The superior physical properties further provide the opportunity for an application in magnetic field assisted hyperthermia[2]. Consequently, synomag® particles possess excellent requirements for a future combination of MPI diagnostic and hyperthermia treatment strategies.

REFERENCES

[1] B. Gleich and J. Weizenecker. Tomographic imaging using the nonlinear response of magnetic particles. *Nature*, 435(7046):1217-1217, 2005. doi: 10.1038/nature03808.

[2] Lartigue, L., et al., Cooperative organization in iron oxide multi-core nanoparticles potentiates their efficiency as heating mediators and MRI contrast agents. *ACS Nano*, 6(12): 10935-10949, 2012.

[3] Gavilán, H., et al., Colloidal Flower-Shaped Iron Oxide Nanoparticles: Synthesis Strategies and Coatings. *Particle & Particle Systems Characterization*, 1700094: 2017.

[4] Kilian, T., et al., Stem cell labeling with iron oxide nanoparticles: impact of 3D culture on cell labeling maintenance. *Nanomedicine*, 11(15): 1957-1970, 2016.

Differential Magnetometry on Fe_2O_3 Nano-Clustered Particles

Leon Abelmann [a,b*], Melissa van de Loosdrecht [b], Bennie ten Haken [b],
Lijun Pan [c], Bum Chul Park [c], Young Keun Kim [c]

[a] *KIST Europe, Saarbrücken, Germany*
[b] *University of Twente, Enschede, The Netherlands*
[c] *Department of Materials Science, Korea University, Seoul, Korea*
[*] *Corresponding author, email: l.abelmann@kist-europe.de, ykim97@korea.ac.kr*

I. Introduction

Modern contrast agents for Magnetic Particle Imaging consist of clusters of superparamagnetic iron-oxide particles, rather than individual particles [1,2]. These multi-granule nanoclusters (MGNCs) have the advantage that the size of clusters can be increased, without sacrificing the superparamagnetic response that is necessary to avoid magnetic attraction and unwanted agglomeration.

Previously, we have investigated the suitability of these nanoclusters for Magnetic Particle Imaging [3]. In this contribution we optimize these particles for use in differential magnetometry, a technique that can for instance be applied to detect sentinel lymph nodes in laparoscopic procedures [4].

II. Material and Methods

This type of magnetic multi-granule nanoclusters (MGNCs) can be easily formed by the simple reaction of $FeCl_3$ in ethylene glycol, which serves as both the solvent and reductant, in the presence of sodium acetate [5]. By adjusting the process condtions, the granule size as well as the number of granules can be adjusted. Two formulations were used, one with an average granule size of 15 nm, and one with 23 nm. The average number of granules per cluster was varied so that the cluster size varies from an average diameter of 25 to 43 nm. The smallest clusters with the bigger granules are composed of only one or two granules.

The magnetic response for differential magnetometry was measured by a home built susceptometer (superparamagnetic quantifier, SpaQ), with a drive field of 1.3 mT at a frequency of 2.5 kHz. The sample volume was 200±10 µL of a 1 mg(Fe)/mL suspension. The bias field was applied with a maximum value of 14 mT.

III. Results

Fig. 1 shows a subset of the range of suspensions investigated. The label "small" (black curves) refers to granules in the order of 15(2) nm, the label "big" (red curves) to granules of about 23(3) nm, as measured by transmission electron microscopy. Of each formulation, two different cluster sizes are shown (continuous and dashed lines). As can be observed, the signal varies considerably with formulation as well as cluster size. The effect of cluster size appears to be much stronger when using bigger granules. Even with this first initial parameter sweep, we can reach signals that are 20% higher than a commercial solution (Resovist™, Bayer Schering Pharma GmbH)) with identical iron content. It should be noted however that the commercial solution was in water, whereas our suspensions are still in ethanol. (Suspensions in water have been prepared, and will be shown at the conference).

The maximum peak height and width of the particle response function at half the maximum signal are shown in table 1. The width of the Resovist curve is significantly larger than that of the nanocluster suspensions.

Table 1: Peak signal at 0 mT and width at half maximum for suspensions with different granule size ("small" vs "big") and cluster size. For comparison, Resovist with identical iron content is shown

	Peak (mV)	FWHM (mT)
Small 30 nm	10±1	2.90±0.05
Small 42 nm	9±1	2.62±0.05
Big 25 nm	13±1	2.92±0.05
Big 34 nm	6±1	2.77±0.05
Big 43 nm	7±1	2.53±0.05
Resovist	10±1	3.55±0.05

2500 Hz

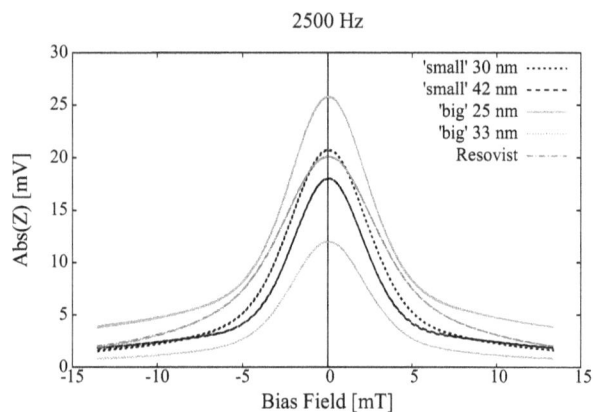

Figure 1: Particle response function for multi-granule nanocluster suspensions with variation in size of the granules (black and red curves) as well as the diameter of the total cluster. For comparison, Resovist with identical iron content is shown in blue.

Fig. 2 shows the transmission electron microscopy image of the suspension with the highest signal ("Big" 25 nm) and the lowest signal ("Big" 34 nm). Apart from the size, there is no apparent difference. Also the coercivities of both suspensions are identical (0.9 kA/m), indicating that the origin of the signal difference might be related to the hydrodynamic radius. Further research is in progress.

Big 25 nm   Big 34 nm

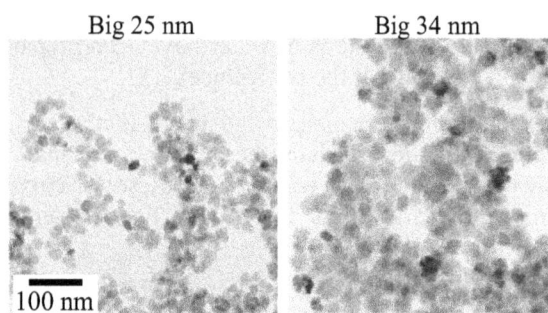

100 nm

Figure 2: Transmission electron micrograph of the suspension with the highest (left) and the lowest signal (right).

IV. Conclusions

When using multi-granule nanoclusters, one can tune the size of the granules relatively independently from the size of the clusters. This offers an extra degree of freedom in tuning magnetic particles for differential magnetometry and Magnetic Particle Imaging. We have shown that the highest signal can be obtained when using bigger granules, but that the relation between cluster size and magnetic signal increases when using big granules.

These promising first results encouraged us to realize suspensions in water by proper surface modification of the nanoclusters, and to further optimize their response.

REFERENCES

[1] F.Ahrentorp, A.Astalan, J.Blomgren, C.Jonasson, E.Wetterskog, P. Svedlindh, A. Lak, F. Ludwig, L.J. Van Ijzendoorn, F. Westphal, C. Gruttner, N. Gehrke, S. Gustafsson, E. Olsson, and C. Johansson. Effective particle magnetic moment of multi-core particles. Journal of Magnetism and Magnetic Materials, 380:221–226, 2015. doi:10.1016/j.jmmm.2014.09.070..

[2] D.Schmidt, F.Palmetshofer, D.Heinke, U.Steinhoff, and F.Ludwig. A phenomenological description of the MPS signal using a model for the field dependence of the effective relaxation time. IEEE Transactions on Magnetics, 51(2), 2015. doi:10.1109/TMAG.2014.2345192.

[3] Pan, L., Park, B. C., Ledwig, M., Abelmann, L., & Kim, Y. K. (2017). Magnetic Particle Spectrometry of Fe3O4 Multi-granule Nanoclusters. IEEE transactions on magnetics, 53(11), [5101004]. DOI: 10.1109/TMAG.2017.2701904

[4] Pouw, J. J., Grootendorst, M., Klaase, J. M., van Baarlen, J., & ten Haken, B. (2016). Ex vivo sentinel lymph node mapping in colorectal cancer using a magnetic nanoparticle tracer to improve staging accuracy: a pilot study. Colorectal disease, 18(12), 1147-1153. DOI: 10.1111/codi.13395

[5] J. Cha, J.S. Lee, S.J. Yoon, Y.K. Kim, and J.-K. Lee. Solid-state phase transformation mechanism for formation of magnetic multi-granule nanoclusters. RSC Advances, 3(11):3631–3637, 2013. doi:10.1039/c3ra21639j.

Continuous-Flow Synthesis of Superparamagnetic Iron Oxide Nanoparticles

Jan Magonov, Klaas Rackebrandt, Kerstin Lüdtke-Buzug*

Institute of Medical Engineering, University of Luebeck, Luebeck, Germany
* Corresponding author, email: luedtke-buzug@imt.uni-luebeck.de

I. Introduction

Superparamagnetic iron oxide nanoparticles (SPIONs) play an important role in many fields of technology, biochemistry and biomedical science. Applications in medicine are, for instance, drug delivery and tumor therapy by hyperthermia. Magnetic Particle Imaging (MPI) makes use of the SPIONs as tracer material [1, 2]. The properties of the tracer material such as the distribution of hydrodynamic and core diameter as well as magnetization and iron content have an impact on the quality of the imaging method. Therefore, it is of interest to synthesize SPIONs with consistent quality. Continuous-flow manufacturing is the keyword for a method that allows a non-stop tracer production in consistent quality. Especially in medical chemistry, this method is a promising approach for the controlled production of pharmaceuticals [3, 4, 5, 6].

In this contribution, a prototype of a miniaturized continuous-flow synthesis line for SPIONs is presented. The prototype device is supposed to enable the SPION production under reliable parameter control. Adjustable parameters are the temperature during the individual synthesis steps, and the flow rate. In this work, the nanoparticle yields obtained with varying flow rates were analyzed with magnetic particle spectroscopy (MPS).

II. Material and Methods

II.I. Synthesis Method

In principle, various synthesis strategies for SPIONs are known, for instance sol-gel preparation, micro-emulsion, gas deposition or co-precipitation [7]. In this work, co-precipitation was chosen. The synthesis of iron oxide nanoparticles by alkaline precipitation is a straightforward method.

Large amounts of aqueous suspensions of nanoparticles can be produced with this method [5]. Precipitation of iron oxide (Fe^{2+} and Fe^{3+}) in the presence of the coating material (Dextran T70) with a base (NH_3, 7.5 %) follows the reaction schemes

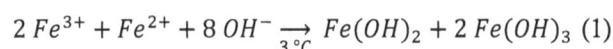

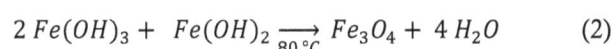

$$2\,Fe^{3+} + Fe^{2+} + 8\,OH^- \xrightarrow{3\,°C} Fe(OH)_2 + 2\,Fe(OH)_3 \quad (1)$$

$$2\,Fe(OH)_3 + Fe(OH)_2 \xrightarrow{80\,°C} Fe_3O_4 + 4\,H_2O \quad (2)$$

The colloidal nanoparticles in aqueous suspension are suitable for medical use due to biocompatibility of dextran. Unfortunately, the synthesized nanoparticles have a broad size distribution. Therefore, typically, further separation steps are required. However, with the approach presented here, the separation cascade should be cut.

II.II. Synthesis Device

The continuous-flow device consists of a syringe pump and a two-step reaction line as shown in Fig. 1.

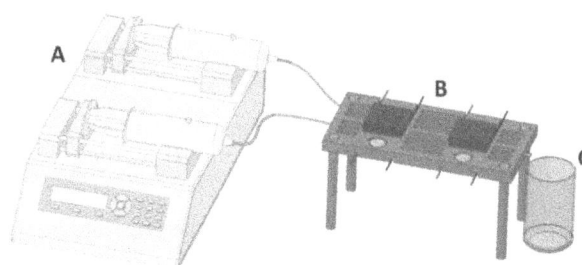

Figure 1: Setup of the synthesis apparatus with syringe-pump (A), reaction line (B) and sample vessel (C).

The iron salts with dextran and the base are placed in two different syringes in the syringe pump. As mentioned before the synthesis follows the principle of the co-precipitation. In the first step of the synthesis line, the solution is cooled, whereas in the second step it is heated up to approx. 80 °C. The yield, i.e. the colloidal nanoparticle suspension, is collected in a sample vessel. In order to prevent the oxidation of the iron by degassing and especially the agglomeration of the particles, the whole synthesis process is subjected to ultrasound vibration.

III. Results

The synthesized SPIONs were evaluated by MPS. With this method the core diameter of the particles in suspension can be estimated. Since the decay of the harmonics in MPS is of importance for imaging quality of MPI, the amplitudes of the harmonics will be compared for different flow rates and validated against Resovist, the commercial gold standard MPI tracer material.

The following parameters for the MPS measurements have been chosen: maximum field strength: 25 mT, measurement period: 5 s, number of repetitions: 12500, frequency 25 kHz. Each measurement was repeated 3 times.

A high reproducibility of SPIONs synthesized with the continuous-flow synthesis device can be obtained. In Fig. 2 the analysis of a series of experiments with a constant flow rate of 0.05 ml/min is shown. All yields obtained with this flow rate show consistent amplitude spectra.

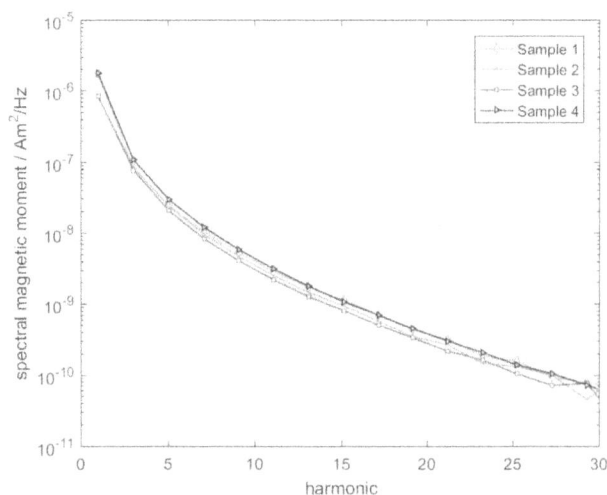

Figure 2: Amplitude spectra of multiple SPIONs synthesized with a flow rate of 0.05 ml/min. Only the odd harmonics are shown in this figure.

In order to investigate the influence of the flow rate on the yield, the synthesis had to be carried out at different flow rates. Fig. 3 shows the amplitude spectra of SPIONs synthesized with different flow rates. The following flow rates were selected for the systematic investigation: 0.05 ml/min, 0.2 ml/min and 0.4 ml/min. Each synthesis experiment has been repeated at least four times. The results are validated against a sample of Resovist.

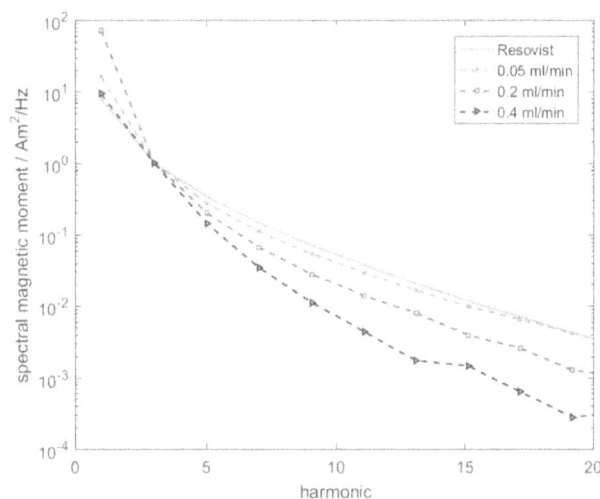

Figure 3: Amplitude spectra of SPIONs synthesized with different flow rates compared with the spectrum of Resovist. The spectra are normalized to the third harmonic.

In order to compare the decay of the spectra, they were normalized to the third harmonic, due to the difference between the iron content of the raw yields of the synthesis line presented here and the iron content of Resovist. It can be shown that increasing of the flow rate leads to a decrease of the amplitude spectra.

IV. Discussion and Conclusion

A continuous-flow synthesis set-up has been presented. In a repetition series of syntheses with the same parameters it was demonstrated that continuous-flow synthesis leads to tracer material suitable for MPI.

Using the same parameters for the synthesis like the reaction temperatures, the concentrations of the reactants and the flow rate high reproducibility is achieved like shown in Fig. 2.

Further, it can be shown that the MPI relevant magnetization properties of the particles are influenced by the flow rate as shown in Fig. 3. It is conjectured that higher flow rates lead to smaller particle cores in the presented setup. With a flow rate of 0.05 ml/min the tracer quality of Resovist can be achieved. However, the first continuous-flow synthesis demonstrator presented here is a prove-of-concept and needs further improvement in future work.

REFERENCES

[1] B. Gleich and J. Weizenecker. *Tomographic imaging using the nonlinear response of magnetic particles*. Nature, 435:121-1217, 2005. doi: 10.1038/nature03808.

[2] T. Knopp and T. M. Buzug. *Magnetic Particle Imaging: An Introduction to Imaging Principles and Scanner Instrumentation*. Springer, Berlin/Heidelberg, 2012. doi: 10.1007/978-3-642-04199-0.

[3] A. Adamo et al. *On-demand continuous-flow production of pharmaceuticals in a compact, reconfigurable system. Science*, 352 (6281), 61-67, 2016. doi: 10.1126/science.aaf1337

[4] S. Laurent et al. *Magnetic iron oxide nanoparticles: synthesis, stabilization, vectorization, physicochemical characterizations, and biological applications*. Chem. Rev.**108**, 2064–2110, 2008. doi:10.1021/cr068445e

[5] A. Baki, et al., *Continuous synthesis of single core iron oxide nanoparticles for MPI tracer development*, International Journal on Magnetic Particle Imaging, 3(1), Article ID 1703004

[6] F. Haseidl et al. *Continuous-Flow synthesis and Functionalization ofMagnetite: Intensified Process for Tailores Nanoparticles*. Chem. Eng. Technol. 11, 2051-2058, 2016. doi: 10.1002/ceat.201600163

[7] K. Lüdtke-Buzug. *Magnetische Nanopartikel: Von der Synthese zur klinischen Anwendung*. Chemie in unserer Zeit 46, 32–39, 2012. doi: 10.1002/ciuz.201200558

Synthesis of Super-Paramagnetic Iron Oxides Nanoparticles Subjected to Magnetic Fields

Ankit Malhotra [a,*], Pauline Kaiser [a], Thorsten M. Buzug [a], and Kerstin Lüdtke-Buzug [a,*],

[a] *Institute of Medical Engineering, University of Lübeck, Lübeck, Germany*
[*] *Corresponding authors, email: {malhotra, luedtke-buzug}@imt.uni-luebeck.de*

I. Introduction

Superparamagnetic iron oxide nanoparticles (SPIONs) have a high potential in the fields of medicine and biology. These nanoparticles have already shown immense use in medical imaging, for instance, in modalities like Magnetic Resonance Imaging (MRI) and Magnetic Particle Imaging (MPI) [1], where they are used as tracer material. MPI is an emerging imaging modality measuring the spatial distribution of SPIONs in a volume. Complementary to MPI these nanoparticles can also be used for MFH (Magnetic Fluid Hyperthermia) [2] and drug delivery [3]. In MFH the SPIONs are used as a medium to deposit energy, which may result in a coagulation of cancer cells. Superparamagnetic nanoparticles can be synthesized straightforwardly and can be varied in core and hull size according to the application. For example, for MPI the ideal core diameter of the nanoparticles should be approximately 20 nm to 30 nm [1, 4]. For MFH the particles should have a hysteresis and must be tailored according to the frequency of the applied magnetic field (AMF), as done by Khandhar et al. [5]. The classic synthesis route for SPIONs is based on the co-precipitation of iron salts in an aqueous solution in the presence of biocompatible coating material. This method is simple and has a high yield of biocompatible particles. However, it does not produce monodisperse particles. Moreover, in this method, the magnetic properties of the SPIONs, which are associated to the particle core size, are difficult to control. There are many methods for modifying the properties of SPIONs, such as the addition of surfactants, reducing agents, and temperature. In this contribution, it is demonstrated that there is one more parameter, which has a significant influence on the synthesis process, a magnetic field applied during synthesis. The effect of an external magnetic field has been shown for nickel nanowires [6] and in preparation of Co-doped α-Fe_2O_3 cubic nanocrystal assemblies [7]. The aim of the work presented here is to show the effect of a static magnetic field on an ultrasound mediated synthesis of the SPIONs with dextran coating. Five different magnetic fields ranging from 200 mT to 400 mT are used.

II. Material and Methods

II.I. Chemicals

Iron (III) chloride ($FeCl_3 \cdot 6H_2O$, ≥ 99 % obtained, Carl Roth GmbH Karlsruhe, Germany), iron (II) chloride ($FeCl_2 \cdot 4H_2O$, ≥ 99 % obtained, Merck KGaA, Darmstadt, Germany), Dextran T70 (AppliChem GmbH, Darmstadt, Germany).

II.II. Synthesis Technique and Characterization

As stated earlier, the nanoparticles are synthesized via alkaline co-precipitation in demineralized water under ultrasonic control [8]. The chemical reaction of the formation of the nanoparticles can be divided in two steps and are described by the following equations:

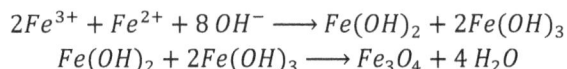

$$2Fe^{3+} + Fe^{2+} + 8\,OH^- \longrightarrow Fe(OH)_2 + 2Fe(OH)_3$$
$$Fe(OH)_2 + 2Fe(OH)_3 \longrightarrow Fe_3O_4 + 4\,H_2O$$

For synthesis, the iron salts and the dextran are dissolved in demineralized water at room temperature inside a flask and placed in an ultrasound bath with a frequency of 42 kHz.

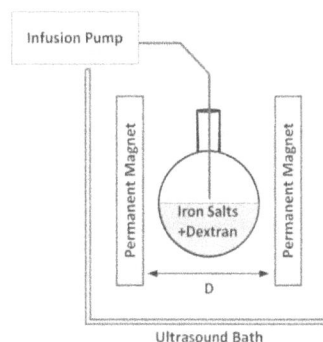

Figure 1. The block diagram of the setup for the synthesis of SPIONs in magnetic field. The setup consists of a pair of permanent magnet which can be shifted in position to vary the field strengths.

A pair of permanent magnets is used to generate the required magnetic field. The distance between the permanent magnets can be appropriately adjusted to attain the required magnetic field strength. The schematic diagram of the experimental setup is shown in Figure 1. In the first part of the chemical reaction, ammonia is dropped into the solution. The flow rate of the ammonia is controlled with the help of an infusion pump (PERFUSOR secura FT, B. Brown). For all the experiments a constant flow rate is set to 15 ml/hr. In the second step after the addition of the ammonia, the solution is slowly heated to a temperature of 80 °C for 30 minutes. For evaluation, the same reaction is also performed without the permanent magnets. The distance (D) between the magnets is altered to adjust different field strengths. The field strength due to the different positions of the permanent magnets is measured by a 3-channel gausmeter (Lake Shore Cryotronics). The effective field strengths obtained at different positions are shown in Table 1.

Table 1. The measured field produced due to positioning of the permanent magnents. The field is measured with 3- channel gauss meter.

Field Strength / mT

D / cm	X	Y	Z	XYZ
2.5	278.47	295.61	32.7	407.44
3	206.89	293.94	21.79	359.61
4	183.13	210.89	15.71	279.75
5	136.73	172.15	11.17	220.13
5.5	149.48	126.45	11.38	196.23

For characterization of the synthesized nanoparticles the magnitude spectrum and the hysteresis curves are obtained by a one dimensional MPS (Magnetic Particle Spectrometer) operating at a frequency of 25 kHz with a magnetic field strength of 20 mT at room temperature [9].

III. Results and Discussion

After the completion of the synthesis process, 10 μL samples of the particles of the different synthesis experiments are measured with the MPS system.

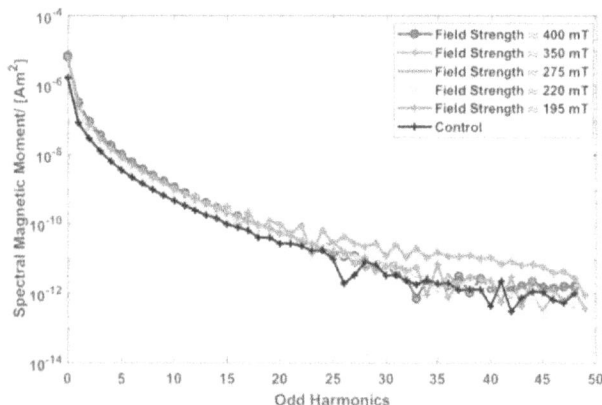

Figure 2. The spectral magnetic moment of all the synthesized samples at different field strengths measured with 1D MPS.

The magnitude and the hysteresis curves obtained are shown in Figure 2 and Figure 3, respectively. The control synthesis without magnetic field is given as well. The amplitude spectrum of the different particles does not change significantly with the field strength. However, there is a significant impact on the hysteresis curves obtained. It

is conjectured that the change in the hysteresis curve is due to an increase in the growth of nanoparticles in comparison to the control measurement. With the exception of the synthesis at 275 mT, the saturation magnetization increase seems to be quite linear to the change of the magnetic field strength.

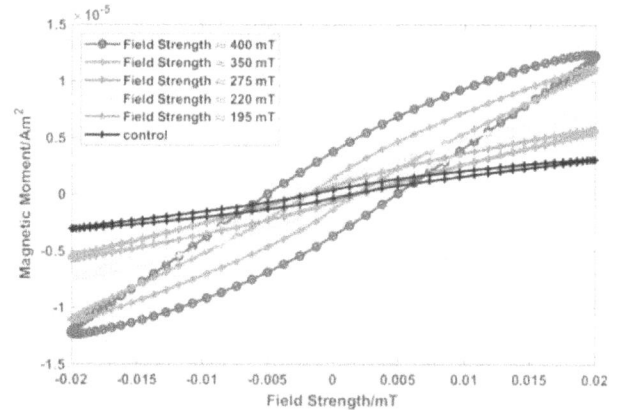

Figure 3. The hystersis curves of all the synthesized samples at different field strengths measured with 1D MPS.

IV. Conclusions

It can be conjectured that due to the presence of a magnetic field during synthesis the growth of the particles can be influenced. In the first experiments presented here, the change in saturation magnetization seems to be proportional to the external magnetic field. Further experiments are required to measure the size distribution of the particles. Additionally, it will be investigated how the growth process is influenced by oscillating and rotating magnetic fields during synthesis.

REFERENCES
[1] Gleich, B. & Weizenecker, J. (2005), 'Tomographic imaging using the nonlinear response of magnetic particles', nature 435, 1214-1217. doi: 10.1038/nature03808.
[2] Lópeza, M.; AntonioTeijeiro & Rivasa, J. (2013), 'Magnetic nanoparticle-based hyperthermia for cancer treatment', Reports of Practical Oncology & Radiotherapy 18(6), 397-400.
[3] Alexiou, C.; Arnold, W.; Klein, R. J.; Parak, F. G.; Hulin, P.; Bergemann, C.; Erhardt, W.; Wagenpfeil, S. & Lübbe, A. S. (2000), 'Locoregional Cancer Treatment with Magnetic Drug Targeting', Cancer Research 60, 6641-6648.
[4] Ferguson, R. M.; Khandhar, A. P. Krishnan & K. M. (2012), 'Tracer design for magnetic particle imaging', Journal of Applied Physics 111(7).
[5] Khandhar, A.; Ferguson, R. M.; Simon, J. A. & Krishnan, K. M. (2012), 'Tailored Magnetic Nanoparticles for Optimizing Magnetic Fluid Hyperthermia', J Biomed Mater Res A. 100(3), 728-737.
[6] Sun, W.; Cheng, J.; Li, L.; Chen, S. & Chang, K. (2017), 'Preparation and magnetic properties of nickel nanowires by reduction in ethylene glycol medium under the influence of magnetic field', IOP Conference Series: Materials Science and Engineering 167, 012030.
[7] Gandha, K.; Mohapatra, J.; Poudyal, N.; Elkins, K. & Liu, J. P. (2017), 'Enhanced coercivity in Co-doped α-Fe_2O_3 cubic nanocrystal assemblies prepared via a magnetic field-assisted hydrothermal synthesis', AIP Advances 7(5), 056324.
[8] Lüdtke-Buzug, K. (2012), 'Magnetische Nanopartikel', Chemie in unserer Zeit 46(1), 32—39.
[9] Biederer, S.; Knopp, T.; Sattel, T. F; Ludtke-Buzug, K.; Gleich, B.; Weizenecker, J.; Borgert, J. & Buzug, T. M. (2009),'Magnetization response spectroscopy of superparamagnetic nanoparticles for magnetic particle imaging', J. Phys. D: Appl. Phys. 42

Comparison of Superparamagnetic Quantifier and Magnetic Particle Spectroscopy

Melissa van de Loosdrecht [a,*], Sebastian Draack [b], Sebastiaan Waanders [a], Erik Krooshoop [a], Frank Ludwig [b], and Bennie ten Haken [a]

[a] *Magnetic Detection and Imaging group, Faculty of Science and Technology, University of Twente, Enschede, the Netherlands*
[b] *Institut für Elektrische Messtechnik und Grundlagen der Elektrotechnik, TU Braunschweig, Braunschweig, Germany*
* Corresponding author, email: m.m.vandeloosdrecht@utwente.nl

I. Introduction

In the design process of superparamagnetic iron oxide nanoparticles (SPIONs) it is inevitable to have a consistent characterization technique. Such a device enables you to check quickly what the effect is of a change in the process. For example, used chemicals and their precursor concentration, temperature, and alkalinity of the medium are factors that influence the produced particles and their magnetic properties [1].

In order to characterize SPIONs, many techniques can be used, including the Superparamagnetic Quantifier (SPaQ) and Magnetic Particle Spectroscopy (MPS). The SPaQ was developed at the University of Twente for the evolution of DiffMag. DiffMag is a procedure to selectively detect SPIONs [2]. In this research, the MPS system of the TU Braunschweig was used [3].

II. Materials and Methods

Both systems make use of Faraday detection, using copper excitation and detection coils. The detector has a gradiometer configuration to compensate for the large excitation signal. The advantages of induction coils are the ease of realization, fast measurements and high signal to noise ratio.

The derivative of the magnetization curve ($m(H)$ curve) is measured in both systems, which is related to the point spread function in MPS [4]. In this contribution, two types of particles (Resovist™ (Bayer Schering Pharma GmbH) and SHP-25 (Ocean Nanotech)) were measured in both devices to evaluate differences in the measured magnetization curves. The differences, both in resulting curve and measurement method, are summarized in Table 1.

III. Results and Discussion

The resulting curves are shown in Fig. 1 and Fig. 2, for the SPaQ and MPS measurements, respectively. The MPS measurements show a clear hysteresis loop, whereas the SPaQ measurements show minor hysteresis. This can be explained by the fact that the entire curve is measured in every period of the sine in de MPS measurements, leading to large influence of particle dynamics. SPaQ measurements, on the other hand, can be considered as quasi-static, due to the small AC amplitude.

The sample influences the height and width of the measured curve. In MPS, the distance between the peaks (e.g. the width of the hysteresis loop) changes as well as a response to particle dynamics.

IV. Applications

Measuring the magnetization curve enables the characterization of SPIONs. Many parameters can be deduced from the curves, such as the core diameter, hydrodynamic diameter, and anisotropy [5]. Additionally, these measurements can provide information about the environment of the particles. As a result, SPIONs can be studied in biological systems, such as blood [6] and lymph nodes.

Characterization of SPIONs in lymph nodes provides information that is useful for the sentinel node biopsy (SNB). SNB is a tool to determine the lymph node status of cancer patients [7]. Consequently, it can be seen if the tumor has metastasized and the patient prognosis and treatment can be personalized. In SNB, a tracer material is injected in or close to the tumor. The tracer will follow the natural path through the lymph nodes and accumulate in the sentinel node. The sentinel node can be found using a dedicated detector, and examined for metastases after surgical removal.

As tracer material, SPIONs can be used in combination with a handheld DiffMag probe [2]. When the SPIONs accumulate in a lymph node, the particles will be (partially) immobilized and their magnetic behavior will change. To evaluate the resulting effect on the DiffMag signal, SPaQ measurements can be utilized. This application is superior in the SPaQ compared to MPS, because of the direct correlation to DiffMag.

A last application of the SPaQ is to use it for *ex-vivo* SNB [8]. In rectal cancer it is recommended to remove all regional lymph nodes, since it reduces the chance of local recurrence [9]. If the SPIONs are injected *in-vivo* during surgery, all lymph nodes can be dissected and measured in the SPaQ *ex-vivo*.

V. Conclusions

In conclusion, both systems are capable of measuring the magnetization curve, which results in invaluable information on particle properties for many applications.

ACKNOWLEDGEMENTS
Financial support by the Netherlands Organization for Scientific Research (NWO), under the research program Magnetic Sensing for Laparoscopy (MagLap) with project number 14322, and by the German Research Foundation DFG via SPP1681 under grant no. SCHI-383/2-1 acknowledged.

REFERENCES

[1]   L. Pan, B. C. Park, M. Ledwig, L. Abelmann, and Y. K. Kim, "Magnetic Particle Spectrometry of Fe3O4 Multi-Granule Nanoclusters," *IEEE Trans. Magn.*, vol. 53, no. 11, pp. 1–4, 2017.

[2]   S. Waanders, M. Visscher, R. R. Wildeboer, T. O. B. Oderkerk, H. J. G. Krooshoop, and B. Ten Haken, "A handheld SPIO-based sentinel lymph node mapping device using differential magnetometry.," *Phys. Med. Biol.*, vol. 61, no. 22, pp. 8120–8134, Nov. 2016.

[3]   S. Draack, T. Viereck, C. Kuhlmann, M. Schilling, and F. Ludwig, "Temperature-dependent MPS measurements," *Int. J. Magn. Part. Imaging; Vol 3, No 1*, Mar. 2017.

[4]   I. Schmale, J. Rahmer, B. Gleich, J. Borgert, and J. Weizenecker, "Point Spread Function Analysis of Magnetic Particles," in *Magnetic Particle Imaging: A Novel SPIO Nanoparticle Imaging Technique*, T. M. Buzug and J. Borgert, Eds. Berlin, Heidelberg: Springer Berlin Heidelberg, 2012, pp. 287–292.

[5]   D. B. Reeves and J. B. Weaver, "Combined Néel and Brown rotational Langevin dynamics in magnetic particle imaging, sensing, and therapy," *Appl. Phys. Lett.*, vol. 107, no. 22, 2015.

[6]   P. D. Pino, B. Pelaz, Q. Zhang, P. Maffre, G. U. Nienhaus, and W. J. Parak, "Protein corona formation around nanoparticles - From the past to the future," *Mater. Horizons*, vol. 1, no. 3, 2014.

[7]   A. E. Giuliano and A. Gangi, "Sentinel node biopsy and improved patient care," *Breast J.*, vol. 21, no. 1, 2015.

[8]   J. J. Pouw, M. R. Grootendorst, J. M. Klaase, J. van Baarlen, and B. ten Haken, "Ex vivo sentinel lymph node mapping in colorectal cancer using a magnetic nanoparticle tracer to improve staging accuracy: a pilot study," *Color. Dis.*, vol. 18, no. 12, 2016.

[9]   C. M. Mery and R. Bleday, "Principles of Total Mesorectal Excision for Rectal Cancer," *Semin. Colon Rectal Surg.*, vol. 16, no. 3, pp. 117–127, 2005.

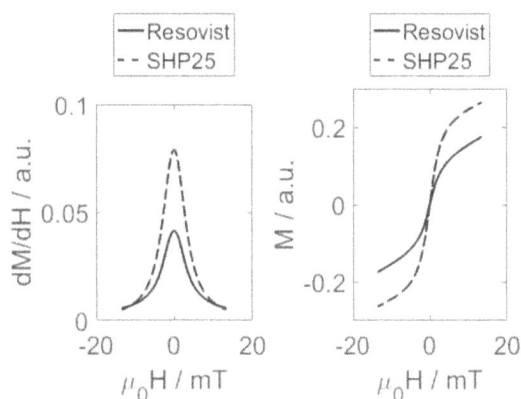

Figure 1: SPaQ results, measured on Resovist^{TM} and SHP-25 samples containing 750 µg iron in a total volume of 150 µl.

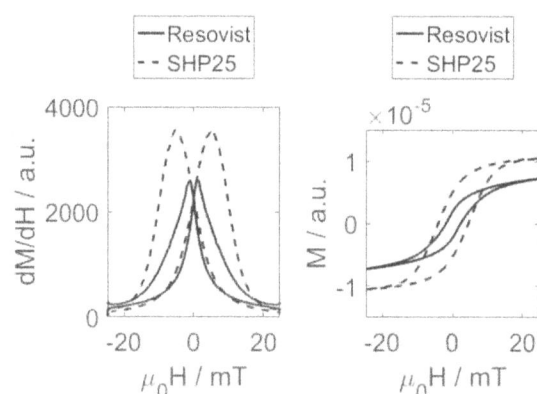

Figure 2: MPS results, measured on Resovist^{TM} and SHP-25 samples containing 750 µg iron in a total volume of 150 µl.

Table 1: Differences between SPaQ and MPS

	SPaQ	MPS
Excitation sequence	Small AC amplitude (1.3 mT)	Large AC amplitude (25 mT)
	DC offset (up to 13.3 mT)	No DC offset
Measurement time	5 seconds	0.5 seconds
Measurement	Quasi-static	Dynamic
Magnetization curve	Minor hysteresis	Hysteresis

From MPI Tracer Materials to Target-Specific *in vivo* Diagnostics

David Heinke [a,*], **Oliver Posth** [b], **Wilfried Reichardt** [c], **Andreas Briel** [a]

a nanoPET Pharma GmbH, Berlin, Germany
b Physikalisch-Technische Bundesanstalt, Berlin, Germany
c Department of Radiology, Medical Physics, University Medical Center Freiburg, Freiburg, Germany
* *Corresponding author (david.heinke@nanopet.de)*

I. Introduction

Since Magnetic Particle Imaging (MPI) was first introduced by Gleich and Weizenecker in 2005 [1], one of the objective targets has been the synthesis of high-performance tracer materials to prove the vast potential of the technology in terms of sensitivity and spatial resolution. The first preclinical MPI scanners for small animal imaging are now commercially available and, as a result, the development of optimal tracer materials that are biocompatible, and thus suitable for *in vivo* application, is becoming increasingly important. Furthermore, it is preferable that these diagnostic materials can be functionalized so that they can be subsequently used in more advanced processes such as in active targeting.

Here, we present the further development of such a diagnostic material, namely a dextran-coated superparamagnetic iron oxide nanoparticle (SPION) having a high MPS performance [2]. In this work, we perform further analysis on the material's colloidal stability, as well as develop suitable formulation and sterilization strategies. Additionally, we conduct biocompatibility studies including cytotoxicity assays. For bioconjugation of e.g. proteins, the particle surface was further modified by carboxymethylation as well as amination.

II. Materials and Methods

The colloidal stability of the SPION suspended in water was determined by dynamic light scattering (DLS). Formulation was achieved through the use of D-mannitol and NaOH in order to adjust the osmolality as well as the pH to physiological values (~300 mosmol/kg, pH 7.4). Subsequently, the formulated SPION was sterilized via autoclaving. Magnetic particle spectra (MPS) were recorded at a drive field having an amplitude of 25 mT/μ_0 and a frequency, f_0 of 25 kHz. Cytotoxicity was evaluated by incubating the formulated and sterilized particles with two different cell lines – mesenchymal stem cells and human keratinocytes – and determining the cell viability via the MTT assay. A first *in vivo* experiment with MR imaging was conducted by injection of the formulated and sterilized particle suspension in the tail vein of a healthy mouse at a dose of 20 μmol Fe/kg body weight (bw). MR images were recorded with a T_2*-weighted FLASH sequence at 9.4 T MRI (Bruker BioSpec 94/20 USR). Surface modification was performed by treatment of the particles with monochloroacetic acid (MCA) at elevated temperatures (70 °C) or by treatment with epichlorohydrin and ammonia. Furthermore, the particles' relaxivity was determined at 0.94 T and 39 °C (minispec mq40, Bruker Biospin).

III. Results

III.I. Formulation and Sterilization

The colloidal stability of the SPION suspended in water was found to be stable over the measured time period of two years, as determined by measurement of the hydrodynamic particle diameter, a parameter that is strongly altered by aggregation processes (see Fig. 1).

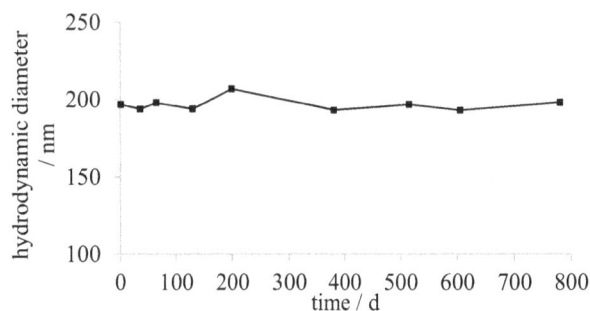

Figure 1: *Colloidal long-term stability of the magnetic nanoparticles evaluated by the change in the hydrodynamic particle diameter measured by DLS.*

After formulation with D-mannitol and NaOH and subsequent sterilization via autoclaving, the particle suspension was found to remain stable for at least 18 days. As shown in Fig. 2 neither the formulation nor the sterilization process altered the MPS performance. Furthermore, after formulation and sterilization, the R_2 relaxivity value remained the same, denoting that the processes did not affect the MR contrast efficacy.

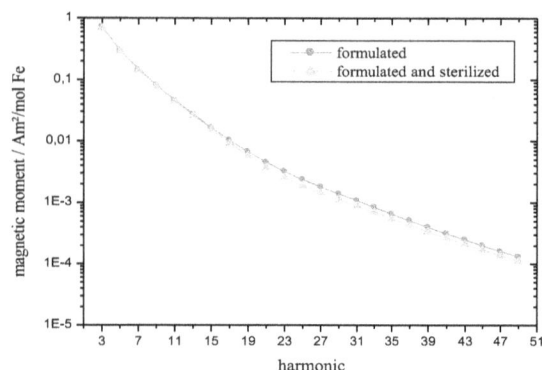

Figure 2: MPS of physiologically formulated nanoparticles measured at 25 mT/μo and f_0 = 25 kHz before and after sterilization by autoclaving.

III.II. Surface modification

Depending on the amount of MCA used for carboxymethylation, the zetapotential of the uncharged dextran-coated particles changed from 0 mV to a value between -2 mV and -24 mV, which is a strong indication of the generation of particles having different amounts of carboxylic acid groups on their surface. To prove that these modified particles are suitable for bioconjugation, NeutrAvidin® protein was coupled to the particle surface via carbodiimide chemistry. Subsequently, these particles were incubated on biotin-coated microplates and the bound particles were made visible by Prussian blue staining. Whereas the non-modified SPIONs (i.e. dextran-coated particles subjected to NeutrAvidin® protein) as control were unable to bind to the plates, binding clearly occurred for the protein-functionalized particles (i.e. the particles that were first carboxymethylated and subsequently treated with NeutrAvidin® protein). Similarly, depending on the amount of epichlorohydrin and ammonia used, particles with positive zetapotentials of +1 to +30 mV were obtained, indicating the presence of amino groups on the particle surface. Neither carboxymethylation nor amination altered the MPS performance of the particles.

III.III. Cytotoxicity

Materials that allow cell viabilities of more than 80 % are generally recognized as biocompatible [3]. As shown in Fig. 3, all analyzed samples tested to a maximum Fe concentration of 2 mM are above this threshold, making them suitable for *in vivo* application.

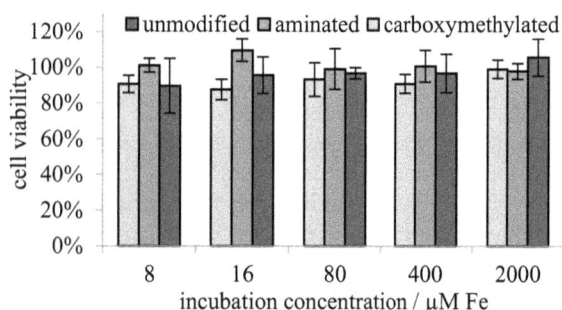

Figure 3: Concentration-dependent cell viability of human keratinocytes after incubation with unmodified, carboxymethylated and aminated SPION as determined by MTT assay.

III.IV. MR imaging

In a first *in vivo* experiment, the animal showed no signs of acute toxicity confirming the biocompatibility of the SPION. Subsequent MRI revealed the rapid particle accumulation in the liver and the excellent contrast efficacy as shown in Fig. 4.

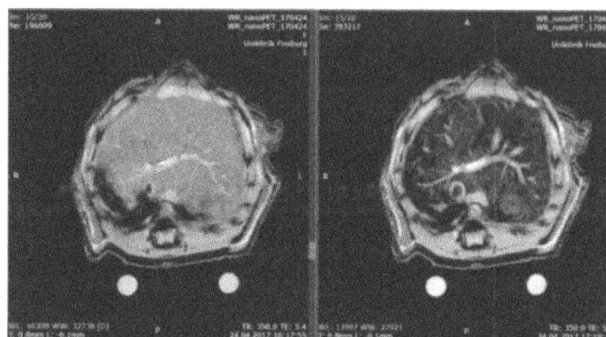

Figure 4: MR imaging of the mouse liver before (left) and 35 min after (right) iv injection of formulated and sterilized nanoparticles at a dose of 20 μmol Fe/kg bw. Depiction in axial orientation of a T_2*-weighted FLASH sequence.

IV. Conclusions

In this work we presented the development of colloidally stable, physiologically formulated and sterilized nanoparticle suspensions as biocompatible MPI tracers for *in vivo* application. Owing to the additional surface modification, these particles can be easily conjugated with diverse biomolecules to produce target-specific tracers for more advanced applications.

ACKNOWLEDGEMENTS

This work was supported by the European Commission Framework Programme 7 under the NanoMag project [grant agreement no 604448].

REFERENCES

[1] B. Gleich and J. Weizenecker. Tomographic imaging using the nonlinear response of magnetic particles. *Nature*, 435(7046):1217-1217, 2005. doi: 10.1038/nature03808.

[2] N. Gehrke, D. Heinke, D. Eberbeck, F. Ludwig, T. Wawrzik, C. Kuhlmann, and A. Briel. Magnetic characterization of clustered core magnetic nanoparticles for MPI, IEEE Trans. Magn., 51, 2015. doi: 10.1109/TMAG.2014.2358275.

[3] M. Mahmoudi, A. Simchi, A. S. Milani and P. Stroeve. Cell toxicity of superparamagnetic iron oxide nanoparticles, Journal of colloid and interface science, 336:510-518, 2009. doi: 10.1016/j.jcis.2009.04.046.

Biocompatible Magnetic Fluids of Modified Co-Ferrite Nanoparticles with Tunable Magnetic Properties

Silvio Dutz [a,*], Norbert Buske [b], Joachim H. Clement [c], Christine Gräfe [c], Frank Wiekhorst [d]

[a] Institute of Biomedical Engineering and Informatics (BMTI), Technische Universität Ilmenau, Ilmenau, Germany
[b] MagneticFluids, Köpenicker Landstr. 203, 12437 Berlin, Germany
[c] Klinik für Innere Medizin II, Abteilung Hämatologie und Internistische Onkologie, Universitätsklinikum Jena, Jena, Germany
[d] Physikalisch-Technische Bundesanstalt Berlin, Berlin, Germany

* Corresponding author, email: silvio.dutz@tu-ilmenau.de

I. Introduction

Magnetite (FeO x Fe_2O_3) particles with diameter around 10 nm have a very low coercivity (Hc) and relative remanent magnetization $M_{rel} = M_r/M_s$. In comparison to this, Co-ferrite (CoO x Fe_2O_3) particles have a very high H_c and M_{rel}, which is very favorable for magnetic recording [1]. Unfortunately, these particles are magnetically too hard to obtain suitable specific heating power (SHP) in magnetic hyperthermia [2] or good tracer performance in magnetic particle imaging (MPI) [3].

For optimization of the magnetic properties, the Fe^{2+} ions of magnetite were substituted by Co^{2+} step by step in our study which results in a Co doped inverse spinel with adjustable Fe^{2+} substitution degree. A Co-concentration of 0% (a = 0) leads to the formation of pure iron oxide particles and a Co-concentration of 25% (a=1) yields pure $CoFe_2O_4$. (Schema 1).

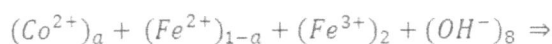

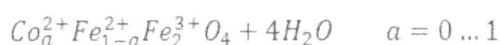

$$(Co^{2+})_a + (Fe^{2+})_{1-a} + (Fe^{3+})_2 + (OH^-)_8 \Rightarrow$$

$$Co_a^{2+}Fe_{1-a}^{2+}Fe_2^{3+}O_4 + 4H_2O \qquad a = 0 \dots 1$$

Schema 1: *Reaction equations for preparation of Co doped inverse spinels.*

II. Material and Methods

The particles were prepared from Co^{2+}, Fe^{2+}, and Fe^{3+} chloride mixtures (0.02 molar) at different "a"-values by co-precipitation with sodium hydroxide under stirring at 100°C for 90 minutes reaction time. The obtained particles were washed with distilled water using magnetic separation technique and stabilized in water with hydrochloric acid (intermediate, with positively charged particles) and with citric acid (final MF, pH = 7, negatively charged particles). All samples were filtrated through a 0.8µm filter.

The structural properties of prepared particles were determined by means of transmission electron microscopy (TEM) and X-ray diffraction (XRD). For the magnetic characterization of the samples (M_s, M_{rel}, and H_c) a vibrating sample magnetometer (VSM) was used. Magnetic heating performance for hyperthermia was investigated in calorimetrical measurements in alternating magnetic fields of different field strength and frequency and MPI performance was tested by means of MPS. The Co-content of the particles was determined by means of inductively coupled plasma optical emission spectrometry (ICP-OES). Biocompatibility was tested with the PrestoBlue Cell Viability Assay using human brain microvascular endothelial cells.

III. Results

For the ferrofluids containing the prepared particles, only a limited dependence of H_c and M_{rel} on the Co content in the particles was found (Figure 1). This confirms a proper and stable dispersion of the particles within the ferrofluid and magnetic properties are determined mainly by hydrodynamic particle size and a possible (but vanishingly low) particle agglomeration.

For dry particle samples, a strong correlation between Co content and resulting H_c and M_{rel} was found. For increasing Co concentrations from 0 to 8.6% (substitution rate "a" from 0 to 0.33) only a slight increase of H_c was found, but from 12 to 25% ("a" from 0.5 to 1) a strong linear increase of H_c results (Figure 1). Within this linear range of dependency, the magnetic properties of the particles, especially H_c, can be tuned easily by changing Co content of the particles.

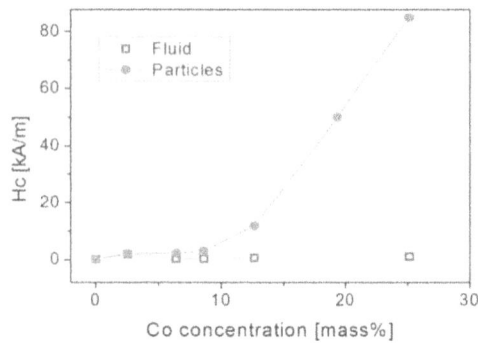

Figure 1: Coercivity of liquid and dry samples as function of Co concentration.

All particles have a size of around 10 nm and the obtained Co content correlates with the applied "a" during preparation. The prepared particles show no increased cytotoxicity compared to iron oxide particles up to a concentration of 25 μg/cm^2. A specific correlation of heating power and MPS performance (intensity and phase) of the particles with the Co content will be presented. Best samples show good performance for application in hyperthermia and MPI.

IV. Discussion

Here prepared particles have an inverse spinel lattice of oxygen atoms with iron (and/or cobalt) in the gaps of the lattice. In the tetrahedral gaps only Fe^{3+} can be located. The octahedral gaps of the lattice contain Fe^{3+} and Fe^{2+}, whereby the Fe^{2+} was substituted step by step by Co^{2+} in our experiments. To verify this hypothesis, the Fe/Co ratio of the ferrites was checked.

Iron and cobalt are chemically very similar elements. Therefore, a strong magnetic interaction at higher ion concentrations and at closest ion contact in the octahedral gaps seems to be possible and caused the strong increase of the coercivity with increasing Co concentration. Similar results were found for the combination of different metal-ferrites using the layer by layer technology [4].

V. Conclusions

We could demonstrate that the magnetic properties of magnetic nanoparticles can be tuned by means of substitution of the Fe^{2+} ions of magnetite by Co^{2+}. In ongoing studies, gels containing the here prepared ferrite particles (immobilized) are tested in magnetic hyperthermia and for MPI. Additionally, further studies on biocompatibility are necessary in order to use the particle for medical or biological applications.

ACKNOWLEDGEMENTS

This work was supported by Deutsche Forschungsgemeinschaft (DFG) (FKZ: DU 1293/6-1 and TR408/9-1).

REFERENCES

[1] C. Gansau and N. Buske, DE Patent 10205332B4 (2002).
[2] S. Dutz and R. Hergt. Magnetic Particle Hyperthermia – A promising tumor therapy? Nanotechnology 25: 452001 (2014).
[3] S. Dutz, D. Eberbeck, R. Müller, M. Zeisberger. Fractionated magnetic multicore nanoparticles for magnetic particle imaging. Springer Proceedings in Physics 140: 79–83 (2012).
[4] J.H. Lee et al. Exchange-coupled magnetic nanoparticles for efficient heat induction. Nature Nanotechnology 6: 418–422 (2011).

Preservation Procedures for Protein-coated Magnetic Nanoparticles and their Interaction with Biological Systems

Andreas Weidner [a], Christine Gräfe [b], Stephanie Wojahn [a], Joachim H. Clement [b], Silvio Dutz [a,*]

[a] Institute of Biomedical Engineering and Informatics, Technische Universität Ilmenau, Ilmenau, Germany
[b] Klinik für Innere Medizin II, Abteilung Hämatologie und Internistische Onkologie, Universitätsklinikum Jena, Jena, Germany
* Corresponding author, email: silvio.dutz@tu-ilmenau.de

I. Introduction

For future medical applications of magnetic nanoparticles (MNP) as drug carrier or MPI tracer in the human body, both effects within the body as well as how to securely handle these systems prior to application have to be elucidated. Therefore, we investigated protein coating of MNP during an in vitro serum incubation, varying the composition of the protein source, as well as the interactions of these incubated hybrid particles with living cells to determine their behavior after application. These interactions are of major importance for the development of long circulating tracer materials for MPI. Furthermore, we investigated ways to sterilize and preserve the particles after production.

II. Material and Methods

For the first part of the study we incubated cytotoxic polyethylenimine (PEI) coated MNP in distinct mixtures of cell medium and fetal calf serum (FCS) for defined times and temperatures to obtain the protein-coated MNP. Before and after the incubation we determined the physical properties of the MNP with different methods like zeta potential measurements, vibrating sample magnetometry (VSM), thermogravimetric analysis (TGA), transmission electron microscopy (TEM) as well as sodium dodecyl sulfate polyacrylamide gel electrophoresis (SDS-PAGE). Additionally, we investigated the effects on cell viability for human brain microvascular endothelial cells (HBMEC) by the CellTiter Glo™ assay and by real time cell analysis. The particle-cell interactions with HBMEC were also studied by means of flow cytometry of fluorochrome-labelled particles [1].

For the second part of the study, incubated MNP have been prepared, incubated as described in [2] and [3] and used within the following preservation and sterilisation methods:

- freezing at -15 °C
- deep freezing at -80 °C
- lyophilisation (with and without PEG or TMAH as additives)
- autoclaving (121 °C for 20 min)
- UV-sterilisation ($\lambda \sim 200$ to 280 nm for 150 to 240 min).

Possible effects on the particles and protein coating like degradation, agglomeration or cross-linking have been investigated by size measurement via dynamic light scattering (DLS). Additionally, the zeta potential was used as an indicator for surface protein load [1]. To determine the composition of the protein coating, a SDS-PAGE and a grey value intensity analysis by means of ImageJ was performed.

III. Results

For the in vitro serum incubation, an influence of the FCS concentration on the formation of the protein corona could be shown. The higher the FCS content, the further the corona evolves until a saturation is reached.

Additionally, we could demonstrate, that the protein coating is able to mask cytotoxic effects. Neither in short-term, nor in long-term viability tests, cytotoxic effects of PEI-coated MNP were observed after formation of a protein coating around the PEI shell. Furthermore, flow cytometry investigations indicated, that the protein coating delayed the particle-cell interaction of cytotoxic PEI-coated MNP.

Concerning the preservation of incubated particles, freezing at -15 °C and thawing the sample after two, four and six weeks, DLS indicates a significant agglomeration and SDS-PAGE reveals an increase in smaller sized proteins. For deep freezing at -80 °C the agglomeration does not appear that strong, but similar degradation effects can be observed. Therefore, both methods are rated as not suit-able for a long-term storage of protein-coated MNP.

Lyophilisation of protein-coated MNP with PEG as additive and redispersion after one, three and six weeks leads to a similar particle size and particle size distribution compared to the original sample, which qualifies this strategy as possible storage method. Plain particles without additive show slight agglomeration and TMAH-supplemented samples show instability and larger agglomerates as well as a fraction of very small protein fragments.

For autoclaving as sterilisation method, the results for DLS and the zeta potential of the samples did not change significantly, but SDS-PAGE reveals alterations in protein integrity. All typical peaks are vanished and only one large agglomeration in the region of 55 kDa could be observed, which is a clear indication for the denaturation and extensive degradation of the proteins in the coating. Thus, the standard autoclaving protocol is not suitable for the sterilisation of protein-coated MNP.

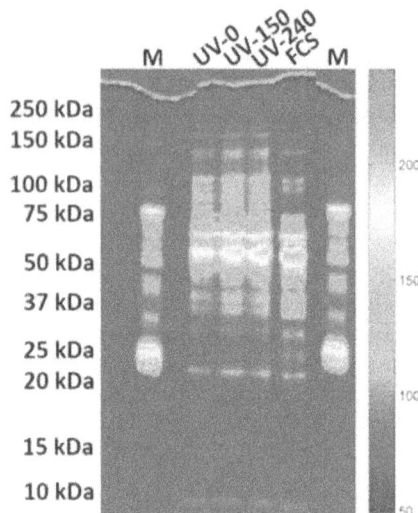

Figure 1: SDS-PAGE of protein-coated MNP before (UV-0) and after (UV-150, UV-240) UV sterilization.

UV sterilisation for 150 and 240 min on the opposite leads to stable zeta potentials of -30 mV as well as very similar results for SDS-PAGE, indicating that there are no major changes in composition and amount of the protein coating (see fig. 1). It can be concluded, that the exposure to UV radiation of 200 to 280 nm for up to 240 minutes, causes no relevant change of protein content and composition. UV sterilisation is therefore a suitable procedure for the sterilisation of protein-coated MNP.

IV. Conclusions

FCS-incubated MNP form a protein corona around them, which can mask cytotoxic effects and hampers particle-cell interaction. By this way, the blood half live of various core materials and particle types might be increased by the described protein coating, which is important for the development of long circulating tracer materials for MPI. Ongoing investigations focus on in vitro and in vivo experiments on the biological fate of protein-coated MNP after cellular uptake.

Furthermore, we found, that only UV sterilisation and lyophilisation with addition of PEG were suitable methods for sterilisation and preservation of the protein-coated MNP.

ACKNOWLEDGEMENTS

This work was supported by Deutsche Forschungsgemeinschaft (DFG) via SPP 1681 (FKZ: DU 1293/4-2, CL202/3-2).

REFERENCES

[1] C. Gräfe, A. Weidner, M. v.d. Lühe, C. Bergemann, F.H. Schacher, J.H. Clement, S. Dutz. Intentional formation of a protein corona on nanoparticles: Serum concentration affects protein corona mass, surface charge, and nanoparticle–cell interaction. Int J Biochem Cell Biol., 2016, 75, 196-202

[2] S. Dutz, J.H. Clement, D. Eberbeck, Th. Gelbrich, R. Hergt, R. Müller, J. Wotschadlo, M. Zeisberger. Ferrofluids of magnetic multicore nanoparticles for biomedical applications. J. Magn. Magn. Mater. 2009, 321/10, 1501–1504

[3] A. Weidner, C. Gräfe, M. v.d. Lühe, H. Remmer, J.H. Clement, D. Eberbeck, F. Ludwig, R. Müller, F.H. Schacher, S. Dutz. Preparation of Core-Shell Hybrid Materials by Producing a Protein Corona around Magnetic Nanoparticles. Nanoscale Research Letters 2015, 10, 28

New MPI Tracer Material – A Resolution Study

Christina Debbeler [a,*], Anselm von Gladiss [a], Thomas Friedrich [a], Thorsten M. Buzug [a],
Kerstin Lüdtke-Buzug [a,*]

[a] *Institute of Medical Engineering, Universität zu Lübeck, Lübeck, Germany*
[*] *Corresponding author, email: {debbeler,luedtke-buzug}@imt.uni-luebeck.de*

I. Introduction

Magnetic particle imaging (MPI) combines high spatial and temporal resolution with excellent sensitivity [1]. The principle of this imaging technique is based on the nonlinear magnetization characteristic of superparamagnetic iron oxide nanoparticles (SPIONs) and does not stress the patient with harmful radiation. The SPIONs response to an oscillating magnetic field allows for a three-dimensional visualization of the particle distribution in space. Being a real-time imaging modality, MPI seems to be ideally suited for applications such as cardiovascular and interventional imaging as well as cellular and targeted imaging.

Parallel to the ongoing efforts in MPI instrumentation development, the advancement of tailored MPI tracer material is impelled as well. Resovist is still being considered as gold standard in MPI research, although it is no longer commercially available. Therefore, tracer development is a crucial step to clinical application scenarios of MPI. New MPI tracer material has to meet highly diverse technical demands, as monodispersity, spherical particle shape, high steepness of the magnetization curve, isotropy and fast relaxation [2,3]. Additionally, biocompatibility is an essential issue in biomedical applications.

The objective of the EU project NanoMag [4] is the standardization, improvement and redefinition of manufacturing technologies as well as analyzing methods of magnetic nanoparticles. In respect to a possible suitability for MPI, newly synthesized particles were analyzed regarding their spatial resolution.

II. Material and Methods

For the spatial resolution study, a multi-dimensional magnetic particle spectroscopy (MPS) device [5,6] and a preclinical MPI scanner (Bruker BioSpin GmbH, Ettlingen, Germany) were used. The investigations presented here are based on a hybrid and a measurement-based approach.

For the hybrid approach, a hybrid system matrix [7] recorded with the multi-dimensional MPS device was used to reconstruct emulated phantoms. Varying magnetic offset fields have been applied in order to emulate different spatial positions [8] resulting in phantoms that consist of four dots (referred to as phantom 1).

The MPS measurements were performed using excitation frequencies of about 25 kHz, 12 mT field strength in both x- and y-direction, offset fields from -16 mT to +16 mT, 10 averages of the receive signal resulting in a single measurement time of 6.5 ms and a sample volume of 10 µl.

For the measurement-based approach, both system matrices and resolution phantom measurements were performed with the preclinical MPI scanner. The resolution phantom (referred to as phantom 2) [9] can be equipped with capillaries positioned in varying spatial distances as seen in Fig. 1.

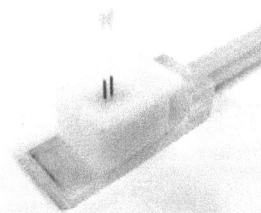

Figure 1: Resolution phantom (phantom 2) used for multi-dimensional MPI measurements. The phantom is equipped with two capillaries and allows a distance variation between different samples.

The MPI scanner measurements feature excitation frequencies of about 25 kHz, 12 mT field strength in both x- and y-direction and 500 averages of the receive signal resulting in a single measurement time of 326 ms. The system matrices have been recorded using 11 x 11 x 1 spatial positions covering a FOV in the range from -5 mT to +5 mT gradient field strength in both x- and y-direction. 0.2 µl of particles have been filled in each capillary.

III. Results

Results of the hybrid approach of three samples and Resovist featuring a distance in the magnetic offset field that corresponds to a spatial distance of 2.3 mm in the MPI scanner are shown in Fig. 2. The four dots of phantom 1 are clearly separable for all four samples at a magnetic offset field distance corresponding to 2.3 mm. Sample B shows a performance slightly worse compared to Resovist. Samples A and C show a slightly better performance.

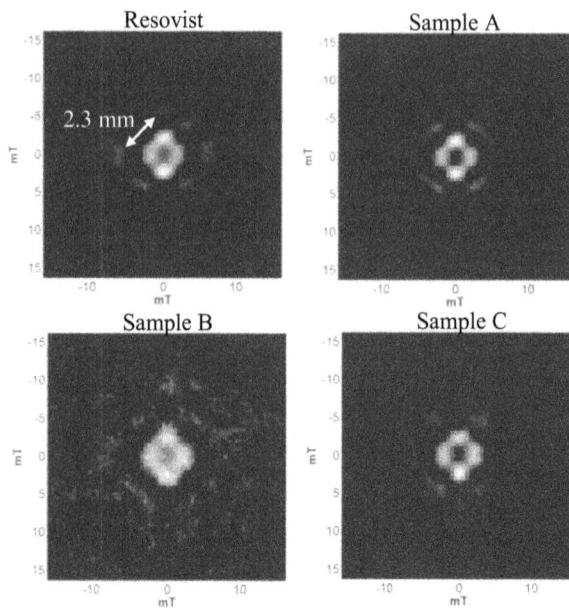

Figure 2: *Reconstruction results using hybrid system matrices and emulated phantoms (phantom 1) with varying magnetic offset field distances between the four dots. The particles can be separated at an offset field distance that would correspond to a spatial distance of 2.3 mm in the MPI scanner.*

The reconstruction results using the MPI scanner measurements of two samples and Resovist can be seen in Fig. 3. The capillaries of the resolution phantom (phantom 2) had a spatial distance of 4 mm. Although the two positions of the capillaries are still clearly separable for all samples, the differentiation between the two points is most distinct for Resovist.

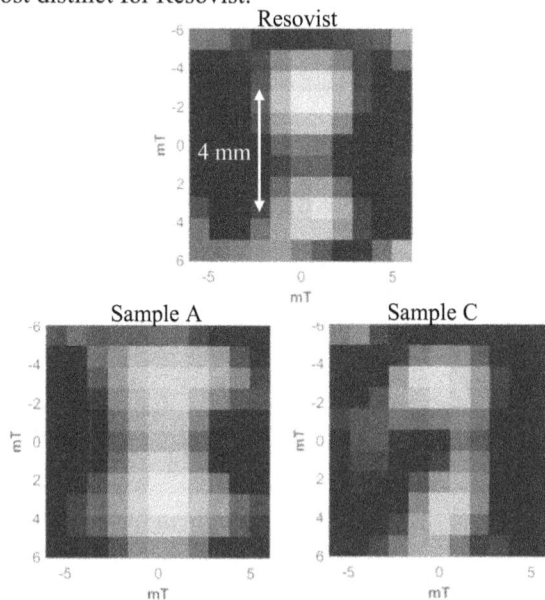

Figure 3: *Reconstruction results of a resolution phantom (phantom 2) measured in the MPI scanner. The samples can clearly be separated at a spatial distance of 4 mm corresponding to a magnetic offset field distance of 5 mT.*

IV. Conclusion

The investigation of more than 40 particle systems with varying characteristic parameters yield some very promising particle systems that might be of great interest for future MPI applications. The image reconstruction results using some of these samples are comparable or even better than using Resovist. Thus, these particles could serve as alternative MPI tracer. Further investigations on the spatial resolution and sensitivity of those particles should be targeted. Additionally, the correlation of particle characteristics and MPI performance should be investigated.

ACKNOWLEDGEMENTS

We acknowledge all NanoMag consortium partners for providing us with magnetic nanoparticles for this study. Especially, we would like to thank Cathrine Frandsen and Miriam Varón from the Department of Physics, Technical University of Denmark, Kongens Lyngby, Denmark, Cordula Grüttner and Anja Johl from Micromod Partikeltechnology GmbH, Rostock, Germany as well as Nicole Gehrke and David Heinke from nanoPET Pharma GmbH, Berlin, Germany, for providing us with the magnetic nanoparticles presented in this contribution. The research leading to these results has received funding from the European Union Seventh Framework Programme (FP7/2007-2013) under grant agreement no 604448 (NanoMag) and the Federal Ministry of Education and Research (BMBF, grant numbers 13GW0069A and 13GW0071D).

REFERENCES

[1] B. Gleich and J. Weizenecker. Tomographic imaging using the nonlinear response of magnetic particles. *Nature*, 435(7046):1217-1217, 2005. doi: 10.1038/nature03808.

[2] K. Lüdtke-Buzug et al. Preparation and Characterization of Dextran-Covered Fe3O4 Nanoparticles for Magnetic Particle Imaging. *Springer IFMBE Proceedings*, 22, 2343—2346, 2008. doi: 10.1007/978-3-540-89208-3_562.

[3] B. D. Cullity and C. D. Graham. Introduction to Magnetic Materials. *John Wiley & Sons*, Hoboken USA, 2008. doi: 10.1002/9780470386323.

[4] F. Ludwig et al. Magnetic, structural and particle size analysis of single- and multi-core magnetic nanoparticles. IEEE Transaction on Magnetics, 50(11):5300204, 2014. doi: 10.1109/TMAG.2014.2321456.

[5] M. Graeser et al. Two dimensional magnetic particle spectrometry. *Physics in Medicine and Biology,* 62(9):3378-3391, 2017. doi: 10.1088/1361-6560/aa5bcd.

[6] X. Chen et al. First measured result of the 3D Magnetic Particle Spectrometer. *International Workshop on Magnetic Particle Imaging,* 123, 2017.

[7] A. von Gladiss et al. Hybrid system calibration for multidimensional magnetic particle imaging. *Physics in Medicine and Biology,* 62(99):3392-3406, 2017. doi: 10.1088/1361-6560/aa5340.

[8] D. Schmidt et al. Imaging Characterization of MPI Tracers Employing Offset Measurements in a two Dimensional Magnetic Particle Spectrometer. *International Journal on Magnetic Particle Imaging,* 1(2), 2016. doi: 10.18416/IJMPI.2016.1604002.

[9] M. Graeser et al. SNR and Discretization Enhancement for System Matrix Determination by Decreasing the Gradient in Magnetic Particle Imaging. *International Journal on Magnetic Particle Imaging,* 3(1), 2017. doi: 10.18416/ijmpi.2017.1703019.

Session 03 - Posters

Reconstruction I

A Comparison of Image-Based System Matrices

Thomas Kampf [a,c,*], Patrick Vogel [a,b], Stefan Herz [b], Martin A. Rückert [a], Thorsten A. Bley [b], Volker C. Behr [a]

[a] Department of Experimental Physics 5 (Biophysics), University of Würzburg, 97074 Würzburg, Germany
[b] Department of Diagnostic and Interventional Radiology, University Hospital Würzburg, 97080 Würzburg, Germany
[c] Department of Diagnostic and Interventional Neuroradiology, University Hospital Würzburg, 97080 Würzburg, Germany
* Corresponding author, email: Thomas.Kampf@physik.uni-wuerzburg.de

I. Introduction

In Magnetic Particle Imaging (MPI) reconstruction methods are often tailored to specific hardware designs [1]. Two different concepts are available: reconstruction using a system matrix (Fourier space) [2] or reconstruction in image space [3, 4]. The first is limited by available compute power, which dictates the usable resolution while for the second specific scanner hardware conditions (accuracy) have to be considered. Compression algorithms and sparse reconstruction can amend these issues at the cost of possibly degraded reconstruction results [5]. An image-based reconstruction concept combining the advantages of both approaches was presented by Vogel et al. [6]. System matrices were built based on hardware-independent raw-images. Different parameters, such as order of signal derivatives, raw-image size, scaling process and parameter picking, are expected to influence the reconstruction quality as well as reconstruction time. The influences of several parameters on the reconstruction will be presented and discussed.

II. Material and Methods

II.I. Simulation environment

The image-based reconstruction concept offers several ways to build image-based system matrices (iSM). The sketch in Fig. 1 gives an overview indicating the different iSM types. All types start with a raw-image built from the measured signal, which was corrected for the receive chain, filtered and the appropriate order of derivative was taken. These data were reordered to the image with high extrinsic resolution [6]:

- Type iSM1 first scales down the raw-image (direct scaling) and takes the pixel values as iSM parameters.
- Type iSM2 takes the inner complex values from the Fourier transformed raw-image as input parameters.
- Type iSM3 uses a Fourier-scaling method to reduce the amount of pixels in the raw-image (Fourier-scaling). iSM3 is the extension of the iSM2, but with an additional inverse Fourier transform.

The data were simulated using a software framework simulating a real Traveling Wave MPI (TWMPI) scanner [7, 8]. The TWMPI system was set up to a gradient strength of about 1 T/m and frequencies of f_1=723.57 Hz and f_2=16823.00 Hz. The simulated field of view (FOV) was set to 29×71 mm^2 with a grid resolution of 1 mm. All datasets have a length of $2 \cdot 10^5$ and were simulated with a sampling rate of 10 MS/s.

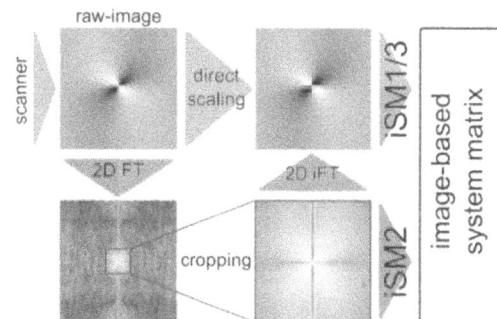

Figure 1: Sketch of the process to build up image-based system matrices: iSM1: the raw-image is directly scaled and the pixels are used as SM parameters. iSM2: the raw-image is Fourier transformed and the complex values are used as SM parameters. iSM3: identical steps as iSM2 but with an additional inverse Fourier transform.

For the visualization of the reconstructed images, a software framework is used to process the data [9].

II.II. Parameter description

In image-based reconstruction, several parameters can be addressed. The order of signal derivatives (see Fig. 2 a) can have dramatic influence on the image quality (edge-detection, size of the point-spread-function, level-of-detail, etc.). The scaling size affects significantly the reconstruction time and the choose of processing the data can influence the reconstruction results.

In the first test, the order of derivatives (d00, d01, d02, d03) applied to the data are investigated. In a second test the influence of the scaling size is studied. The third test examines the difference of all three iSM types.

III. Results

In Fig. 2 (b) the raw-images of the point-spread functions (PSF) are shown and the graph gives the eigenvalues for the corresponding system matrices (type: iSM1, scale-size: 70×70 px², matrix size: 4900×2059). In Fig. 2 (c) the eigenvalues of iSMs with different scale-size are plotted. Fig. 2 (d) compares the eigenvalues of the all three types of image-based system matrices.

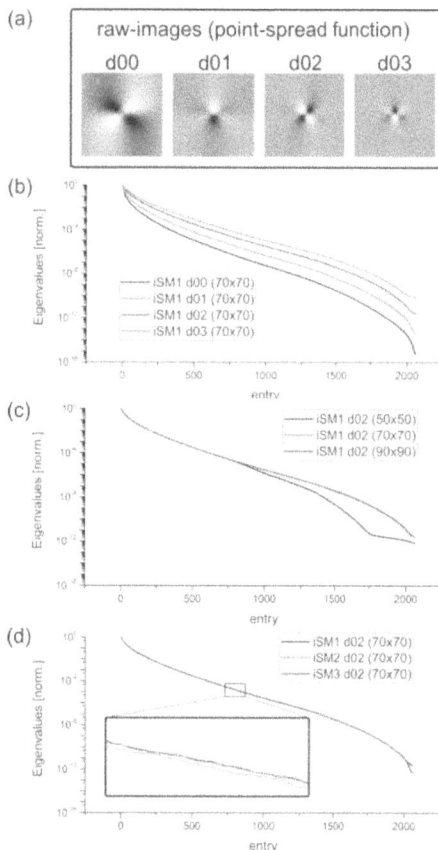

Figure 2: *Results of the eigenvalue investigations of different iSM parameters: (a) order of derivatives, (b) scale-size and (c) comparison of equivalent iSMs.*

For the comparison of the image quality, a sample consisting of the 'TWMPI' lettering is simulated (Fig. 3). To all data noise was added and they were bandpass-filtered (20 kHz…400 kHz). For reconstruction a singular-value-decomposition (SVD) is used to calculate the pseudo inverse. All types of iSM used the iSM1 setting and a scale-size of 70×70 px². The regularization value for every reconstruction is chosen to: d00: $\lambda = 1 \cdot 10^{11}$, d01: $\lambda = 1 \cdot 10^{8}$, d02: $\lambda = 1 \cdot 10^{5}$ and d03: $\lambda = 3 \cdot 10^{4}$.

The most influence on the quality of the reconstruction has the selection of the derivative (Fig. 3), where the second derivative shows the best quality for a noisy sample.

IV. Discussion

The eigenvalue investigation in Fig. 2 shows several effects of the chosen parameters:
1. With increasing order of derivatives of the signal the eigenvalue spread decreases. However, the noise in every step also is increased by factor of $2\pi f$.

2. The scale size (the amount of parameters available for the iSM) requires at least twice the amount of points, which have to be encoded: 2500×2059 vs. 4900×2059 vs. 8100×2059 (Fig. 2 (b)).
3. All three types of iSM seem to have the same performance from the eigenvalue-spread (see Fig. 2 d).

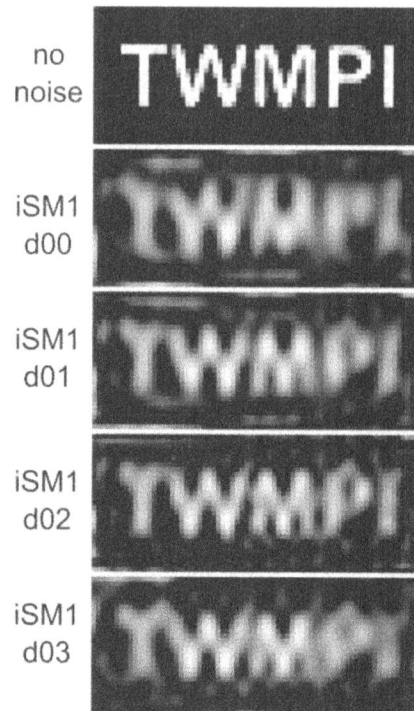

Figure 3: *Comparison of iSMs with different orders of derivatives on the quality of the reconstruction of noisy input data are shown. The best result is achieved using the second derivative.*

V. Conclusions

Since the image-based system matrix (iSM) reconstruction was introduced, several types of iSMs are possible. In this abstract, the influence of several parameters on the image quality of noisy data sets was investigated. The best result is achieved using the second derivative (d02) at a scaling-size of 70×70 px² on the input signal.

REFERENCES

[1] T. Knopp, et al., Magnetic Particle Imaging: from proof of principle to preclinical applications, *Phys. Med. Biol.*, vol. 62(14), pp. R124-R178, 2017. Doi: 10.1088/1361-6560/aa6c99

[2] J. Rahmer, et al., Signal encoding in MPI: properties of the system function, *BMC Med Imag.*, vol. 9(4), 2009. Doi:10.1186/1471-2342-9-4

[3] P. Goodwill, et al., The x-space formulation of the MPI process: 1-D signal, resolution, bandwidth, SNR, SAR, and Magnetostimulation, *IEEE TMI*, vol. 29(11), pp. 1851-9, 2010. Doi:10.1109/TMI.2010.2052284

[4] P. Vogel & S. Lother, et al., MRI meets MPI: a bimodal MPI-MRI tomograph, *IEEE TMI*, vol. 33(10), pp. 1954-9, 2014. Doi:10.1109/TMI.2014.2327515

[5] Lampe, et al., Fast reconstruction in magnetic particle imaging, Phys. Med. Biol., vol. 57(4), pp. 1113-34, 2012. Doi:10.1088/0031-9155/57/4/1113

[6] P. Vogel, et al., Flexible and Dynamic Patch Reconstruction for Traveling Wave MPI, *Int. Journal on MPI*, vol. 2(2):1611001, 2016. Doi: 10.1088/0031-9155/61/18/6620

[7] P. Vogel, et al., 3D-GUI Simulation Environment for MPI, *Proc. on IWMPI (Lübeck)*, p. 95, 2016.

[8] P. Vogel, et al., Traveling Wave Magnetic Particle Imaging, *IEEE TMI*, vol. 33(2), pp. 400-7, 2014. Doi: 10.1109/TMI.2013.2285472

[9] P. Vogel, et al., Low-Latency Real-time Reconstruction for MPI Systems, *Int. Journal on MPI*, vol. 3(2):1707002, 2017. Doi: 10.18416/ijmpi.2017.1707002

On the Formulation of the Magnetic Particle Imaging System Function in Fourier Space

Marco Maass [a,*] and Alfred Mertins [a]

[a] Institute for Signal Processing, University of Lübeck, Lübeck, Germany
* Corresponding author, email: maass@isip.uni-luebeck.de

I. Introduction

Several publications on magnetic particle imaging (MPI) are based on the Langevin theory of paramagnetism to describe the imaging process [1-4]. However, although some reconstruction methods require the Fourier transform of the Langevin function and its derivative, in practice, due to the lack of a closed-form expression, they are approximated either numerically or via the Lorentzian function, which works quite well in practice. Nevertheless, we here give a closed-form solution for the Fourier transform of the Langevin function and derive the temporal and spatial Fourier transformed versions of the system function according to the Langevin model.

II. Fourier transform of the Langevin function

The Langevin function has the following uniformly convergent series expansion:

$$\mathcal{L}(x) = \coth(x) - \frac{1}{x} = \sum_{k=1}^{\infty} \frac{2x}{k^2\pi^2 + x^2}$$
$$= \frac{1}{i}\sum_{k=1}^{\infty}\left(\frac{1}{k\pi - ix} - \frac{1}{k\pi + ix}\right). \tag{1}$$

First, we derive the Fourier transform of $\mathcal{L}'(x) \in L^1(\mathbb{R})$. We obtain

$$\hat{\mathcal{L}}_d(\omega_x) = \mathcal{F}[\mathcal{L}'(x)] = \sum_{k=1}^{\infty}\left(\mathcal{F}\left[\frac{1}{i}\left(\frac{1}{k\pi - ix}\right)'\right] - \mathcal{F}\left[\frac{1}{i}\left(\frac{1}{k\pi + ix}\right)'\right]\right)$$
$$= \begin{cases} \frac{2\pi|\omega_x|}{e^{\pi|\omega_x|}-1}, & \text{if } |\omega_x| > 0 \\ 2, & \text{if } \omega_x = 0, \end{cases} \tag{2}$$

where $\omega_x = 2\pi f_x$ denotes the spatial frequency along the x-dimension. With an approach similar to (2), we can calculate the Fourier transform of $\frac{\mathcal{L}(x)}{x}$, which is not in $L^1(\mathbb{R})$, but in $L^2(\mathbb{R})$. This yields

$$\hat{\mathcal{L}}_n(\omega_x) = \mathcal{F}\left[\frac{\mathcal{L}(x)}{x}\right] = -2\ln(1 - e^{-\pi|\omega_x|}) \in L^1(\mathbb{R}). \tag{3}$$

It should be explicitly noted that the Fourier transform of $\mathcal{L}(x)$ only exists in the sense of the distribution theory, because $\mathcal{L}(x)$ is neither in $L^1(\mathbb{R})$ nor in $L^2(\mathbb{R})$. The distributional Fourier transform of $\mathcal{L}(x)$ is given by

$$\hat{\mathcal{L}}(\omega_x) = \mathcal{F}[\mathcal{L}(x)] = 2\pi i \, \text{sgn}(\omega_x)\frac{1}{1 - e^{\pi|\omega_x|}} \tag{4}$$

for $\omega_x \neq 0$. The Fourier transform of the Langevin function has a singularity at $\omega_x = 0$. However, it can be easily verified that $\mathcal{L}(x)$ can be expressed as

$$\mathcal{L}(x) = \frac{1}{2}(\text{sgn}(x) * \mathcal{L}'(x)), \tag{5}$$

where $*$ denotes the convolution operation. The function $\text{sgn}(x)$ can be seen as a temperate distribution from S' in the spatial domain which also has a distributional expression in the Fourier domain given by $\frac{2}{i\omega_x}$ [5]. Both distributions are to be understood in the sense that the Fourier transform and its inverse have to be evaluated with help of the Cauchy principal value (p.v.). It can be proofed that this makes the last term in (4) itself a distribution, which can be evaluated with the p.v..

III. 1D MPI Fourier representation of the Langevin-Model

One-dimensional MPI can be described by the simplified model [1]

$$u(t) = \frac{d}{dt}\left[\int_{-\infty}^{\infty} c(x)M_0\mathcal{L}(\beta G(x_{FFP}(t) - x))dx\right]$$
$$= \frac{d}{dt}\Phi(t) = \left[\int_{-\infty}^{\infty} c(x)\,s(x,t)dx\right] \tag{6}$$

with $\beta = \frac{\mu_0 m}{k_B T}$ and $M_0 = \mu_0 pm$, where $u(t)$ denotes the measured voltage signal, $c(x)$ is the spatial SPIOs distribution, p denotes the coil sensitivity, μ_0 the vacuum permeability, k_B the Boltzmann's constant, T the temperature of the SPIOs, and m the magnetic moment of one nanoparticle. All parameters in (6) that are independent of $c(x)$ are included in $s(x,t)$, the so-called system function. The spatial position of the FFP at time point t is given by $x_{FFP}(t) = -G^{-1}H^D(t)$, where $H^D(t)$ denotes the magnetic drive field and G denotes the applied gradient strength of the static gradient field. Commonly, one chooses $H^D(t) = -A\cos(2\pi f t)$, which is a periodic function in $T_D = \frac{1}{f}$. For the sake of clarity, we omit the constant factor M_0 in the following. The Fourier series coefficients of $u(t)$ are given by

$$\hat{u}_k = \frac{1}{T_D}\int_{-T_D/2}^{T_D/2}\frac{d}{dt}\Phi(t)e^{-i\omega_k t}dt = \frac{i\omega_k}{T_D}\int_{-T_D/2}^{T_D/2}\Phi(t)e^{-i\omega_k t}dt, \tag{7}$$

where $\omega_k = 2\pi k f$. A convolution in the spatial domain is a multiplication in the frequency domain:

$$h(x) = \int_{-\infty}^{\infty} c(u)\mathcal{L}\big(\beta G(x-u)\big)du$$

$$\hat{h}(\omega_x) = \hat{c}(\omega_x)\frac{1}{|\beta G|}\,\hat{\mathcal{L}}\left(\frac{\omega_x}{\beta G}\right). \qquad (8)$$

We are now interested in the Fourier series expansion of $g(t) = h(x_{\text{FFP}}(t))$. In a first step, $h(x_{\text{FFP}}(t))$ is represented by the inverse Fourier transform [6] along x:

$$h\big(x_{\text{FFP}}(t)\big) = \frac{1}{2\pi}\int_{-\infty}^{\infty} \hat{h}(\omega_x)\,e^{i\omega_x x_{\text{FFP}}(t)}d\omega_x. \qquad (9)$$

Then, we derive the Fourier series coefficients of $g(t)$:

$$\hat{g}_k = \frac{1}{T_D}\int_{-\frac{T_D}{2}}^{\frac{T_D}{2}} h(x_{\text{FFP}}(t))e^{-i\omega_k t}dt$$

$$= \frac{1}{2\pi}\int_{-\pi}^{\pi} h\left(x_{\text{FFP}}\left(\frac{z}{2\pi f}\right)\right)e^{-ikz}dz \qquad (10)$$

$$= \frac{1}{(2\pi)^2}\int_{-\pi}^{\pi}\left(\int_{-\infty}^{\infty}\hat{h}(\omega_x)\,e^{i\omega_x x_{\text{FFP}}\left(\frac{z}{2\pi f}\right)}d\omega_x\right)e^{-ikz}dz.$$

$$= \frac{1}{2\pi}\int_{-\infty}^{\infty}\hat{h}(\omega_x)\left(\frac{1}{2\pi}\int_{-\pi}^{\pi}e^{-i\left(-\omega_x x_{\text{FFP}}\left(\frac{z}{2\pi f}\right)+kz\right)}dz\right)d\omega_x.$$

We now consider the function

$$P(\omega_x, k) = \frac{1}{2\pi}\int_{-\pi}^{\pi}e^{-i\left(-\omega_x x_{\text{FFP}}\left(\frac{z}{2\pi f}\right)+kz\right)}dz$$

$$= \frac{1}{2\pi}\int_{-\pi}^{\pi}e^{-i\left(-\frac{\omega_x A}{G}\cos(z)+kz\right)}dz. \qquad (11)$$

The integration problem can be solved with help of the Jacobi-Anger expansion:

$$e^{i\omega\cos(z)} = \sum_{n=-\infty}^{\infty} i^n J_n(\omega)e^{inz}, \qquad (12)$$

where $J_n(\omega)$ denotes the n-th Bessel function of first kind. With (12) it follows

$$P(\omega_x, k) = i^k J_k\left(\frac{\omega_x A}{G}\right). \qquad (13)$$

Finally, we obtain for (10)

$$\hat{g}_k = \frac{i^k}{2\pi|\beta G|}\int_{-\infty}^{\infty}\hat{c}(\omega_x)\hat{\mathcal{L}}\left(\frac{\omega_x}{\beta G}\right)J_k\left(\frac{\omega_x A}{G}\right)d\omega_x. \qquad (14)$$

It should be noted that the product of $\hat{\mathcal{L}}(\omega_x)$ and $J_k(\alpha\omega_x)$ is always in $L^1(\mathbb{R})$ for $k > 0$ and $\alpha \neq 0$. Next, we derive the Fourier representation of the MPI system equation (7) as

$$\hat{u}_k = \frac{i^{k+1}\omega_k}{2\pi|\beta G|}M_0\int_{-\infty}^{\infty}\hat{c}(\omega_x)\hat{\mathcal{L}}\left(\frac{\omega_x}{\beta G}\right)J_k\left(\frac{\omega_x A}{G}\right)d\omega_x$$

$$= \frac{1}{2\pi}\int_{-\infty}^{\infty}\hat{s}_k(-\omega_x)\hat{c}(\omega_x)d\omega_x = \int_{-\infty}^{\infty}s_k(x)c(x)dx, \qquad (15)$$

where $\hat{s}_k(\omega_x)$ with $k \in \mathbb{N}$ and $\omega_x \in \mathbb{R}$ is the 2D frequency-domain representation of the spatio-temporal system function. Another term needed is the inverse Fourier transform of $J_k(\omega_x)$ along ω_x. The result can be derived as [7]

$$j_k(x) = \mathcal{F}^{-1}[J_k(\omega_x)] = \begin{cases} \frac{i^k T_k(x)}{\pi\sqrt{1-x^2}} & \text{for } |x| < 1 \\ 0 & \text{else,} \end{cases} \qquad (16)$$

where $T_k(x)$ denotes the k-th Chebyshev polynomial of the first kind. Finally, we want to show that the Fourier representation

$$\hat{s}_k(\omega_x) = \frac{(-i)^{k+1}\omega_k M_0}{|\beta G|}\hat{\mathcal{L}}\left(\frac{\omega_x}{\beta G}\right)J_k\left(\frac{\omega_x A}{G}\right) \qquad (17)$$

is consistent with the closed-form solution for $s_k(x)$. Let us remove the spatial Fourier transform to get

$$s_k(x) = \frac{(-i)^{k+1}\omega_k M_0 G}{A}\int_{-\frac{A}{G}}^{\frac{A}{G}}\mathcal{L}\big(\beta G(x-u)\big)j_k\left(\frac{Gu}{A}\right)du \quad =$$

$$-i2fM_0\mathcal{L}(\beta Gx) * \frac{G\,k\,T_k\left(\frac{Gx}{A}\right)}{A\sqrt{1-\left(\frac{Gx}{A}\right)^2}}$$

$$= i2fM_0\mathcal{L}(\beta Gx) * \frac{\partial}{\partial x}\left(U_{k-1}\left(\frac{Gx}{A}\right)\sqrt{1-\left(\frac{Gx}{A}\right)^2}\right) \qquad (18)$$

$$= i2fM_0\beta G\mathcal{L}'(\beta Gx) * U_{k-1}\left(\frac{Gx}{A}\right)\sqrt{1-\left(\frac{Gx}{A}\right)^2},$$

where $U_n(x)$ denotes the n-th Chebyshev polynomial of the second kind, which is equivalent to the closed-form solution from [1].

IV. Conclusions

The description developed in this contribution can be extended to two- and three-dimensional MPI in a similar way with some minor assumptions. We hope this will help us to prove some systemically made observations in MPI, like the nonlinear frequency mixing [8], which connects the spatial frequency in two and more dimensions with the temporal frequency. However, the proof of the nonlinear frequency mixing is still pending.

ACKNOWLEDGEMENTS

This work was supported by the German Research Foundation under grant number ME 1170/7-1.

REFERENCES

[1] J. Rahmer, J. Weizenecker, B. Gleich, and J. Borgert. Signal encoding in magnetic particle imaging: properties of the system function. *BMC Medical Imaging*, 9(4), 2009. doi:10.1186/1471-2342-9-4.

[2] P. W. Goodwill and S. M. Conolly. Multidimensional X-Space Magnetic Particle Imaging. *IEEE Trans. Med. Imag.*, 30(9):1581–1590, 2011. doi:10.1109/TMI.2011.2125982.

[3] J.J. Konkle, P. W. Goodwill, O. M. Carrasco-Zevallos, and S. M. Conolly. Projection reconstruction magnetic particle imaging. *IEEE Trans. Med. Imag.*, 32(2):338-347, 2013. doi: 10.1109/TMI.2012.2227121.

[4] T. Knopp, S. Biederer, T. F. Sattel, M. Erbe, and T. M. Buzug. Prediction of the Spatial Resolution of Magnetic Particle Imaging Using the Modulation Transfer Function of the Imaging Process. *IEEE Trans. Med. Imag.*, 30(6):1284-1294, 2011. doi: 10.1109/TMI.2011.2113188.

[5] D.C. Champeney. *A handbook of Fourier Theorems*. Cambridge University Press, New York, 1987. doi: 10.1017/CBO9781139171823

[6] S. Bergner, T. Möller, D. Weiskopf, and D. J. Muraki. A Spectral Analysis of Function Composition and its Implications for Sampling in Direct Volume Visualization. *IEEE Trans. Vis. Comput. Graphics*, 12(5):1353-1360, 2006. doi: 10.1109/TVCG.2006.113.

[7] H. O. Beća. An orthogonal set based on Bessel functions of the first kind. *Univ. Beograd. Publ. Elektrotehn. Fak. Ser. Mat. Fiz.*, 1980.

[8] T. Knopp and T. M. Buzug. *Magnetic Particle Imaging: An Introduction to Imaging Principles and Scanner Instrumentation.* Springer, Berlin/Heidelberg, 2012. doi: 10.1007/978-3-642-04199-0.

Spectral Filtering for Chebyshev Reconstruction Algorithms in Magnetic Particle Imaging: A Case Study for Reconstruction on Lissajous Nodes

Stefano De Marchi [a], Wolfgang Erb [b,*], Francesco Marchetti [c]

[a] *Department of Mathematics "Tullio Levi-Civita", University of Padova, Italy*
[b] *Department of Mathematics, University of Hawai'i at Mānoa, USA*
[c] *Department of Woman's and Children's Health, University of Padova, Italy*
[*] *Corresponding author, email: erb@math.hawaii.edu*

I. Introduction

Chebyshev spectral methods evolve to a principle tool in reconstruction algorithms for Magnetic Particle Imaging (MPI) if the data acquisition process is based on Lissajous sampling trajectories. In this case, the rows of the MPI imaging operator have resemblances to tensor products of Chebyshev polynomials ([1]) and a sparse and efficient reconstruction scheme can be build upon the Chebyshev transform [2]. Further, the self-intersection and the boundary points of the Lissajous curve can be used directly as nodes for a spectral interpolation scheme based on multivariate Chebyshev polynomials [3,4].

The usage of Chebyshev series to approximate the particle distribution gives a sparse representation of the system matrix and, even more, a fast direct reconstruction scheme [2]. A well-known drawback of spectral methods is the emerging of Gibbs artifacts in the reconstruction if the underlying particle density has sharp edges. For Chebyshev reconstructions based on measurements at Lissajous node points such artifacts were observed in [4].

In [5], a mathematical description of the Gibbs effect and classical as well as adaptive spectral filtering techniques were presented to handle these artifacts and to improve the Chebyshev-based reconstruction process in MPI. In this work, we use the spectral filters investigated in [5] for a case study in MPI. We show how adaptive and non-adaptive filtering schemes can be applied to improve the Chebyshev based MPI reconstruction on Lissajous nodes.

II. Material and Methods

For a bivariate particle distribution f on a normalized field of view $[-1,1]^2$ we assume that we have an approximate reconstruction of the form

$$S_N(f)(x,y) = \sum_{k,l=0}^{N} c_{k,l}(f) T_{k,l}(x,y), \qquad (1)$$

where $T_{k,l}(x,y) = \cos(k \arccos(x)) \cos(l \arccos(y))$ denote tensor product Chebyshev polynomials of the first kind. If the distribution f has sharp edges, the coefficients $c_{k,l}(f)$ decay slowly as k and l decrease. The sharp cut-off of the

expansion at the frequencies k,l = N causes striping artifacts in the approximation close to the location of the discontinuities of f, the so-called Gibbs phenomenon.

II.I. Classical spectral filtering

A standard procedure to avoid these striping artifacts is the usage of spectral filters. The resulting filtered approximation of f has the form

$$S_N^\sigma(f)(x,y) = \sum_{k,l=0}^{N} \sigma_k \, \sigma_l c_{k,l}(f) T_{k,l}(x,y),$$

in which the multipliers σ_k guarantee a smooth cut-off of the coefficients at frequency N. One example of such a spectral filter, the raised cosine filter, is given by

$$\sigma_k = \frac{1}{2}\left(1 + \cos\left(\pi \frac{k}{N}\right)\right). \qquad (2)$$

In physical space, such a filtering process can be regarded as convolution of f with a polynomial mollifier.

II.II. Adaptive spectral filtering

Classical spectral filters as the cosine filter given above act globally on the function f and do not take into account the physical position of the discontinuities.

For a possible improvement of the reconstruction quality, the following adaptive filter has been considered in [5]:

$$\sigma_k^p = exp\left(\frac{(k/N)^p}{(k/N)^2-1}\right) \text{if k<N and} \sigma_k^p = 0 \text{else.}$$

Here p is a function depending on the distance d(x,y) of a point (x,y) to its closest discontinuity in the image and

$$p(x,y) = \eta\big(Nd(x,y)\big)^\beta,$$

where $\eta>0$ and $\beta>0$ denote tuning parameters that have to be chosen appropriately. To obtain the location of the discontinuities of f, we used the Canny edge detector.

III. Results

As underlying data we use MPI measurements performed on the phantom described in [4]. In the reduction concept presented in [4], the measurements and the reconstruction of the distribution of magnetic particles are conducted on the node points $\mathbf{LS}^{(66,64)}$ of a non-degenerate Lissajous curve $\gamma^{(33,32)}$. The parameters 33 and 32 are the frequency dividers of the Lissajous curve. For the reconstruction a proper weighting of the node points and an additional Tikhonov regularization as described in [4] are used. Once the reconstruction is done on the points $\mathbf{LS}^{(66,64)}$, a full polynomial interpolant with a Chebyshev expansion of the form (1) is computed. Here, N = 66 corresponds to the maximal polynomial degree in the expansion (1). In the upper part of Figure 1, the reconstruction on $\mathbf{LS}^{(66,64)}$ and the corresponding polynomial interpolant are shown. In the upper right image, the Gibbs phenomenon is visible in form of striping artifacts.

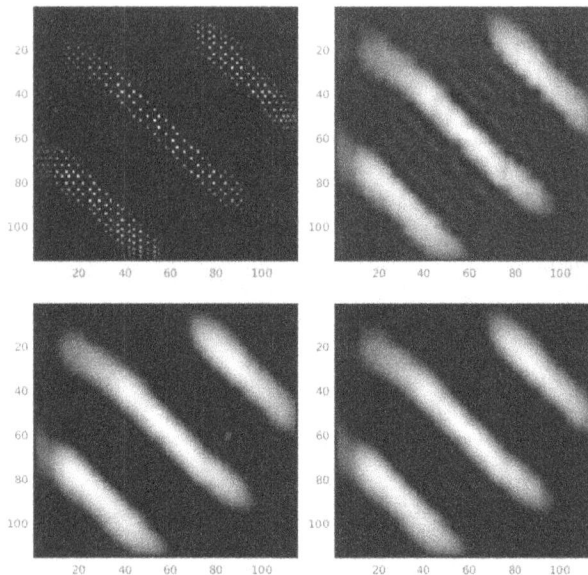

Figure 1: Chebyshev reconstruction of MPI measurements on discrete Lissajous samples. In order to reduce Gibbs effects in the Chebyshev reconstruction (upper right), we apply classical (lower left) and adaptive spectral filters (lower right)

To reduce these artifacts, we apply first the classical cosine filter (2) to the polynomial interpolant (Figure 1, lower left). In this way, the Gibbs effect vanishes. By applying the spatially adaptive spectral filter described in Section II.II. using the parameters η=0.6 and β=0.25 a second filtered reconstruction is obtained (Figure 1, lower right). As a precalculation step for the adaptive filter, the edges of the particle distribution were derived by using the Canny edge detector [6] to the classically filtered spectral interpolant. A more detailed illustration of the adaptive filtered reconstruction is given in Figure 2.

IV. Discussion and Conclusion

For particle distributions with sharp edges, the application of spectral filters improves the quality of Chebyshev reconstructions algorithms in Magnetic Particle Imaging considerably. Classical filters as the raised cosine filter are simple and cheap to implement and are able to eliminate the Gibbs artifacts in the reconstruction entirely. For the adaptive spectral filtering the results are currently only partly satisfactory. Although the spatial adaptivity

promises a further improvement of the image quality, in our experiments this could be verified only in some minor aspects. The choice of parameters in Figure 1 leads to an adaptive filtered reconstruction which is considerably better than in the unfiltered case. On the other hand, compared to the classical filter the computational efforts are slightly larger and the striping artifacts are still visible in the reconstruction. Here, further research for the design of suitable adaptive spectral filters is necessary.

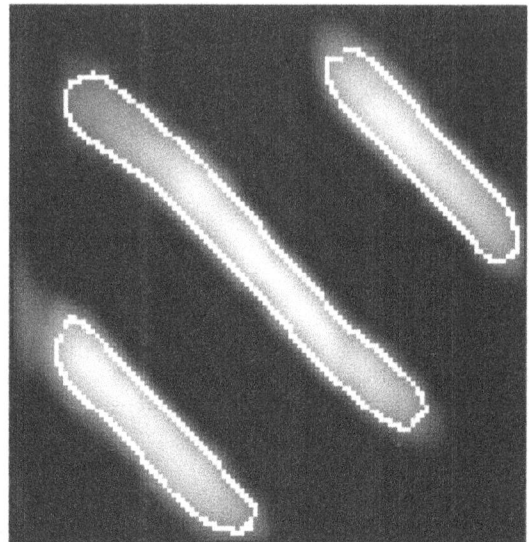

Figure 2: Chebyshev reconstruction of MPI data on Lissajous nodes with adaptive spectral filtering. The discontinuities of the Canny edge detector are marked in white.

ACKNOWLEDGEMENTS
The authors gratefully acknowledge the support of RITA (Rete Italiana di Approssimazione) for this research.

REFERENCES
[1] J. Rahmer, J. Weizenecker, B. Gleich and J. Borgert. Signal encoding in magnetic particle imaging. *BMC Medical imaging*, 9, 4, 2009. doi: 10.1186/1471-2342-9-4.
[2] L. Schmiester, M. Möddel, W. Erb and T. Knopp. Direct Image Reconstruction of Lissajous-Type Magnetic Particle Imaging Data Using Chebyshev-Based Matrix Compression. *IEEE Trans ComplImaging*, 3(4), 671-681, 2017. doi: 10.1109/TCI.2017.2706058.
[3] P. Dencker and W. Erb. Multivariate polynomial interpolation on Lissajous-Chebyshev nodes *J. Approx. Theory 219* (2017), 15-45
[4] C. Kaethner, W. Erb, M. Ahlborg, P. Szwargulski, T. Knopp and T.M. Buzug. Non-Equispaced System Matrix Acquisition for Magnetic Particle Imaging based on Lissajous Node Points *IEEE Transactions on Medical Imaging 35, 11* (2016), 2476-2485
[5] S. De Marchi, W. Erb and F. Marchetti. Spectral filtering for the reduction of the Gibbs phenomenon for polynomial approximation methods on Lissajous curves with applications in MPI *Dolomites Res. Notes Approx. 10* (2017), 128-137
[6] J. Canny. A computational approach to edge detection *IEEE Trans. Pattern Analysis and Machine Intelligence 8 (6)* (1986), 679-698

An Alternative X-space Based Image Reconstruction without Partial FOV Processing

Semih Kurt[a,*], Yavuz Muslu[a,b], Damla Sarica[a,b], Omer Burak Demirel[a,b], Emine Ulku Saritas[a,b,c]

[a]Department of Electrical and Electronics Engineering, Bilkent University, Ankara, Turkey
[b]National Magnetic Resonance Research Center (UMRAM), Bilkent University, Ankara, Turkey
[c]Neuroscience Program, Sabuncu Brain Research Center, Bilkent University, Ankara, Turkey
*Corresponding author, email: semih.kurt@ug.bilkent.edu.tr

I. Introduction

In Magnetic Particle Imaging (MPI), image reconstruction is performed typically via system function [1-3] or x-space reconstructions [4, 5]. X-space reconstruction requires speed compensation of the received signal, gridding to the field free point (FFP) position, and a DC recovery algorithm [6]. Here, we propose a new x-space based reconstruction technique that does not require the partial field-of-view (pFOV) processing steps. The proposed technique leverages the fact that the FFP speed is identical at the centers of pFOVs. It is geared towards rapid imaging applications that utilize small pFOV sizes due to the safety limits of drive fields. Here, we provide a brief theoretical explanation of this technique, and verify the technique via simulations and imaging experiments.

II. Material and Methods

II.I. Theory

This work is aimed at trajectories that utilize a 1D drive field that rapidly scans a small pFOV, while slow shifting focus fields enable the coverage of a wider FOV. Here, we take advantage of the fact that the FFP speed is identical at the central positions of all pFOVs. We refer to the proposed reconstruction as pFOV center image (PCI).

Using the mathematical expression for the lost first harmonic term [3, 6], we have previously shown that the DC loss in an x-space-reconstructed image can be expressed in convolution form as follows [7]:

$$\hat{\rho}_{DC}(x) = \frac{4}{\pi W}\left(\hat{\rho}(x) * \sqrt{1 - \left(\frac{2x}{W}\right)^2}\right) \quad (1)$$

Here, $\hat{\rho}(x)$ is the ideal x-space MPI image, $\hat{\rho}_{DC}(x)$ is the x-space image that would be reconstructed using only the first harmonic, W is the total extent of each pFOV, and $\sqrt{1 - (2x/W)^2}$ is a space variant velocity term.

A "raw PCI image", $\hat{\rho}_{rpci}(x)$, can then be formed by directly assigning the time-domain signal corresponding to pFOV centers to each pixel. It can be shown that this image is equal to:

$$\hat{\rho}_{rpci}(x) = \alpha\left(\hat{\rho}(x) - \hat{\rho}_{DC}(x)\right) \quad (2)$$

Here, α is a constant related to the speed of the FFP while passing through the pFOV center. Combining Eqs. 1-2, this image also can be written as:

$$\hat{\rho}_{rpci}(x) = \alpha\left(\hat{\rho}(x) * h_{pci}(x)\right) \quad (3)$$

where

$$h_{pci}(x) = \delta(x) - \frac{4}{\pi W}\sqrt{1 - \left(\frac{2x}{W}\right)^2} \quad (4)$$

Importantly, $h_{pci}(x)$ is a fully known kernel, as it is independent of nanoparticle type and depends only on W. Using $\hat{\rho}_{rpci}(x)$, the ideal image can be recovered via deconvolution by this known kernel. Here, a regularized deconvolution with a Laplacian operator was utilized to retain image smoothness (using *deconvreg* in MATLAB). For comparison purposes, standard x-space reconstruction with DC recovery was also implemented [6].

II.II. Simulations

Simulations were performed in MATLAB using a custom MPI toolbox. The parameters were chosen to match experimental parameters given in Section II.III: (-4.8, 2.4, 2.4) T/m selection field gradients in (x, y, z) directions, 10 mT drive field at 9.7 kHz along the z-direction, and 25 nm nanoparticle diameter. A 5x5 cm² phantom featuring vasculature was utilized (Fig. 1a). A Cartesian trajectory with a pFOV size of 8.33 mm and 90% overlap among pFOVs along the z-direction, and 51 lines along the x-direction was utilized to cover the 5x5 cm² FOV. The fundamental harmonic was filtered out.

II.III. Imaging Experiments

Imaging experiments were performed on our in-house FFP scanner with (-4.8, 2.4, 2.4) T/m selection field gradients in (x, y, z) directions, using 10 mT drive field at 9.7 kHz along the z-direction. A Cartesian trajectory was utilized with a pFOV size of 8.33 mm and 90% overlap among pFOVs along z-direction, and 9 lines along the x-direction. The total imaging FOV was 6.5x0.8 cm², with a total scan time of 4 min 49 sec. Perimag nanoparticles (Micromod

GmbH, Germany) with 30 mmol Fe/L concentration were prepared in 3-mm diameter vials, separated at 9 mm distance (see Fig. 2a).

III. Results

III.I. Simulation Results

Figure 1 shows the simulation results. For this vasculature phantom and under ideal conditions, PCI and standard x-space reconstruction results match perfectly, as expected.

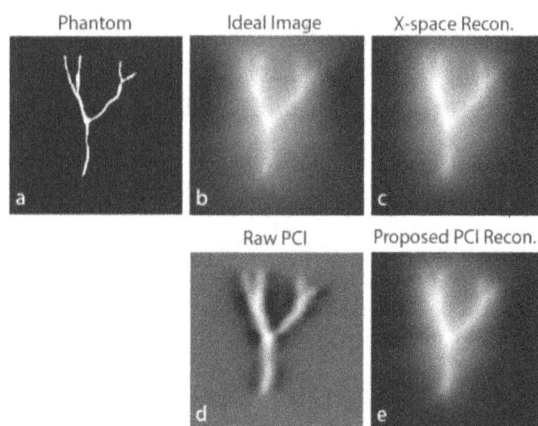

Figure 1: Simulation results. (a) Vasculature phantom (5x5 cm²). (b) Ideal x-space MPI Image (particle distribution convolved with 3D PSF). (c) Standard x-space reconstructed image. (d) Raw PCI image (i.e., $\hat{\rho}_{rpci}(x)$). (e) Proposed PCI reconstruction result.

III.II. Experimental Results

Figure 2 shows the experimental imaging results. As seen in Fig. 2b, the standard x-space image suffers from a few artifacts: the pFOV boundaries are visible as periodic vertical dark stripes, and DC-recovery algorithm causes a pile up of image intensity along the scanning direction (left-right) in certain lines. These artifacts are caused by nanoparticle relaxation effects that delay the signal and interferences at harmonic frequencies due to hardware imperfections. The proposed PCI technique, on the other hand, provides significantly improved image quality that is free of these artifacts. The robustness of the PCI reconstruction stems from the fact that the time-domain MPI signal has the highest signal-to-noise ratio (SNR) at pFOV centers. The speed compensation in standard x-space causes division by small speed values at the edges of pFOVs, which in turn may cause amplification of both noise and interferences. Due to regularized deconvolution, however, the resulting PCI image is slightly blurred when compared to the standard x-space image.

IV. Discussion

The proposed PCI reconstruction has advantages in terms of both computational simplicity and robustness against interferences. Unlike the standard x-space reconstruction, it does not require speed compensation, gridding, or DC recovery. One disadvantage of the proposed method is that it requires the pFOV overlap percentage to be large, so that the pFOV centers are closely spaced. While this seems limiting at first, a rapid drive field combined with a slow shifting focus field automatically leads to trajectories that

feature large pFOV overlaps. Because drive field safety limits force pFOV sizes to be ~1 cm for human torso imaging, MPI scans will have to incorporate numerous overlapping pFOVs. Hence, obviating the need for pFOV processing steps provide a more straightforward reconstruction. In addition, the PCI technique can also be generalized to include signals at other positions, which can further boost the SNR.

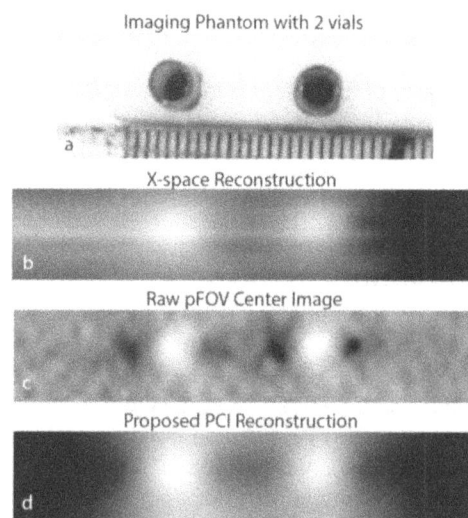

Figure 2: Experimental results on in-house FFP scanner. (a) Imaging phantom with 2 vials. (b) Standard x-space reconstructed image suffers from artifacts due to relaxation and signal interferences. (c) Raw pFOV center image (i.e., $\hat{\rho}_{rpci}(x)$). (d) Proposed PCI reconstruction result.

V. Conclusions

We presented an alternative x-space based reconstruction technique for MPI. The proposed technique utilizes the highest SNR regions of the MPI signal to overcome artifacts due to relaxation and interference effects.

ACKNOWLEDGEMENTS

This work was supported by the European Commission through an FP7 Marie Curie Career Integration Grant (PCIG13-GA-2013-618834), by the Turkish Academy of Sciences through TUBA-GEBIP 2015 program, and by the Science Academy through BAGEP award.

REFERENCES

[1] B. Gleich and J. Weizenecker.Tomographic imaging using the nonlinearresponse of magnetic particles. *Nature*,435(7046):1217-1217, 2005. doi: 10.1038/nature03808.

[2] J. Weizenecker, *et al*. A simulation study on the resolution and sensitivity of magnetic particle imaging. *Phys Med Biol*,52(21):6363-6374, 2007.

[3] J. Rahmer, *et al*. Signal Encoding in magnetic particle imaging: properties of the system function. *BCM Medical Imaging*,9:4, 2009.

[4] P. W. Goodwill and S.M. Conolly. The X-space formulation of the magnetic particle imaging process: 1-D signal, resolution, bandwidth, SNR, SAR, and magnetostimulation. *IEEE Trans Med Imaging*,29(11):1851-1859, 2010.

[5] P. W. Goodwill and S.M. Conolly. Multidimensional X-Space Magnetic Particle Imaging. *IEEE Trans Med Imaging*,30 (9):1581-1590, 2011. doi: 10.1109/TMI.2011.2125982.

[6] K. Lu, *et al*. Linearity and Shift Invariance for Quantitative Magnetic Particle Imaging. *IEEE Trans Med Imaging*,32 (9):1565-1575, 2013. doi: 10.1109/TMI.2013.2257177.

[7] D. Sarica, *et al*. DC Shift Imaging for X-Space MPI Reconstruction. *Proc of the 6th International Workshop on Magnetic Particle Imaging*, Lubeck, Germany, p.80, 2016.

Joint Multiresolution Magnetic Particle Imaging and System Matrix Compression

Marco Maass [a,*], Christian Mink [a], and Alfred Mertins [a]

[a] *Institute for Signal Processing, University of Lübeck, Lübeck, Germany*
[*] *Corresponding author, email: maass@isip.uni-luebeck.de*

I. Introduction

Magnetic particle imaging (MPI) is a tracer-based medical imaging method that is based on the nonlinear magnetization characteristics of super-paramagnetic iron oxide nanoparticles (SPIOs) [1]. With different accelerated and static magnetic fields, the MPI-scanner generates a small area in which the magnetic fields neutralize each other. The area is called the field free point (FFP). The FFP is normally periodically moved on a pre-defined trajectory over the whole field of view (FOV). The change of magnetization leads to an induced voltage in a receive coil, where, due to the nonlinear magnetization characteristics of the SPIOs, only SPIOs from the vicinity of the FFP contribute significantly to the measured signal. For MPI-scanners with a Lissajous FFP-trajectory, the system response normally has to be measured. For this, a probe of SPIOs material is placed on different spatial positions, and the responses are saved in a so-called system matrix. With help of the system matrix, the inverse problem of estimating the SPIOs' distribution from the voltage signal can be solved. Unfortunately, the system matrix can be very dense and huge in size. For a dense matrix, the reconstruction process can be very slow. In [2], it was observed that the system matrix of MPI-scanners with a FFP traveling along a Lissajous-trajectory can be highly compressed by the discrete cosine transform (DCT) followed by thresholding. Recently, a work for matrix compression was published on a non-Euclidian grid, where the Chebyshev transform becomes orthogonal and the compression performance is even improved [3]. In this work, we develop a multiresolution representation for the system matrix. In particular, we use a combination of the DCT-II and the discrete wavelet transform (DWT) for the joint system-matrix compression and multiresolution reconstruction.

II. Material and Methods

The reconstruction problem in MPI can be described as a linear inverse problem by

$$Sc \approx f , \qquad (1)$$

where $S \in \mathbb{C}^{M \times N}$ denotes the system matrix, $c \in \mathbb{R}_+^N$ is the positive unknown particle distribution, and $f \in \mathbb{C}^M$

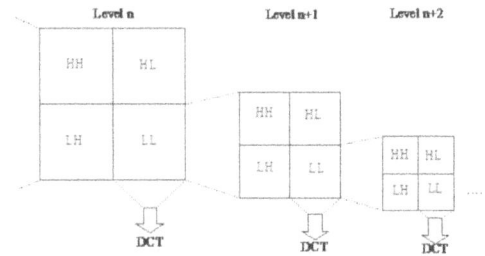

Figure 1: The spatial dimension of the system matrix is decomposed by the discrete wavelet transform to form a multiresolution pyramid. In HH both dimensions are highpass filtered, in LH/HL one of the dimensions is highpass and the other is lowpass filtered, and in LL both dimensions are lowpass filtered.

contains the frequency components of the voltage signal. Following the work in [2], the reconstruction problem in (1) can also be expressed in a transform domain as

$$S_T c_T = S T T^{-1} c \approx f , \qquad (2)$$

where $T \in \mathbb{R}^{N \times N}$ describes an invertible transform, S_T is the system matrix in the transform domain, and c_T the particle distribution in the transform domain. The idea is to choose T in such a way that the matrix $S_T = ST$ has many small components that become zero after thresholding. It is well known that the DCT-I and -II are such kinds of transform for MPI system matrices. Unfortunately, the DCT is a global transform on the spatial domain and offers no strategy for a multiresolution analysis (MRA). One transform to apply a MRA is the DWT [4], which can also be represented as a linear transform T. Nevertheless, the DWT is not as sparsifying as the DCT for MPI system matrices. The good news is that the lowpass filtered and downsampled coefficients of the system matrix can be interpreted as a coarser version of the system matrix. By combining the advantages of both transforms, we develop an MRA for MPI system matrices. The system matrix will be decomposed level-wise by the d-dimensional DWT with respect to the dimensionality $d \in \{1,2,3\}$ of the particle distribution, followed by a DCT of the lowpass filtered coefficients of the system matrix. For demonstration purposes, a two-dimensional decomposition is shown in Fig. 1. For each stage of the two-dimensional DWT, the system matrix will be decomposed into four submatrices. The lowpass filtered version of the system matrix will then be transformed with the DCT to the compressive domain and is also the basis for the next level of the decomposition to form a spatial pyramid. The formulation is independent of the used reconstruction method. Thus, the introduced formulation of the system matrix can be included in different solvers. We considered the Tikhonov regularized least square reconstruction problem

$$c^\ell = \underset{c \in \mathbb{R}_+^{K_\ell}}{\arg \min} \left\| S_T^\ell T_\ell^{-1} c - f \right\|_2^2 + \lambda^2 \|c\|_2^2 \quad (3)$$

with $S_T^\ell \in \mathbb{C}^{M \times K_\ell}$ being the compressed system matrix on the decomposition stage ℓ, $\lambda > 0$, and $T_\ell^{-1} \in \mathbb{R}^{K_\ell \times K_\ell}$ representing the DWT+DCT transform of the ℓ-level, where $K_0 = N = N_x N_y N_z$ denotes the number of voxels of the particle distribution. The number of voxels of each subspace problem in (3) is $K_\ell = \left\lceil \frac{N_x}{2^\ell} \right\rceil \left\lceil \frac{N_y}{2^\ell} \right\rceil \left\lceil \frac{N_z}{2^\ell} \right\rceil$ where $\lceil \cdot \rceil$ means the ceiling operator. We started the reconstruction on the coarse level L_{max} and ended on the finest level 0. The SPIOs distribution from the coarser resolution will be used as input for the next finer resolution stage by inserting it into the low-resolution components of the finer stage and the unknown high-resolution components initialized with zeros for the iterative reconstruction. The reconstruction problem is solved by a variation of the fast iterative shrinkage-thresholding [5], where we replaced the ℓ_1-constraint by a non-negativity and an ℓ_2-constraint. We tested the approach on the simulated Lissajous-trajectory MPI system matrix dataset which was also used in [6]. For the simulated dataset, the first 62 frequency components were deleted. To speed up the reconstruction, the system matrix was globally thresholded, so that every sublevel system matrix retained 99.7% of its energy. The DWT was implemented in a non-expansive form with biorthogonal 9/7-wavelets for arbitrary signal length in lifting structure [4]. We reconstructed the SPIOs distribution with ($\lambda = 0.35$) and without ($\lambda = 10^{-4}$) energy normalization of the rows of the subsystem matrix. Both regularization parameters were selected by hand. As stopping criterion, an upper limit for the relative change of the objective function was set.

III. Results

Due to the limited space, we exemplarily show only one example of SPIOs-distribution reconstruction on different levels in Fig. 2. It can be recognized that the structure of the 250x250-pixel distribution is also identifiable inside the low-resolution reconstructions. It can be observed that the 63x63-pixel reconstruction still has a good separation between the particle spots and that the shapes are quite similar to the 250x250 high-resolution version. The 32x32-pixel reconstruction, however, has significant artifacts and deformations of the particle spots.

IV. Discussion

The presented method offers a combination of two matrix compression techniques and gives rise to an MRA. It has the ability to first reconstruct the particle distribution on a coarse level, and, if more computational power is at hand,

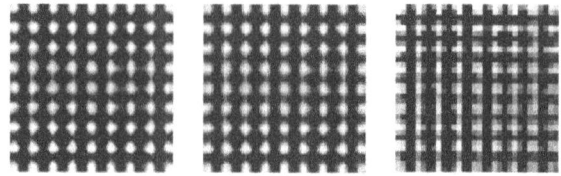

Figure 2: The SPIOs reconstruction with energy normalization of the MRA from left to right: 250x250, 63x63, and 32x32 pixels. The images are clipped to [0, 2^{level}] for visualization.

a high-resolution reconstruction can be performed. The compression is not a necessary part of this method. The method can also be used for a fast reconstruction inside a multiresolution analysis without compression of the system matrix. A possible application of the developed method could be to find the support of the SPIOs distribution inside the FOV and to exclude regions without particle distribution earlier on the finer grid, where the linear system's condition is typically worse. In addition, an interesting scenario for the approach with its joint local and global transforms could be the use inside a compressed-sensing framework for the reconstruction of SPIO distributions. Since the DWT and DCT offer compression for both the system matrix and the image to be reconstructed, our developed transform offers us the best of two worlds: A good compressive transform for the system matrix and a good compressive transform for the particle distribution, which is highly promising for this purpose.

V. Conclusions

We developed an MRA formulation for MPI based on the DWT and the DCT-II. We were able to show the efficiency of our approach, which offers the possibility to proceed step-wise from a coarse level to a high-resolution reconstruction of the SPIOs distribution. Our future research will be directed toward developing a compressed sensing based reconstruction of the particle distributions using our MRA formulation of the system matrix.

ACKNOWLEDGEMENTS

This work was supported by the German Research Foundation under grant number ME 1170/7-1.

REFERENCES

[1] B. Gleich and J. Weizenecker. Tomographic imaging using the nonlinear response of magnetic particles. *Nature*, 435(7046):1217-1217, 2005. doi: 10.1038/nature03808.

[2] J. Lampe, C. Bassoy, J. Rahmer, J. Weizenecker, H. Voss, B. Gleich and J. Bogert. Fast reconstruction in magnetic particle imaging. *Phys. Med. Biol.*, 60(10):4033-4044, 2015. doi: 10.1088/0031-9155/60/10/4033.

[3] L. Schmiester, M. Möddel, W. Erb and T. Knopp. Direct Image Reconstruction of Lissajous-Type Magnetic Particle Imaging Data Using Chebyshev-Based Matrix Compression. *IEEE Trans. Comput. Imag.*, 3(4):671-681, 2017. doi: 10.1109/TCI.2017.2706058.

[4] S. Mallat. *A Wavelet Tour of Signal Processing: The Sparse Way.* Academic press, 2008.

[5] A. Beck and M. Teboulle. A Fast Iterative Shrinkage-Thresholding Algorithm for Linear Inverse Problems. SIAM J. Imaging Sci., 2(1): 183–202, 2009. doi:10.1137/080716542.

[6] M. Maass, M. Ahlborg, A. Bakenecker, F. Katzberg, H. Phan, T. M. Buzug and A. Mertins. A trajectory study for obtaining MPI system matrices in a compressed-sensing framework. *Intern. J. Magnetic Particle Imaging*, 3(2):1706005, 2017. doi: 10.18416/ijmpi.2017.1706005.

Influence of Excitation Signal Coupling on Reconstructed Images in MPI

Anselm von Gladiss [a,*], Matthias Graeser [b,c], Thorsten M. Buzug [a]

[a] *Institute of Medical Engineering, University of Lübeck, Lübeck, Germany*
[b] *Section for Biomedical Imaging, University Medical Center Hamburg-Eppendorf, Hamburg, Germany*
[c] *Institute for Biomedical Imaging, Hamburg University of Technology, Hamburg, Germany*
[*] *Corresponding author, email: {gladiss,buzug}@imt.uni-luebeck.de*

I. Introduction

Magnetic Particle Imaging (MPI) is an emerging medical imaging technology that visualises superparamagnetic nanoparticles in a field of view (FOV). The particles are excited by oscillating sinusoidal magnetic fields H_{D_i} in different spatial directions $i \in \{x, y, z\}$ forming a trajectory as in Fig. 1. A receive signal can be detected whose spectrum contains the excitation frequency and higher harmonics [1].

A system matrix can be used to reconstruct the spatial distribution of the particles inside the FOV. System matrix reconstruction relies on the stability and consistency of a system. This means, that e. g. the driven trajectory must be the same for both system matrix acquisition and measurements.

Recently, it has been proposed to reconstruct MPI measurements with a hybrid system matrix that has not been acquired in the scanning device but in a magnetic particle spectrometer (MPS) [2]. Although this is an important step towards reducing the calibration time in MPI and therefore increasing the efficiency of MPI scanning devices, new requirements have to be met, as the driven trajectory in both the MPS and the MPI scanning device must be the same.

I.I. Excitation Signal Coupling

According to Faraday's law of induction the excitation signal from one sending coil may couple into another sending coil causing a twisted trajectory as displayed in Fig. 1. Conventional multidimensional MPI scanner set-ups feature orthogonal sending coils that should prevent signal coupling. In practice, coupling may occur due to accuracy limitations in hardware assembly. Then, the magnetic drive field H_{D_i} features not only one frequency as in Eq. 1, but is superposed by the coupled signals $H_{D\kappa_{ij}}$ of other spatial directions j. Here, the effective field coupling ratio κ_{ij} defines the coupling ratio from sending coil j into i:

$$\kappa_{ij} = H_{D\kappa_{ij}}/H_{D_i} \qquad (1)$$

A software decoupling can be implemented that monitors the current on the sending coils and identifies coupled signals. The cancellation signal $H_{\mathrm{canc}\kappa_{ij}}$ is generated with a phase shift of $\Delta\phi = -180°$ and fed back into the signal path in order to cancel out the coupling signal $H_{D\kappa_{ij}} \to 0$.

This contribution discusses the influence of signal excitation coupling for system matrix reconstruction. The software decoupling is used to manipulate the trajectory by introducing an additional signal that corresponds to signal coupling.

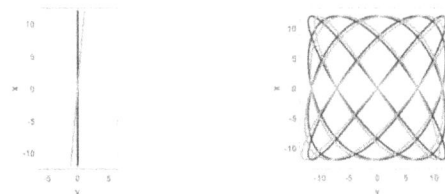

(a) Sinusoidal excitation   (b) Lissajous trajectory

Figure 1: Influence of field coupling on the trajectory in MPI for (a) 1D and (b) 2D excitation. Introducing a field coupling of $\kappa_{yx} = 10\%$ in y-direction, the trajectory is twisted (grey) in comparison to the original one (black).

II. Material and Methods

The measurements have been carried out using a multidimensional MPS [3]. The currents on the sending coils are monitored by a software decoupling unit that ensures a maximum effective field coupling of $\kappa_{ij} \leq 0.1\%$. Also, an accuracy of 99.9% for the amplitudes of the excitation signals with a maximal phase error of 0.2° is guaranteed.

It has been shown that an MPS can be used to acquire a hybrid system matrix [2]. Furthermore, phantoms can be emulated with an MPS [4]. The phantom is discretised into distinct spatial positions that are emulated by the MPS. The addition of the receive signals at those positions corresponds to a phantom measurement in an MPI scanning device.

II.I. Measurements

First, two hybrid system matrices with 1D excitation in x-direction have been acquired. One of them will serve as a system matrix in the reconstruction, the other one will be used to emulate the phantom. Then, the same excitation frequency has been introduced in y-direction with a magnetic field strength corresponding to a magnetic field coupling from sending coil x into y of $\kappa_{yx} = 1\%$ and $\kappa_{yx} = 10\%$. Hybrid system matrices with 2D excitation have been acquired the same way introducing the same field coupling as in the 1D case.

The phantoms are emulated by choosing single spatial positions out of the system matrices that feature a defined field coupling. As a reference, the same phantom is emulated using one system matrix that has been acquired without field coupling. Out of the 1D excitation measurements, a 2 dot phantom in the centre of the FOV is emulated. A 9 dot grid has been emulated using the 2D excitation measurements. The images are reconstructed by solving an underdetermined linear system of equations as described in [5] using a regularised Kaczmarz algorithm and the hybrid system matrix featuring no field coupling.

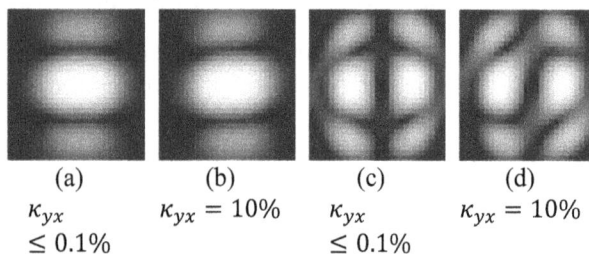

(a)	(b)	(c)	(d)
κ_{yx} $\leq 0.1\%$	$\kappa_{yx} = 10\%$	κ_{yx} $\leq 0.1\%$	$\kappa_{yx} = 10\%$

Figure 2: *Frequency components of system matrices. (a) and (b) were obtained using 1D, (c) and (d) using 2D excitation. For (b) and (d) a field coupling of $\kappa_{yx} = 10\%$ has been introduced from sending coil x to y.*

III. Results

Fig. 2 shows frequency components of the hybrid system matrices, i. e. system functions. Fig. 2 (a) and (c) display the reference system function for 1D and 2D excitation without field coupling. In contrast, Fig. 2 (b) and (d) show the same system functions after introducing a field coupling of $\kappa_{yx} = 10\%$. These system functions with coupling are twisted in comparison to their reference. Furthermore, wave peaks that are clearly separated disperse when introducing coupling in 2D excitation. In Fig. 3, the reconstruction results of the emulated phantoms are displayed. The 2 dot phantom is not reconstructed as 2 dots but as two lines. After twisting the excitation trajectory background noise increases. Furthermore, the centre of the reconstructed lines begins to blur. This effect increases with increasing emulated coupling. The single dots of the 9 dot grid are reconstructed into a point cloud consisting of one bright pixel, the centre, and neighbouring pixels (see Fig. 3 (d)). As for 1D excitation, the background noise increases when introducing field coupling. Furthermore, the reconstruction of the dots blurs out. For a high coupling factor of $\kappa_{yx} = 10\%$, the centres of different point clouds move by one pixel (e. g. lower left corner).

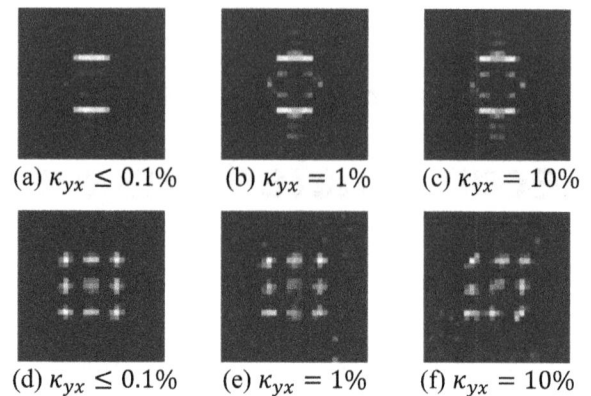

(a) $\kappa_{yx} \leq 0.1\%$	(b) $\kappa_{yx} = 1\%$	(c) $\kappa_{yx} = 10\%$
(d) $\kappa_{yx} \leq 0.1\%$	(e) $\kappa_{yx} = 1\%$	(f) $\kappa_{yx} = 10\%$

Figure 3: *Reconstructed images of emulated phantoms. (a)-(c): 2 dot phantom using 1D excitation. (d)-(f): 9 dot grid phantom using 2D excitation. (a) and (d) are the reconstruction references without field coupling. After introducing field coupling κ_{yx}, background noise appears in the reconstructed images.*

IV. Discussion

Although a twist in the 1D system function can be identified (see Fig. 2 (b)), this twist is not visible in the reconstructed images (see Fig. 3 (c)). As the spatial resolution in y direction is poor when exciting only in the direction of x, this twist in the y direction cannot be observed in the reconstructed images. The twist of the 2D system function in Fig. 2 (d) can also be seen in Fig. 3 (f). In this work, the field coupling has only been emulated from sending coil x into y. In a real scenario, signal coupling may also occur from sending coil y into x which will increase the mismatch between the driven trajectories and therefore, deteriorate the reconstructed images.

V. Conclusions

It has been shown, that a small coupling of $\kappa_{yx} = 1\%$ has a large effect on the reconstructed images in terms of image quality. After introducing coupling signals, background noise appears in the reconstructed images. Furthermore, the reconstructed dots are starting to blur out and shift. In order to reduce the calibration time in MPI, it is important to be able to measure the system matrix in a dedicated device [2]. Then, the driven trajectory including the coupled signals must be the same as in the imaging device in order to avoid artefacts in the reconstructed images.

ACKNOWLEDGEMENTS

The authors thankfully acknowledge the financial support by the German Research Foundation (DFG, grant number BU 1436/10-1) and the Federal Ministry of Education and Research (BMBF, grant number 13GW0069A).

REFERENCES

[1] B. Gleich and J. Weizenecker. *Nature*, 2005. doi: 10.1038/nature03808.

[2] A. von Gladiss, M. Graeser, et al. *PMB*, 2017. doi: 10.1088/1361-6560/aa5340.

[3] M. Graeser, A. von Gladiss, et al. *PMB*, 2017. doi: 10.1088/1361-6560/aa5bcd.

[4] D. Schmidt, M. Graeser, et al. *IJMPI*, 2016. doi: 10.18416/IJMPI.2016.1604002.

[5] T. Knopp, J. Rahmer, et al. *PMB*, 2010. doi: 10.1088/0031-9155/55/6/003.

Deconvolution Kernel for 1D X-Space MPI

Aileen Cordes [a,*], Thorsten M. Buzug [a]

[a] *Institut für Medizintechnik, Universität zu Lübeck, Lübeck, Germany*
* *Corresponding author, email: {cordes,buzug}@imt.uni-luebeck.de*

I. Introduction

According to the x-space formulation, a one-dimensional magnetic particle imaging (MPI) process can be described as a linear, space invariant system [1, 2, 3]. In terms of signal processing, the image $g(x)$ obtained by simple regridding can be formulated as a convolution of the original nanoparticle distribution $f(x)$ with a point-spread function (PSF) $h(x)$

$$g(x) = f(x) * h(x) = \int_{-\infty}^{+\infty} f(\xi)h(x-\xi)d\xi. \quad (1)$$

In [1] it could be shown, that the PSF is given by the derivative of the Langevin function which is visualized in Fig 1a.

According to equation (1), the regridding process does not result in the correct distribution $f(x)$ of nanoparticles. Because the PSF is a non-negative function, each point in the image grid receives positive contributions from all other points of the original image. Positive values are assigned to image pixels even outside the object. To compensate for the blurring effects, adequate reconstruction strategies that include a suitable deconvolution of the image must be applied. According to the convolution theorem, the necessary filtering can either be formulated as a multiplication in the spectral domain

$$f(x) = \mathcal{F}^{-1}\left\{\mathcal{F}\{g(x)\}\frac{1}{\mathcal{F}\{h(x)\}}\right\} \quad (2)$$

or as a convolution in the spatial domain

$$f(x) = \int_{-\infty}^{+\infty} g(\xi)\hat{h}(x-\xi)d\xi, \quad (3)$$

where $\mathcal{F}$ represents the one-dimensional Fourier transform and $\hat{h}(x) := \mathcal{F}^{-1}\left\{\frac{1}{\mathcal{F}(h(x))}\right\}$. Applying equation (3) means that those areas in the image that are blurred by simple regridding are considered right from the beginning. The PSF is compensated for by negative values of $\hat{h}(x)$.

In this contribution, an explicit expression for the respective deconvolution kernel in the spatial domain is derived.

II. Material and Methods

II.I. Derivation of $\hat{h}(x)$

It can be shown that the Fourier transform of the derivative of the Langevin function is given by

$$H(\omega) := \mathcal{F}\{\dot{\mathcal{L}}[x]\} = \frac{1}{\sqrt{2\pi}}\int_{-\infty}^{+\infty}\left(\frac{1}{x^2} - \frac{1}{\sinh^2(x)}\right)e^{-i\omega x}dx$$

$$= \begin{cases} \sqrt{\frac{\pi}{2}}\left(\omega \coth\left(\frac{\pi\omega}{2}\right) - |\omega|\right) & \omega \neq 0 \\ \sqrt{2/\pi} & \omega = 0 \end{cases}. \quad (4)$$

Using the definition $\coth(x) = 1 + \frac{2}{e^{2x}-1}$, the reciprocal of $H(\omega)$ can then be expressed as follows

$$\frac{1}{H(\omega)} = \begin{cases} \frac{e^{\pi|\omega|}-1}{\sqrt{2\pi}|\omega|} & \omega \neq 0 \\ \sqrt{\pi/2} & \omega = 0 \end{cases}. \quad (5)$$

Finally, the inverse Fourier transform of $\frac{1}{H(\omega)}$ is sought.

However, one has to keep in mind that $\frac{1}{H(\omega)}$ is not a square integrable function because

$$\lim_{\omega \to -\infty}\frac{e^{\pi|\omega|}-1}{\sqrt{2\pi}|\omega|} = \lim_{\omega \to +\infty}\frac{e^{\pi|\omega|}-1}{\sqrt{2\pi}|\omega|} \to \infty. \quad (6)$$

Therefore, a rectangular weighting function, which acts as a low-pass filter, is applied

$$\int_{-\infty}^{\infty}\frac{e^{\pi|\omega|}-1}{2\pi|\omega|}e^{i\omega x}rect(-\epsilon,\epsilon)d\omega = \int_{-\epsilon}^{\epsilon}\frac{e^{\pi|\omega|}-1}{2\pi|\omega|}e^{i\omega x}d\omega. \quad (7)$$

The band limitation describes a regularization of the reconstruction problem and results in a sufficiently smooth filter in the spatial domain

$$\hat{h}(x) = \quad (8)$$

$$\begin{cases} \frac{1}{2\pi}\left(2\ln|x| - \ln(\pi^2 + x^2) - 2\Re\{Ei((\pi+ix)\epsilon) - Ei(ix\epsilon)\}\right) & x \neq 0 \\ \frac{1}{2\pi}(2Ei(\pi\epsilon) - 2(\gamma + \ln(\pi)) - \ln(\epsilon^2)) & x = 0 \end{cases},$$

where $Ei(x)$ is the exponential integral function

$$Ei(x) = \int_{-\infty}^{x}\frac{e^t}{t}dt. \quad (9)$$

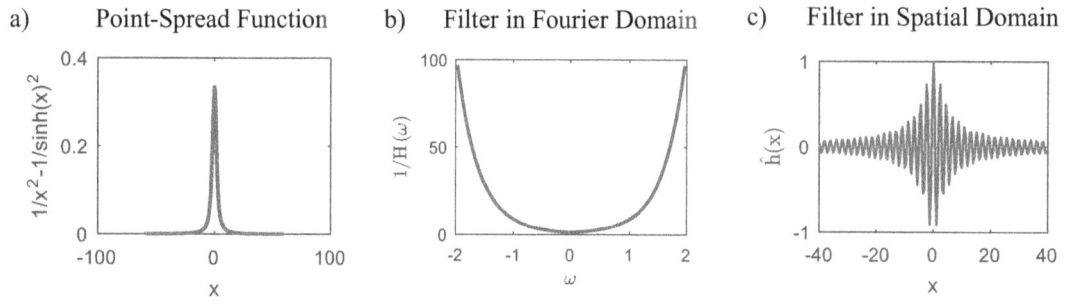

Figure 1: *a) Derivative of the Langevin function* $\dot{\mathcal{L}}(x)$ *. b) Filter in Fourier Domain: Reciprocal of the Fourier transform of the derivative of the Langevin function (see equation (5)).*
c) Filter in spatial domain: Inverse Fourier transform of $1/H(\omega)$ *(see equation (8)).*

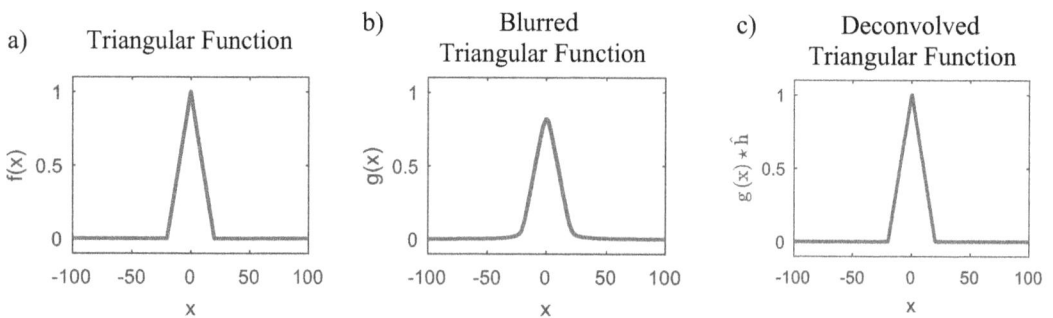

Figure 2: *a) Triangular function* $tri(-20,20)$ *(see equation (11)).b) Triangular function convolved with the derivative of the Langevin function. c) g(x) convolved with the filter in the spatial domain* $\hat{h}(x)$.

γ is the Euler-Mascheroni-Constant

$$\gamma = \lim_{n \to \infty} \left[\sum_{k=1}^{n} \frac{1}{k} - \ln(n) \right] \approx 0.5772 \qquad (10)$$

and $\Re$ denotes the real part.

II.II. Validation

In order to demonstrate that the high-pass filter $\hat{h}(x)$ defined in equation (8) is working properly, a triangular function

$$f(x) = tri(-20,20) = \begin{cases} 1 - \left|\frac{x}{20}\right| & |x| \le 20 \\ 0 & |x| > 20 \end{cases} \qquad (11)$$

is convolved with the derivative of the Langevin function. Subsequently, the resulting low-pass filtered signal $g(x)$ is convolved with $\hat{h}(x)$ according to equation (3) to compensate for the blurring due to the convolution with $\dot{\mathcal{L}}[x]$.

III. Results and Discussion

An analytical expression for the deconvolution kernel $\hat{h}(x)$ in the spatial domain could be derived. As shown in Fig. 1c, $\hat{h}(x)$ is a highly oscillating even function that acts as high-pass filter. The high-pass nature of $\hat{h}(x)$ can also be seen in frequency space (Fig. 1b). A multiplication of $\mathcal{F}\{g(x)\}$ with $1/H(\omega)$ according to equation (2) results in a suppression of low frequencies.

Fig. 2 demonstrates that an application of the filter function $\hat{h}(x)$ on a blurred triangular function $g(x) = f(x) * \dot{\mathcal{L}}[x]$ allows the recovery of the original signal $f(x)$. The error that arises from the rectangular weighting function in

equation (7) is negligible. Although one has to keep in mind that the spectral weighting increases the noise in the high frequency band, incorporating the deconvolution kernel $\hat{h}(x)$ into MPI reconstruction algorithms may therefore improve the spatial resolution of one-dimensional MPI signals.

IV. Conclusions

Since the blurring of an image obtained by simple regridding is due to an inherent convolution with a PSF, the image can be further processed to increase the spatial resolution. The respective deconvolution kernel in the spatial domain is given by equation (8). The application of $\hat{h}(x)$ allows for the compensation of the blurring effects due to the PSF.

ACKNOWLEDGEMENTS
Funding by the Federal Ministry of Education and Research via the Project SAMBA-PATI (FKZ: 13GW0069A) is gratefully acknowledged.

REFERENCES
[1] P.W. Goodwill and S. M. Conolly. The X-Space Formulation of the Magnetic Particle Imaging Process: 1-D Signal, Resolution, Bandwidth, SNR, SAR, and Magnetostimulation. *IEEE Transactions on Medical Imaging*, 29(11):1851-1859, 2010. doi: 10.1109/TMI.2010.2052284.
[2] M. Grüttner, T. Knopp, J.Franke, M. Heidenreich, J. Rahmer, A. Halkola, C. Kaethner, J. Borgert and T. M. Buzug. On the formulation of the image reconstruction problem in magnetic particle imaging. *Biomedizinische Technik/ Biomedical Engineering*, 58(6):583-591, 2013. doi: 10.1515/bmt-2012-0063.
[3] P.W. Goodwill, K. Lu, B. Zheng and S. M. Conolly. An x-space magnetic particle imaging scanner. *Rev. Sci. Instrum.*, 83(3):033708, 2012. doi: 10.1063/1.3694534.

Reusing System Matrices of Patches in Magnetic Particle Imaging via Mirroring

Mandy Ahlborg [a,*], Christian Kaethner [a], Patryk Szwargulski [b,c], Tobias Knopp [b,c] and Thorsten M. Buzug [a]

[a] Institute of Medical Engineering, Universität zu Lübeck, Lübeck, Germany
[b] Section for Biomedical Imaging, University Medical Center Hamburg-Eppendorf, Hamburg, Germany
[c] Institute for Biomedical Imaging, Hamburg University of Technology, Hamburg, Germany
* Corresponding author, email: ahlborg@imt.uni-luebeck.de

I. Introduction

In Magnetic Particle Imaging (MPI), the amplitude of the drive field and the gradient strength of the selection field define the size of the field of view (FOV). However, the amplitude and thus the FOV size are limited, because a peripheral nerve stimulation can occur dependent on the drive field frequency [1].

To enlarge the imaging area, one possible solution is the use of imaging patches [2], i.e. several FOVs covering the area of interest. In [3], different possibilities of reconstructing overlapping Lissajous patches with respect to the image quality have been investigated. One challenge using Lissajous patches is the necessity to acquire a system matrix for each patch. On the one hand, the measurement of the system matrices is time consuming. On the other hand, a joint reconstruction [4] demands a large amount of memory. It could be shown in [5] that reusing matrices is possible if the field imperfections of the MPI system are negligible.

In this contribution, it is investigated how system matrices can be reused if the MPI magnetic fields are not homogenous/linear.

II. Material and Methods

The selection field in MPI has a mirror symmetric appearance. Typically, closed bore MPI systems have a symmetry axis in every dimension. Special topologies, such as the 2D single sided scanner [6], may have less symmetry axes (see Fig. 1). If a simple reuse of one central system matrix by a spatial shift is insufficient due to field imperfections, we propose to reuse a system matrix acquired at one patch position by mirroring to the other positions. Considering the system matrix $S_k(r) \in \mathbb{R}$ with $S_k \in \mathbb{C}^R$, $S(r) \in \mathbb{C}^K$, R the number of spatial positions and K the number of frequency components, two adaptions of a system matrix are necessary to reuse it for another patch: (i) a spatial mirroring (see Sec. II.I) and (ii) a phase correction to cope for the resulting time shift (see Sec. II.II). The proposed method is validated with simulation data and a proof of concept is given with one measured data set.

II.I. Spatial Mirroring

If two patches are mirrored along one or more axes, the spatial positions in the system matrix must be rearranged accordingly. Thus, for each position r the corresponding mirrored position $\tilde{r}$ has to be calculated. The modified system matrix $\check{S}$ is then given by

$$\check{S}(\tilde{r}) = S(r). \tag{1}$$

In the subsequent image reconstruction, the mirroring of the system matrix causes a mirrored particle distribution.

II.II. Phase correction

A spatial mirroring changes the spatio-temporal correlation between the particles and the trajectory. This results in a phase shift of size π in the receive signal for each mirroring axis.

The use of orthogonal orientated drive fields causes that a phase correction is not only dependent on the frequency component, but also on the excitation direction [7].

Using the assumptions of [7], the phase correction of the system matrix can be calculated as follows:

For a mirroring in x-direction, the correction for the receive channel in x-direction is carried out as

$$\check{S}_k = \bar{S}_k(-1)^k. \tag{2}$$

For a mirroring in x-direction, the correction for the receive channel in y-direction is carried out as

$$\check{S}_k = \bar{S}_k(-1)^{k+1}. \tag{3}$$

For a mirroring in y-direction, the correction for the receive channel in x-direction is carried out as

$$\check{S}_k = S_k(-1)^k. \tag{4}$$

For a mirroring in y-direction, the correction for the receive channel in y-direction is carried out as

$$\check{S}_k = S_k(-1)^{k+1}. \tag{5}$$

Here, $\bar{S}_k$ represents the complex conjugation of all system matrix entries.

Since a measured system matrix also contains the complex transfer function of the system, a direct application of the correction via complex conjugation is not feasible. In [3], it was proposed to introduce a correction term. Subsequently, a measured system matrix can be phase corrected via multiplication with $e^{-2\phi}$.

II.III. Simulations

The simulation of the single-sided scanner gradient field is based on the specifications mentioned in [6]. For the particle model, the Langevin function with a particle core diameter of 30 nm is used. The image reconstruction is performed using a non-weighted Kaczmarz method with a Tikhonov regularization. The phantom consists of 5×5 points such that both patches are needed to cover the whole information.

II.IV. Experiments

For the experiment a pre-clinical MPI scanner (Bruker Biospin MRI GmbH, Ettlingen, Germany) is used. The gradient strength is 1.25 Tm^{-1} in x and y directions. The excitation frequencies are f_x = 24.509 kHz and f_y = 26.042 kHz and the field amplitude is 10mT for both channels. For each patch, the size of the system matrix is chosen to be approximately 4 mm larger than the FOV. Undiluted Resovist is chosen as a tracer. Four patches arranged in a grid-like structure are used. The measured object is a phantom with a C-like structure, which covers all four patches. The reconstruction is performed individually for each patch with a non-weighted Kaczmarz method with a Tikhonov regularization and a cut-off as post-processing [3].

III. Results

Fig. 1 shows the results of simulation data for different possible scenarios: (i) the phantom, (ii) reconstruction of a FOV covering the whole area of interest, (iii) reconstruction of patches with individual system matrix, (iv) reconstruction of patches with a reused system matrix without adaption and (v) reconstruction of patches with an adapted system matrix.

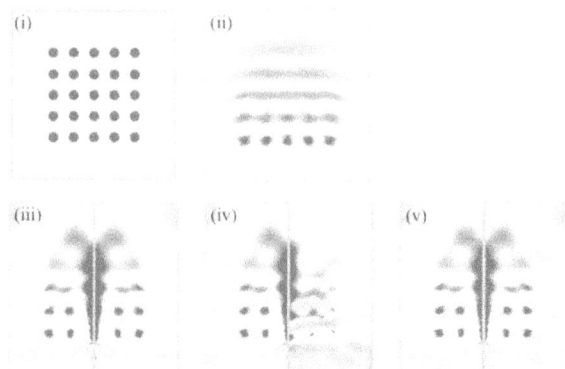

Figure 1: *Simulation results for a single sided scanner.*

Fig. 2 shows the results for the measured data set: (i) reconstruction of patches with individual system matrix, (ii) reconstruction of patches with a reused system matrix without adaption and (iii) reconstruction of patches with an adapted system matrix.

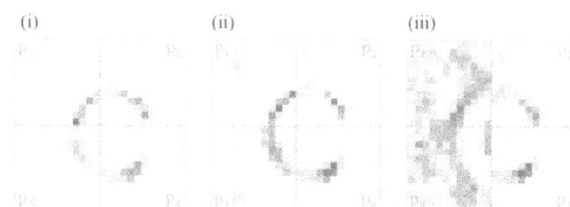

Figure 2: *Experimental results of a Bruker scanner. P4 is used for the reconstructions in (ii) and (iii).*

IV. Discussion

If there are strong imperfection in the magnetic fields, as in the simulation data for the single sided scanner, a spatial mirroring with an additional phase correction is necessary to obtain correct image reconstruction results. This indicates that for MPI scanners with just slight field inhomogeneities a reuse of system matrices may be superior to a simple system matrix shift. However, since the phase correction cannot be applied directly for measured data containing the complex valued transfer function, strong artifacts occur in the corresponding patches (P1 and P3). In y-direction, where no complex conjugation is necessary for a mirrored system matrix, the results are very similar to the ones where individual system matrices are used. Thus, the approach shows promising results, but further research is necessary to evaluate the influence of the transfer function.

V. Conclusions

In this work, it is proposed to use symmetry properties of magnetic fields in order to reuse the system matrix of one patch for the image reconstruction of all patches by mirroring. It has been shown that the proposed method works for simulation data, but has to be adapted for experimental data with unknown transfer function.

ACKNOWLEDGEMENTS

MA and TMB like to thank the Federal Ministry of Education and Research (13GW0071D, 13GW0069A, 01DL17010A). TK and PS thankfully acknowledge the financial support by the German Research Foundation (KN 1108/2-1) and the Federal Ministry of Education and Research (05M16GKA).

REFERENCES

[1] E. U. Saritas et al. Magnetostimulation Limits in Magnetic Particle Imaging. *TMI*, 32(9):1600 – 1610, 2013. doi: 10.1109/TMI.2013.2260764.

[2] J. Rahmer et al. Results on Rapid 3D Magnetic Particle Imaging with a Large Field of View. *ISMRM*, 19:629, 2011.

[3] M. Ahlborg et al. Using data redundancy gained by patch overlaps to reduce truncation artifacts in magnetic particle imaging. *Phys Med Biol.*, 61(12):4583, 2016, doi: 10.1088/0031-9155/61/12/4583.

[4] T. Knopp et al. Joint reconstruction of non-overlapping magnetic particle imaging focus-field data. *Phys Med Biol.*, 60(8):L15-21, 2015, doi: 10.1088/0031-9155/60/8/L15.

[5] T. Knopp et al. Reusing System Matrices at different Focus Field Positions in Magnetic Particle Imaging. *Biomed. Eng.*, 60, S1, 2015.

[6] K. Gräfe et al. System matrix recording and phantom measurements with a single-sided magnetic particle imaging device. *TMI*, 51(2):6502303, 2015, doi: 10.1109/TMAG.2014.2330371.

[7] A. Weber und T. Knopp: Symmetries of the 2D magnetic particle imaging system matrix. *Phys Med Biol.*, 60(10):4033 – 4044, 2015, doi: 10.1088/0031-9155/60/10/4033.

Improving Generalization Properties of Measured System Matrices by Using Regularized Total Least Squares Reconstruction in MPI

Janna Flötotto [a], Tobias Kluth [a,*], Martin Möddel [b,c], Tobias Knopp [b,c], Peter Maass [a]

[a] Center for Industrial Mathematics, University of Bremen, Bremen, Germany
[b] Section for Biomedical Imaging, University Medical Center Hamburg-Eppendorf, Hamburg, Germany
[c] Institute for Biomedical Imaging, Hamburg University of Technology, Hamburg, Germany
* Corresponding author, email: tkluth@math.uni-bremen.de

I. Introduction

In magnetic particle imaging (MPI) the relationship between particle concentration and measured potential is modeled by a Fredholm integral equation of the first kind. The integral kernel is still determined in a time-consuming calibration scan for each MPI tracer. The challenging part of modeling MPI appropriately is finding the correct integral kernel which describes the magnetic response of the tracer. Existing models are promising but they are not able to reach the quality of measured system functions [4]. One possible reason is the magnetization dynamics which can substantially change in different environments limiting the generalization property of measured system functions. The dynamic behavior of the particle's magnetization is affected by Brownian and Néel relaxation mechanisms [8]. For Resovist it was reported that the behavior is mainly determined by Néel relaxation while Brownian relaxation may influence its behavior in suspension depending on the frequency of the applied field [5]. An experimental validation of the Brownian relaxation model using low frequencies in one-dimensional sinusoidal excitation patterns [6] emphasize its relevance. Relaxation in MPI applied magnetic fields has also been shown to be relevant in terms of a distinction of different kinds of tracers [7]. All this emphasizes the limited generalization property of measured system matrices.

Methods taking measurement errors in the system matrix into account, e.g., total least squares [2], can improve results for measured and "semi"-modeled system matrices (fitted transfer function) [3]. In this contribution we focus on measured system matrices obtained from particles in different viscous environments and investigate the generalization property of these system matrices. Image reconstructions from regularized total least squares (TLS) are compared with regularized least squares solutions (LS).

II. Regularized total least squares (TLS)

We assume that the spatial domain $\Omega \subset \mathbb{R}^3$ is discretized in the given voxel basis $\{\phi_i\}_{i=1,\dots,N}$ corresponding to the positions used in the calibration process. A solution $c \in \mathbb{R}_+^N$ is obtained from potential measurements $\hat{v} \in \mathbb{C}^M$ (multiple receive coils concatenated in Fourier space) by solving the problem $\hat{S}c = \hat{v}$ for the measured system matrix $\hat{S} \in \mathbb{C}^{M \times N}$. Potential particle errors and noise in measured system matrices motivate the incorporation of deviations in the system matrix during the reconstruction process. The following consideration is based on the TLS approach [2] where an error in the linear operator is assumed. The extended problem becomes finding the concentration function $c \in \mathbb{R}_+^N$ and a deviation matrix $\delta\hat{S} \in \mathbb{C}^{M \times N}$ which fulfill

$$(\hat{S} + \delta\hat{S})c = \hat{v}.$$

The simultaneous reconstruction of the concentration and the deviation matrix is a nonlinear inverse problem. A solution to the problem is obtained by minimizing the following Tikhonov-type functional

$$J_{\gamma,\beta}^{TLS}(c, \delta\hat{S}) = \frac{1}{2}\left\|(\hat{S} + \delta\hat{S})c - \hat{v}\right\|_2^2 + \frac{\beta}{2}\left\|\delta\hat{S}\right\|_F^2 + \frac{\gamma}{2}\|c\|_2^2$$

where $\|\cdot\|_F$ denotes the Frobenius norm and $\gamma, \beta > 0$. γ and β weight the data fidelity term with respect to the penalty term. The functional is minimized by using an alternating algorithm resulting in the following iteration steps:

$$c^{i+1} = \arg\min_{c \in \mathbb{R}_+^N} J_{\gamma,\beta}^{TLS}(c, \delta\hat{S}^i)$$

$$\delta\hat{S}^{i+1} = \arg\min_{\delta\hat{S} \in \mathbb{C}^{M \times N}} J_{\gamma,\beta}^{TLS}(c^{i+1}, \delta\hat{S})$$

$$= \frac{1}{\beta + \|c^{i+1}\|^2}(\hat{v} - \hat{S}c^{i+1})(c^{i+1})^T.$$

The first step is performed by using the regularized Kaczmarz algorithm provided in [1]. The explicit formulation in the second step results directly from the normal equation.

We test the capability of the TLS approach to compensate errors in the system matrix due to a change of viscosity. This is done in experiments using the preclinical MPI system (Bruker) at the University Medical Center Hamburg-Eppendorf. The particle's Brownian rotation is changed by using glycerin-water-Resovist suspensions with different viscosities $\eta > 0$. For each viscosity a system matrix and a phantom is measured. The measurements are obtained using a 2D-excitation in x/z-plane with excitation frequencies of 24.51kHz and 25.25kHz. In both directions amplitudes of $12mT/\mu_0$ are used. The selection field has a gradient strength of $2T/m/\mu_0$ in z-direction and $1T/m/\mu_0$ in x- and y-direction. The field of view has a size of 26mm $\times$ 14mm and is discretized in 1mm $\times$ 1mm pixels. The phantom is a glass capillary with an inner diameter of 1.3mm filled with the tracer suspension with viscosity $\eta^{\dagger} = 26.8mPas$ positioned orthogonal to the x/z-plane. The x- and z-receive channels are used for reconstruction after post processing the system matrix and measurements by applying SNR-thresholding (SNR $\geq$ 2) without additional background subtraction.

III. Results

Reconstructions c_η from viscosity-η system matrices, $\eta > 0$, are illustrated in Figure 1. Regularized LS reconstructions are computed by the regularized Kaczmarz algorithm provided in [1]. In the LS case artifacts arise when system matrix and phantom have different viscosities. This might be caused by the change of the relaxation behavior due to Brownian rotation which has a structured smoothing effect on the reconstruction. When applying the TLS reconstruction approach a small increase of the amplitude can be observed but also a better localization of the phantom as the structural distortion of the reconstruction is suppressed. We observed an increase of the amplitude in TLS reconstructions depending on the particular choice of the regularization parameter. But the relative difference $d_i = \left\| c_{\eta^{\dagger}} - c_{\eta_i} \right\|_2 / \left\| c_{\eta^{\dagger}} \right\|_2$, $i = 1, 2$, to the reference reconstruction obtained from the viscosity-$\eta^{\dagger}$ system matrix can be decreased by using TLS (LS: $d_1 = 1.4, d_2 = 2.25$; TLS: $d_1 = 0.73, d_2 = 0.54$).

IV. Discussion

On the one hand the present results confirm an influence of the Brownian rotation on the image reconstruction. On the other hand they indicate that the TLS approach allowing an additional degree of freedom in the reconstruction can improve the reconstruction of structural information. But quantitative information in the reconstruction might be lost due to a priori assumptions on the solution encoded in the particular choice of β. Dealing with errors in the system matrix becomes relevant in in-vivo experiments when magnetization behavior can change due to environmental conditions. Particularly for these applications the development of an efficient parameter choice rule is highly desirable. Furthermore, future research may also include taking into account the reconstructed matrix deviation to improve models for MPI.

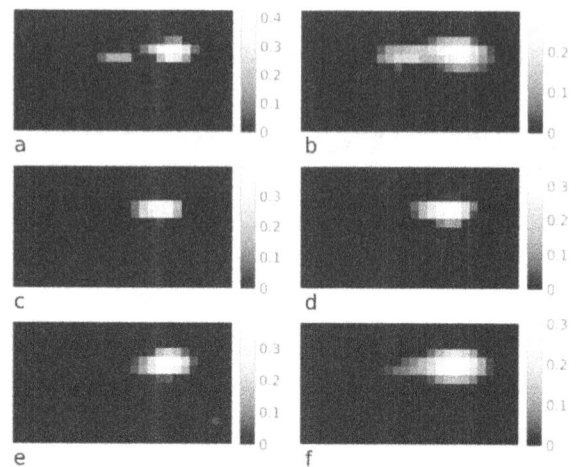

Figure 1: Normalized phantom ($\eta^{\dagger} = 26.8mPas$) reconstructions ($c_\eta / \left\| c_\eta \right\|_2$) by using regularized TLS (left column) and regularized LS (right column). System matrices with viscosities $(a, b)\ \eta_1 = 7.2mPas$, $(c, d)\ \eta^{\dagger} = 26.8mPas$, and $(e, f)\ \eta_2 = 51.8mPas$ are used. Here $\beta = 6 \cdot 10^3$ and γ is as follows: $(a, b)1.08 \cdot 10^{10}$, $(c, d)1.64 \cdot 10^{10}$, $(e, f)0.91 \cdot 10^{10}$.

ACKNOWLEDGEMENTS

T. Kluth is supported by the Deutsche Forschungsgemeinschaft (DFG) within the framework of GRK 2224/1. P. Maass acknowledges funding from the German Federal Ministry of Education and Research (BMBF, project no. 05M16LBA).

REFERENCES

[1] A. Dax. On row relaxation methods for large constrained least squares problems. SIAM Journal on Scientific Computing, 14(3):570–584, 1993.

[2] G. H. Golub, P. C. Hansen, and D. P. O'Leary. Tikhonov regularization and total least squares. SIAM Journal on Matrix Analysis and Applications, 21(1):185–194, 1999.

[3] T. Kluth and P. Maass. Model uncertainty in magnetic particle imaging: Nonlinear problem formulation and model-based sparse reconstruction. International Journal on Magnetic Particle Imaging, 3(2):ID 1707004, 10 pages, 2017.

[4] T. Knopp, S. Biederer, T. F. Sattel, J. Rahmer, J. Weizenecker, B. Gleich, J. Borgert, and T. M. Buzug. 2D modelbased reconstruction for magnetic particle imaging. Medical Physics, 37(2):485–491, 2010.

[5] F. Ludwig, D. Eberbeck, N. Löwa, U. Steinhoff, T. Wawrzik, M. Schilling, and L. Trahms. Characterization of magnetic nanoparticle systems with respect to their magnetic particle imaging performance. Biomedizinische Technik/Biomedical Engineering, 58(6):535–545, 2013.

[6] M. Martens, R. Deissler, Y. Wu, L. Bauer, Z. Yao, R. Brown, and M. Griswold. Modeling the brownian relaxation of nanoparticle ferrofluids: Comparison with experiment. Medical Physics, 40(2), 2013.

[7] J. Rahmer, A. Halkola, B. Gleich, I. Schmale, and J. Borgert. First experimental evidence of the feasibility of multi-color magnetic particle imaging. Physics in medicine and biology, 60(5):1775, 2015.

[8] D. B. Reeves and J. B. Weaver. Approaches for modeling magnetic nanoparticle dynamics. Critical Review in Biomedical Engineering, 42(1):85–93, 2014.

Temporal Polyrigid Registration for Patch-based MPI Reconstruction of Moving Objects

Jan Ehrhardt[a,*], Mandy Ahlborg[b], Hristina Uzunova[a], Thorsten M. Buzug[b], Heinz Handels[a]

[a] Institute of Medical Informatics, Universität zu Lübeck, Lübeck, Germany
[b] Institute of Medical Engineering, Universität zu Lübeck, Lübeck, Germany
* Corresponding author, email: ehrhardt@imi.uni-luebeck.de

I. Introduction

I.I. Motivation

Magnetic Particle Imaging (MPI) allows the detection of magnetic material, in particular superparamagnetic nano-particles, by remagnetization via magnetic fields. One application of this technique is medical imaging where the particles are applied as tracer directly into the blood stream. Despite that, a number of imaging sequences for the acquisition of MPI images were developed. The size of the field of view (FOV) is limited compared to other medical imaging techniques. One of the main reasons is the planned use on living individuals because potential tissue heating or stimulation of nerves limit the applicable field amplitudes. A proposed approach to cope with this problem is a patch-wise acquisition of the required region of interest (ROI). This technique uses a successive measurement of several FOVs with varying positions to cover the entire ROI [1,2]. The patches are acquired in an overlapping manner in order to use redundant information for the reduction of truncation artifacts [3].

Because the relative position of the acquired patches is known, the reconstruction of the ROI is straightforward for static objects. However, the application on living organisms implies the occurrence of motion during image acquisition, and therefore a patch-wise reconstruction has to account for object motion during the acquisition process. Fig. 1 visualizes the influence of object motion on a reconstructed image. Composing an image from multiple patches is a known problem in image processing and referred to as mosaicking or stitching. Classic algorithms account for camera movement between successive acquired patches, and have e.g. medical applications in endoscopic imaging [4]. The compensation of object motion in a static acquisition system has applications in tomographic imaging, like CT and MRI, and some interesting approaches directly connect image reconstruction and motion compensation, e.g. by using compressive sensing techniques [5].

In this work, we follow a registration-based approach, i.e. we use the reconstructed image patches to predict the underlying object motion and to generate a "plausible" image of the entire ROI. Registration-based approaches

have been used before for an improved reconstruction of 4D CT or 4D MRI images [5,6]. These techniques apply a two-step approach: estimate the underlying object motion, and use the estimated motion to generate improved images. In contrast, this work uses an integrated approach, i.e. image and object motion are estimated simultaneously.

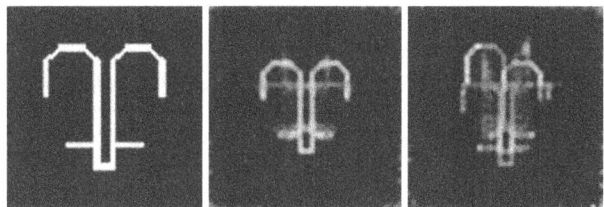

Figure 1: *Phantom image (left) and a simulated patch-wise MPI reconstruction using four overlapping image patches without object motion (middle) and with object motion (right).*

II. Material and Methods

II.I. Methods

Given N overlapping patches p_i of image regions Ω_i, and acquired at time points $\tau_i \in [0, T]$, we aim to find the particle concentration $c_0 : \Omega \to \mathbb{R}$ in the entire ROI $\Omega = \bigcup_i \Omega_i$ and the associated spatial-temporal object motion $\phi : \Omega \times [0, T] \to \Omega$ during acquisition. Assuming rigid object motion, the following minimization problem

$$J(c_0, \phi) = \sum_{i=1,\dots,N} \int_{\Omega_i} \left\| c_0 \circ \phi_{\tau_i} - c_{p_i} \right\|^2 dx \qquad (1)$$

aims for solving both simultaneously. The transformation ϕ is parameterized as time-varying poly-rigid transformation using the Log-Euclidean framework [7], i.e. $\phi(x, \tau) = \phi_\tau(x, 1)$ where $\phi_\tau(x, 1)$ is the solution of the forward integration $\frac{d}{ds}\phi_\tau(x, s) = \frac{\sum_i w_i(\tau)(t_i + A_i(x - st_i))}{\sum_i w_i(\tau)}$ over unit time. A_i are matrix logarithms of the searched rotation matrices and t_i the translations, see e.g. [7] for more details. Arbitrary numbers of temporal key-point transformations can be chosen, however, a natural choice is to use patch acquisition times τ_i and weights $w_i(\tau) = \exp\left(-\frac{\|\tau - \tau_i\|^2}{2\sigma^2}\right)$.

The resulting transformation $\phi(x,\tau)$ is a diffeomorphism, i.e. C^∞ with respect to spatial position and time. The parameter σ regularizes the temporal smoothness and can be used to encode prior knowledge about the underlying object motion. Eq. (1) is solved alternately with respect to c_0 and ϕ ($i.e.\{A_i,t_i\}_{i=1}^N$) by a second order gradient descent.

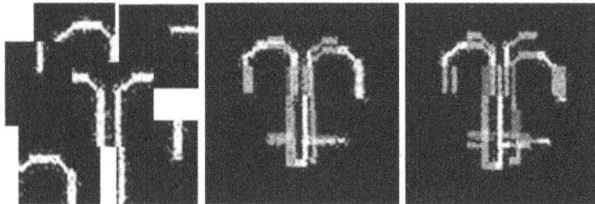

Figure 2: *Simulated images with sinusoidal object motion: Examples of generated patches (left), and reconstructions without motion compensation for $\alpha = 2$ (middle) and $\alpha = 4$ (right).*

II.II. Material

To evaluate our approach we use simulated data based on the phantom shown in Fig. 1 (left). In a first study, we split the image space into 9 overlapping patch regions and generate noisy successive observations during a sinusoidal object motion with amplitude α: $(\delta x,\delta y)=(\alpha*\sin(2\pi\tau/T),\alpha*\cos(2\pi\tau/T))$. Fig. 2 shows generated patches and reconstructions without motion compensation. Note, that some of the patches include only a few structures.

In a second study, the image space is split into 4 overlapping patches and MPI images are simulated using the framework described in [3]. Object motions up to 15% of the patch size were applied before patch acquisition, see Fig. 1 for reconstructions with and without motion. Truncation artefacts at patch borders are clearly visible.

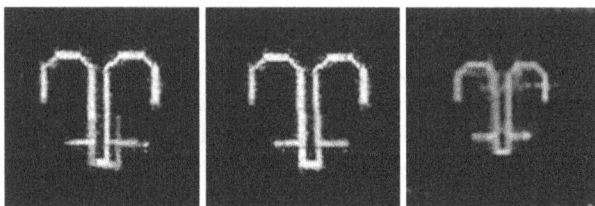

Figure 3: *Reconstructed images with sinusoidal object motion ($\alpha = 4$) using $\sigma = 0.1\Delta\tau$ (left) and $\sigma = 0.8\Delta\tau$ (middle) (compare with Fig.2 right), and reconstructed image of the simulated MPI data (right) (compare with Fig. 1 right).*

III. Results

In the first experiment, we use noisy image patches generated under sinusoidal motion with different motion amplitudes ($\alpha = 2,3,4$ pixel). Reconstruction quality for $\alpha = 4$ and two different regularization parameters is shown in Fig. 3. The temporal regularization particularly improves the registration of patches with little structural information as visible in Fig. 3 left and middle.

In the second experiment, the proposed algorithm is applied to simulated MPI data. As visible in the results presented in Fig. 3 right, an accurate co-registration of the image patches is possible despite the presence of truncation artefacts at the patch borders.

Quantitative results of both experiments are presented in Table 1. We computed the mean intensity difference between reconstructed image and ground truth relative to the maximum image intensity.

	Study 1 (Phantom)			Study 2 (MPI)
	$\alpha=2$	$\alpha=3$	$\alpha=4$	
Without motion compensation	9,9%	12,5%	13,9%	5,3%
with motion compensation	6,1%	6,5%	7,1%	3,4%

Table 1: *Mean relative intensity difference between the reconstructed image and the phantom image (study 1) or the MPI reconstruction without object motion (study2).*

IV. Discussion and Conclusions

The results show that a motion corrected reconstruction of patch-wise acquired MPI data is possible – at least in the presence of rigid object motion. As shown in the two studies, the image can be reconstructed successfully even in the presence of relatively large motion amplitudes and sparse image structures (see Fig. 2), and despite truncation artefacts at the patch borders. Crucial for this robustness of the presented approach is the temporal smoothness constrain imposed by the temporal polyrigid transformation model. A limitation of this work is the missing investigation of the influence of patch overlap and rotational motion components, this will be addressed in future work. Further, the extension of the approach to deformable object motions is possible within the same framework using spatially varying polyrigid or polyaffine transformations [7]. However, such an extension increases the number of parameters to estimate and might require larger patch overlaps.

ACKNOWLEDGEMENTS

TMB and MA thankfully acknowledge the financial support by the Federal Ministry of Education and Research (BMBF, grant numbers 13GW0069A, 13GW0071D, 01DL17010A, and 13GW0230B).

REFERENCES

[1] Lu K, Goodwill P W, Saritas E U, Zheng B and Conolly S M 2013 Linearity and shift invariance for quantitative magnetic particle imaging IEEE Trans. Med. Imaging 32 1565–75

[2] Rahmer J, Gleich B, Bontus C, Schmale I, Schmidt J, Kanzenbach, Woywode O, Weizenecker J and Borgert J 2011 Results on rapid 3d magnetic particle imaging with a large field of view Proc. of the Int. Society for Magnetic Resonance in Medicine vol 19 p 629

[3] Ahlborg, M., Kaethner, C., Knopp, T., Szwargulski, P., & Buzug, T. M. (2016). Using data redundancy gained by patch overlaps to reduce truncation artifacts in magnetic particle imaging. Physics in medicine and biology, 61(12), 4583-4598.

[4] Vercauteren, T., Perchant, A., Malandain, G., Pennec, X., & Ayache, N. (2006). Robust mosaicing with correction of motion distortions and tissue deformations for in vivo fibered microscopy. Medical image analysis, 10(5), 673-692.

[5] Forman, C., Piccini, D., Grimm, R., Hutter, J., Hornegger, J., & Zenge, M. O. (2015). Reduction of respiratory motion artifacts for free-breathing whole-heart coronary MRA by weighted iterative reconstruction. Magnetic resonance in medicine, 73(5), 1885-1895.

[6] Ehrhardt, J., Werner, R., Säring, D., Frenzel, T., Lu, W., Low, D., and Handels, H. (2007). An optical flow based method for improved reconstruction of 4D CT data sets acquired during free breathing. Medical Physics, 34(2), 711-721.

[7] Arsigny, V., Pennec, X., & Ayache, N. (2005). Polyrigid and polyaffine transformations: a novel geometrical tool to deal with non-rigid deformations–application to the registration of histological slices. Medical image analysis, 9(6), 507-523.

Session 04 - Talks

Methods I

Direct Image Projection Estimation in MPI Using Projected System Matrices

Jochen Franke [a,b,*], **Michael Herbst** [a]

[a] *Bruker BioSpin MRI GmbH, Ettlingen, Germany*
[b] *Physics of Molecular Imaging Systems, University RWTH Aachen, Germany*
[*] *Corresponding author, email: Jochen.Franke@Bruker.com*

I. Introduction

Magnetic Particle Imaging (MPI) is an extremely fast 3D+t imaging modality, capable to acquire with approx. 46 volumes per second [1] signal related quantitatively to the iron concentration. However, image reconstruction is computational expensive and thus depicts nowadays the bottleneck in the real-time capability of MPI. To allow for e.g. MPI based image guided interventions, fast feedback and thus fast image reconstruction with a short dead time is a prerequisite to allow for precise steering of e.g. a catheter. The real-time capability was addressed e.g. in [2], allowing 3D reconstructions with an latency off approx. 2 s. Rather than to investigate reconstructed 3D datasets, cardiologists are often used to work with (orthogonal) slice views or even projections such as in X-ray DSA. For this and many other applications, fast reconstruction with minimal latency of projection estimates might be sufficient even on the expense of reduced spatial resolution.

Therefore, we propose a fast and direct projection estimation reconstruction by using projected system matrices rather than projecting in the fully reconstructed image space.

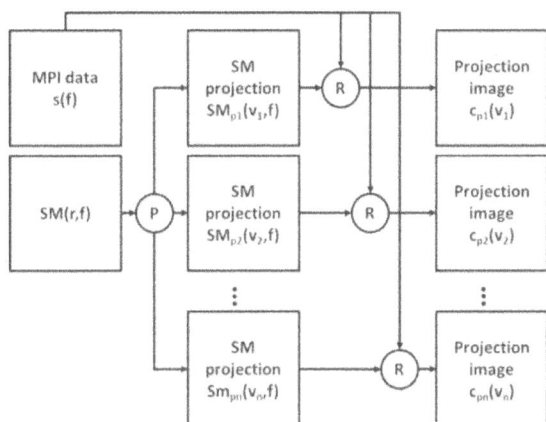

Figure 1: Schematics of direct projection estimate reconstruction using projected system matrices. Prior to the image reconstruction, the system matrix gets projected in the desired direction(s). The reconstruction of projection estimates of different directions can be parallelized.

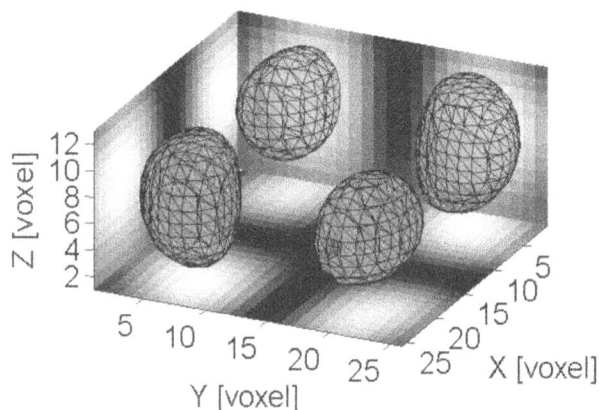

Figure 2: 3D iso-surface representation of on frequency component (75.1 kHz) of the used 3D system matrix (SM3D) and its three orthogonal 2D projections (SMxy, SMxz, SMyz).

II. Material and Methods

II. I. Theory

Direct projection estimate reconstruction is facilitated by computation of at least one projected system matrix prior to the reconstruction process. A schematic of this reconstruction framework is presented in Fig. 1. System matrices projection could be performed in the spatial domain:

$$SM_{projection}(x, y, f) = \sum_z SM(x, y, z, f) \quad (1)$$

Here, the projection along the spatial dimension z spanned up by a 3D system matrix is illustrated exemplarily. System matrix projection in the spatial domain is, however, not restricted to orthogonal projections along the matrix dimensions and not restricted to a single projection step.

In case of a multi-parameter approach [3], a system matrix could be also projected in the parameter domain:

$$SM_{projection}(x, y, z, f) = \sum_p SM(x, y, z, f, p) \quad (2)$$

With this, the information of all system matrices spanning up the parameter space, gets compressed into one system matrix. Furthermore, projection in the parameter domain as well as spatial domain can be combined.

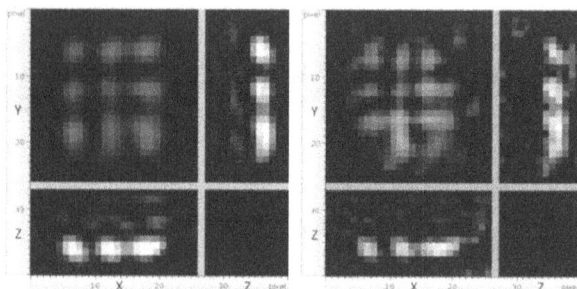

Figure 3: Reconstruction results of a resolution phantom (in-plane 4×4 dot phantom). LEFT) Reconstructed 3D dataset, projected in the image space into three orthogonal directions. RIGHT) Direct projection estimate reconstruction, using three in the spatial dimensions orthogonally projected system matrices.

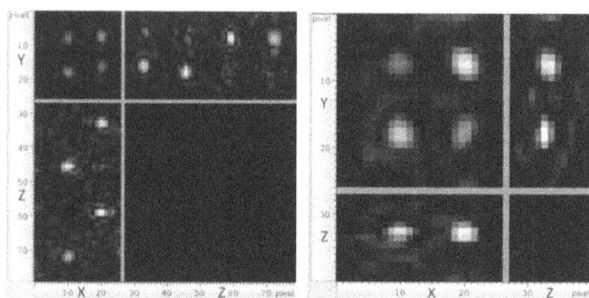

Figure 4: Reconstruction results of an in-plane 2×2 dot phantom. LEFT) Multi-parameter reconstruction using an appended system matrix consisting of four individual 3D system matrices. The parameter space is appended along the z-direction. RIGHT) Direct reconstruction using the appended system matrix, projected along the parameter dimension. Both results are displayed as orthogonal image projections.

II.II. Experiments

Two experiments were performed on a MPI-Scanner (MPI 25/20FF, Bruker BioSpin MRI GmbH). Both, the object data as well as the 3D system matrices were measured using a 3D Lissajous trajectory ($DF_{x/y/z} = 14/14/14$ mT, $SF_{x/y/z} = 1.25/1.25/2.5$ T/m, detection bandwidth $= 1.25$ MHz, $f_{x/y/z} = 24.51/26.04/25.25$ kHz).

Exp.1: A resolution phantom (in-plane 4×4 dot phantom), filled with Perimag®, was imaged in the scanner. Data were reconstructed in the software platform ParaVision (Bruker BioSpin MRI GmbH) using a Kaczmarz algorithm in a sparse domain (system matrices: SM_{xy} 26×26, SM_{xz} 26×13, SM_{yz} 26×13 or SM_{3D} 26×26×13 voxel, SNR threshold = 10, iterations = 3, average = 1, relative regularization = 10^{-5}), while the SNR values were computed for each SM individually. For comparison, the full 3D reconstruction was projected in image space afterwards.

Exp. 2: A phantom (in-plane 2×2 dot phantom), filled with 4 different probes, Perimag®, FeO2-powder, Resovist® and a magnetic nailpolish, were imaged in the scanner simultaneously. Data were reconstructed using a Kaczmarz algorithm in a sparse domain. Reconstruction parameters: system matrices: $SM_{projection}$ 26×26×13 voxel or the appended SM_{mp} 26×26×13×4 voxel (containing four

dedicated system matrices of the respective four probes), SNR threshold = 10, iterations = 3, average = 1, relative regularization = 10^{-5}. Both results were projected in image space afterwards (c.f. Fig. 4), while the fully reconstructed parameter space (c.f. Fig. 4 left) was appended in the z-direction.

III. Results and Discussion

As depicted in Fig. 1, direct reconstruction of individual image projection estimates can be computed in parallel. Fig. 2 shows one frequency component of a full 3D system matrix and its three orthogonal projections as used in Exp. 1. By projecting system matrices, the computational effort for image reconstruction is highly reduced. Even in the case of the reconstruction of three independent orthogonal projections, the equations used for reconstruction are reduced in the case of Exp. 1 by a factor of 5.8 compared to the 3D reconstruction. With the usage of the same frequency selection, a maximum equation reduction factor of 6.5 would be possible comparing the three orthogonal projections and a full 3D reconstruction. Additionally, the three projections were reconstructed in parallel reducing the computation time to less than 21 ms. Fig. 3 shows state of the art reconstruction with projections in the image space next to the proposed direct reconstruction of projection estimates. Fig. 4 presents the results of Exp. 2. featuring a direct reconstruction of projections in the parameter domain.

IV. Conclusions

With this contribution, we have shown the feasibility of a direct image projection estimation by using projected system matrices. Orthogonal projections in the spatial domain as well as projection in the parameter domain have been presented. It is evident, that the reduction of equations due to system matrix projection will lead to only an approximation to image projections with reduced spatial resolution and on the expense of image artifacts. However, the computational effort is highly reduced and the projected system matrices depict a higher SNR compared to its source system matrix. In case of parameter-space projection, with a single SM only the total iron concentration distribution of all tracer types without the capability of tracer type discrimination can be reconstructed. This proposed approach allows for direct and real-time reconstruction of image projections with repetition rates up to 46 sets of orthogonal projections per second and thus enables real-time feed-back for e.g. image guided interventions.

REFERENCES

[1] B. Gleich and J. Weizenecker. *Tomographic imaging using the nonlinear response of magnetic particles.* Nature, 435(7046):1217-1217, 2005. doi: 10.1038/nature03808.

[2] T. Knopp and M. Hofmann. *Online reconstruction of 3D magnetic particle imaging data.* Phys Med Biol. 2016 Jun 7;61(11):N257-67. doi: 10.1088/0031-9155/61/11/N257

[3] J. Rahmer et al. *First experimental evidence of the feasibility of multi-color magnetic particle imaging.* Phys Med Biol. 2015 Mar 7;60(5):1775-91. doi: 10.1088/0031-9155/60/5/1775.

Fast Multi-Resolution Imaging using Adaptive Feature Detection

Nadine Gdaniec [a,b*], Patryk Szwargulski [a,b] and Tobias Knopp [a,b]

[a] Section for Biomedical Imaging, University Medical Center Hamburg-Eppendorf, Hamburg, Germany
[b] Institute for Biomedical Imaging, Hamburg University of Technology, Hamburg, Germany
* Corresponding author, email: n.gdaniec@uke.de

I. Introduction

Magnetic particle imaging (MPI) is an imaging technique to determine the distribution of magnetic nano-particles with the help of magnetic fields. A volume of about $20 \times 20 \times 10 \text{ mm}^3$ can be acquired in a short acquisition time of 21.54 ms [1]. The size of the field of view (FOV) is limited due to physiological constraints. The FOV can be increased by lowering the magnetic field gradient, which has the drawback of lowering the spatial resolution of the final image. An alternative for enlarging the FOV is spatially shifting the imaging volume stepwise with the help of focus fields [2]. The acquisition time increases with the region of interest and reduces the temporal resolution.

To improve the temporal resolution for larger volumes, imaging at multiple gradient strengths together with a joint reconstruction is proposed in this work. A low-resolution overview scan is performed and high-resolution scans are performed at selected locations afterwards. The data are reconstructed jointly for a final image with information from low- and high-resolution scans. This abstract is based on an article published in [3]. A similar approach was used for reconstruction of large FOV's with high resolution in Traveling Wave Magnetic Particle Imaging in [4].

II. Material and Methods

II.I. Sparse Scan Protocol

The state-of-the art dense multi patch scan protocol divides the full region of interest Ω into L_D divisions Ω^{DF}. Each division is captured by one patch. The proposed multi-scale imaging protocol reduces the number of patches and is schematically shown in Fig. 1 for vascular imaging. It divides Ω into a low-resolution (LR) region $\Omega^{\text{LR}} \subseteq \Omega$ and a high-resolution (HR) region $\Omega^{\text{HR}} \subseteq \Omega$. An overview scan with a low gradient strength G^{LR} is acquired at the beginning to cover the entire region of interest, i.e. $\Omega = \Omega^{\text{LR}}$. A low-resolution image LR representing the particle distribution is reconstructed from these data. A binary mask of the LR image is determined by applying a threshold-based segmentation. The number of patches L_S and patch positions of the HR scans are calculated based on

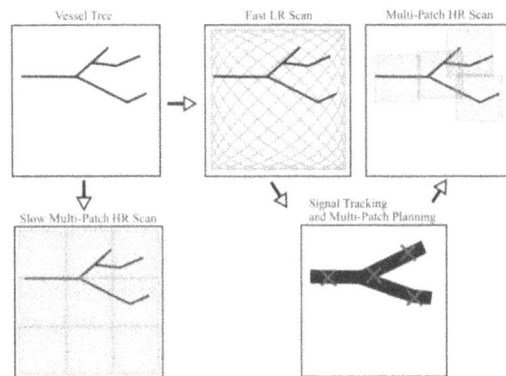

Figure 1: Schematic scan protocol. The vessel tree (top left) acquired with the conventional dense multi-patch scan protocol (bottom left) and the proposed sparse multi-scale imaging protocol (right). Based on a low-resolution scan (top middle), structures for a series of high-resolution scans are identified.

an algorithm that recursively determines the center of mass of decreasing parts of the binary mask.

Finally, the HR patches are acquired at the determined spatial locations using a high gradient strength G^{HR}. In practice, the scan protocol will be highly application specific and should be adjusted to the needed setting.

II.II. Reconstruction

The relation between the particle concentration vector $c \in \mathbb{R}^N$ with N pixels and the measurement vector $u \in \mathbb{C}^K$, with the frequency components K is described by $Sc = u$, with the system matrix $S \in \mathbb{C}^{N \times K}$. The particle concentration is obtained by solving the linear system. This results in $L_S + 1$ equations, i.e. one from the overview scan and L_S from the HR scans. A joint reconstruction of the stacked linear system $S_{\text{joint}}^{\text{HR}} c^{\text{HR}} = u_{\text{joint}}^{\text{HR}}$ with $S_{\text{joint}}^{\text{HR}} = \left(S_1^{\text{HR}}, S_2^{\text{HR}}, \dots, S_{L_S}^{\text{HR}} \right)^T$ and $u_{\text{joint}}^{\text{HR}} = \left(u_1^{\text{HR}}, u_2^{\text{HR}}, \dots, u_{L_S}^{\text{HR}} \right)^T$ was proposed in [5]. It is also possible to solve the linear system

$$\begin{pmatrix} S^{\text{LR}} \\ S_{\text{joint}}^{\text{HR}} \end{pmatrix} c^{\text{combined}} = \begin{pmatrix} u^{\text{LR}} \\ u_{\text{joint}}^{\text{HR}} \end{pmatrix}.$$

This way, locations not captured by the HR scans are reconstructed using information from the LR scan.

II.IV. Experimental setup

Measurements were performed using a preclinical MPI scanner (Bruker Biospin, Ettlingen, Germany) with 12 cm bore size and a 3D focus-field generator. The system matrices required for reconstruction were measured prior to the experiment using a delta sample filled with undiluted Resovist. All system matrices have a voxel size of 1 mm in each direction. The imaging sequence was performed using a drive-field amplitude of 12 mT/μ_0. The overview scan was measured using the gradient strength $G^{LR} = 1$ T/$(m\mu_0)$ and the HR scans with $G^{HR} = 2$ T/$(m\mu_0)$. The adaptive multi-scale imaging sequence was evaluated using the vessel phantom shown in Fig. 2. It consists of four glass capillaries with gaps and branches with an inner diameter of 0.7 mm filled with diluted Resovist with a concentration of 250 mmol(Fe)/L.

III. Results

Reconstruction results are shown in Fig. 2. Beside a reconstruction of the low-gradient measurement and a joint reconstruction of the high-gradient measurements, we also reconstructed the low- and high-gradient measurements jointly. Additionally, the dense multi-patch reconstruction result is shown. In the low-gradient reconstruction result only the main branch is visible. By selectively adding high gradient patches at the predefined locations, the spatial resolution is partially improved. The reconstruction result using all high-gradient patches recovers the full structure of the phantom. The fragmentation in the left and the right side are visible, whereas the gaps are not fully resolved. The reconstruction results of the high-gradient scans and the joint multi-gradient scans have a similar quality in terms of SNR and spatial resolution.

IV. Discussion

The proposed adaptive multi-gradient acquisition allows measuring a large object in a fraction of time compared to a dense multi-patch protocol. The gain in imaging speed was 2.25 (4 Scans instead of 9). A higher gain is expected for 3D imaging by exploiting the sparsity in the third dimension. The multi-gradient scan protocol was designed for angiographic applications. It can work for non-sparse particle distributions as well, like liver imaging [6] for

detecting lesions. Furthermore, the LR overview scan can be used as static background for instrument tracking with high resolution through a vessel tree. To reduce the computational effort of the joint reconstruction [5] a fast algorithm [7] using an implicit formulation of the system matrix can be developed.

V. Conclusions

MPI is a tomographic imaging method with high spatio-temporal resolution. One key challenge when upscaling current small animal scanners to human-sized scanners is the limitation of the FOV while maintaining the high spatio-temporal resolution. Within this work, we addressed the issue with a multi-gradient imaging sequence. Only important regions are scanned with high resolution. By combining LR and HR scans during image reconstruction, it is possible to derive a single image of the particle distribution capturing the entire FOV with anisotropic spatial resolution in only a fraction of time.

ACKNOWLEDGEMENTS

The authors thankfully acknowledge financial support by the German Research Foundation (DFG, grant number KN 1108/2-1)) and the Federal Ministry of Education and Research (BMBF, grant number 05M16GKA).

REFERENCES

[1] J.Weizenecker, B. Gleich, J. Rahmer, H. Dahnke, and J. Borgert. Three-dimensional real-time in vivo magnetic particle imaging. *Physics in Medicine and Biology*, vol. 54, no. 5, pp. L1-L10, 2009.

[2] B. Gleich and J. Weizenecker. Tomographic imaging using the nonlinear response of magnetic particles. Nature, 435(7046):1217-1217, 2005. doi: 10.1038/nature03808.

[3] N. Gdaniec, P. Szwargulski, and T. Knopp. Fast multiresolution data acquisition for magnetic particle imaging using adaptive feature detection. *Medical Physics*, doi: 10.1002/mp.12628

[4] P. Vogel, T. Kampf, M. A. Rückert, V. C. Behr. Flexible and Dynamic Patch Reconstruction for Traveling Wave Magnetic Particle Imaging, IJMPI, vol. 2, no. 2, pp. 1611001, 2016

[5] T. Knopp, K. Them, M. Kaul, and N. Gdaniec. Joint reconstruction of non-overlapping magnetic particle imaging focus-field data. *Physics in Medicine and Biology*, vol. 60, no. 8, pp. L15-21, 2015.

[6] J. Dieckhoff, M. Kaul, T. Mummert, C. Jung, J. Salamon, G. Adam, T. Knopp, F. Ludwig, C. Balceris, and H. Ittrich. In vivo liver visualizations with magnetic particle imaging based on the calibration measurement approach. *Physics in Medicine and Biology*, vol. 62, no. 9, p. 3470, 2016.

[7] P. Szwargulski, M. Hofmann, N. Gdaniec, and T. Knopp. Fast implicit reconstruction of focus field data in MPI. *6th International Workshop on Magnetic Particle Imaging* (IWMPI 2016), 2016, p. 176.

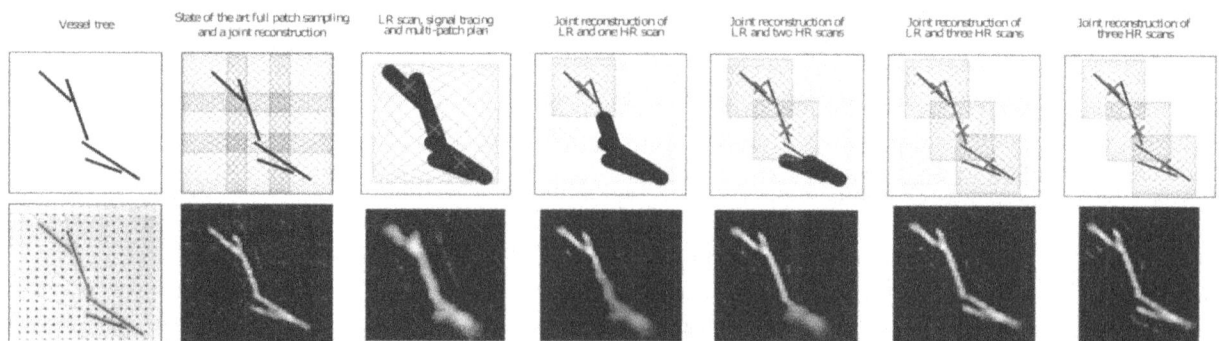

Figure 2: Schematic illustration of patches and reconstructed image data. The schematic vessel tree phantom and an image is shown in the first column. The next column indicates the dense scan protocol planning and the corresponding reconstructed image. The following columns indicate the patches (top row) used for reconstruction of the images (bottom row).

Fast System Calibration for MPI Using a Rotating Coded Calibration Scene

Serhat Ilbey [a,b,*], Can Barış Top [a], Emine Ulku Saritas [b,c], H. Emre Güven [a]

[a] ASELSAN Research Center, 06370 Ankara, Turkey
[b] Department of Electrical and Electronics Engineering, Bilkent University, Ankara, Turkey
[c] National Magnetic Resonance Research Center (UMRAM), Bilkent University, Ankara, Turkey
[*] Corresponding author, email: silbey@aselsan.com.tr

I. Introduction

Image reconstruction in Magnetic Particle Imaging (MPI) [1] can be done either by using the system matrix approach [2], or directly from the time-domain data in the X-space method [3]. In the former, a time-consuming system calibration procedure is necessary to obtain the system matrix [4]. For a full calibration, the signals received from a superparamagnetic iron oxide (SPIO) sample are measured at each voxel position in the field-of-view (FOV). Typically, the mechanical movement of a robot arm to translate a sample between two grid points takes more than 1.3 seconds [5], causing lengthy calibration scans.

To decrease the amount of time required to obtain the system matrix, compressed sensing methods have been proposed. It is shown that the rows of the system matrix are sparse in discrete cosine transform (DCT), discrete Fourier transform (DFT), and Chebyshev transform domains [6]. Using this property, calibration measurements are taken at random voxel positions [7] and the system matrix is reconstructed using algorithms such as Fast Iterative Shrinkage Thresholding (FISTA) or Alternating Direction Method of Multipliers (ADMM) [8].

In this study, we introduce a rotating and translating Coded Calibration Scene (CCS) approach, which features multiple SPIO samples at random voxel positions instead of a single point source. During the calibration measurements, the CCS is rotated 360° around different rotation centers. We show that for the same number of measurements, the system matrix reconstructed via a CCS yields significantly better image quality with respect to the standard sparse system matrix reconstruction method using single voxel measurements.

II. Material and Methods

II.I. MPI System Parameters and Fast Calibration

For the simulations, a 40 mm x 20 mm numerical phantom with 100 x 50 pixels resolution was used (Fig. 1). Selection field gradients were 1.875 T/m and 3.75 T/m in the y- and

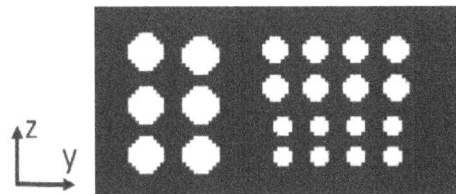

Figure 1: *Numerical phantom (40 mm x 20 mm). Diameters of the discs are: 4, 2.8, and 2 mm.*

z-directions, respectively. The drive fields had 36 mT amplitude with 26.04 kHz and 25.25 kHz frequencies in the y- and z-directions, respectively. The SPIO magnetization was modeled with the Langevin function [1], assuming 30-nm diameter monodisperse SPIOs. The received signal was filtered using an ideal band-pass filter passing frequency components between 30 kHz and 1 MHz. The signal-to-noise ratio (SNR) from a single pixel acquisition data was set to 20 dB.

In this study, we analyzed the effect of different acceleration rates (~2x, ~4.6x and ~13.9x) for the system calibration, where acceleration is defined as the ratio of the total number of pixels over the number of measurements. The CCS was a square with 250 x 250 pixels, 40% of which were filled in a uniformly-random fashion. Measurements were taken at 1° angular steps. For ~2x acceleration, the CCS was rotated fully around its center at seven different y-positions along the midline of the FOV, making a total of 2520 measurements. Similarly, for ~4.6x acceleration, the CCS was rotated fully at three different positions, while a calibration with a single full rotation resulted in ~13.9x acceleration.

II.II. Reconstruction of the System Calibration Matrix

To reconstruct the system matrix from the acquired data, the below problem is solved using ADMM:

$$\underset{A}{argmin} \quad \|DA^T\|_1$$

$$subject\ to \quad \|AX - B\|_2 < \epsilon_c \tag{1}$$

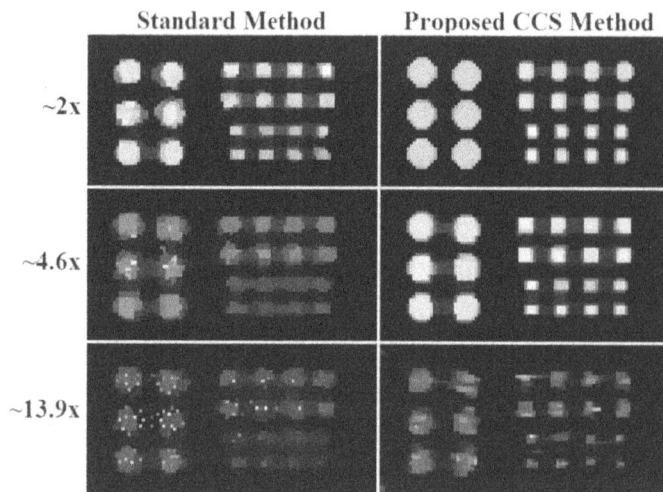

Figure 2: *Reconstructed images with system matrices obtained via the standard method (left) and with the rotating and translating coded calibration scene (right). From top to bottom: ~2x, ~4.6x, and ~13.9x accelerations.*

where, **A** is the reconstructed system matrix, **D** is the DCT matrix. The columns of **X** correspond to the rotated/translated versions of the CCS, whereas the columns of **B** correspond to the CCS measurements.

For image reconstruction, we used ADMM, minimizing the total variation and l_1 norm of the reconstructed images. Details of the specific algorithm can be found in [9].

III. Results

Reconstructed images obtained with the rotating CCS and the standard sparse system calibration matrix reconstruction methods are shown in Fig. 2. Visual inspection of the results suggests significantly better image quality using the proposed method at equal acceleration rates. This is also supported by the quantitative Structural Similarity Index Measure (SSIM) and Peak SNR (PSNR) metrics, shown in Table 1.

Table 1: *SSIM and PSNR of the reconstructed images*

Method	Metric	Acceleration		
		~2x	~4.6x	~13.9x
Standard Method [7]	SSIM	0.71	0.50	0.41
	PSNR	15.8	12.4	10.1
Proposed CCS Method	SSIM	0.95	0.83	0.46
	PSNR	22.2	17.8	11.4

IV. Discussion

In this study, we used a rotating CCS filled at a 40% rate, and translated the CCS linearly along a single direction. We showed that the proposed method outperforms the standard acceleration method. An optimized filling rate and a translation trajectory might result in further improvements in image quality. As the SNR of a CCS measurement is higher than that of a standard single point source, measurements can be obtained during continuous rotation/translation of the CCS, which can decrease the calibration time substantially. Optimization and implementation of the technique are subjects of future studies.

V. Conclusions

In this work, we introduced a fast system calibration method via rotating and translating a coded calibration scene (CCS). The proposed method results in significant improvements in image quality over standard methods.

ACKNOWLEDGEMENTS

This work was supported by the Scientific and Technological Research Council of Turkey (Project numbers: 9050103, 115E677). The work of EUS was supported in part by the European Commission through FP7 Marie Curie Career Integration Grant (PCIG13-GA-2013-618834), by the Turkish Academy of Sciences through TUBA-GEBIP 2015 program, and by the BAGEP Award of the Science Academy.

REFERENCES

[1] B. Gleich and J. Weizenecker. Tomographic imaging using the nonlinear response of magnetic particles. *Nature*, 435(7046):1217-1217, 2005. doi: 10.1038/nature03808.

[2] T. Knopp, J. Rahmer, T. F. Sattel, S. Biederer, J. Weizenecker, B. Gleich, J. Borgert, and T. M. Buzug. Weighted iterative reconstruction for magnetic particle imaging. *Phys. Med. Biol.*, vol. 55, no. 6, pp. 1577–1589, 2010. doi:10.1088/0031-9155/55/6/003.

[3] P. W. Goodwill, E. U. Saritas, L. R. Croft, T. N. Kim, K. M. Krishnan, D. V. Schaffer, and S. M. Conolly. XSpace MPI: Magnetic Nanoparticles for Safe Medical Imaging. *Adv. Mater.*, vol. 24, pp. 3870–3877, 2012. doi: 10.1002/adma.201200221.

[4] J. Weizenecker, B. Gleich, J. Rahmer, H. Dahnke, and J. Borgert. Three-dimensional real-time in vivo magnetic particle imaging. *Phys. Med. Biol.*, vol. 54, no. 5, pp. L1–L10, 2009. doi: 10.1088/0031-9155/54/5/L01

[5] A.v. Gladiss, M. Graeser, P. Szwargulski, T. Knopp and T. M. Buzug. Hybrid system calibration for multidimensional magnetic particle imaging. *Phys. Med. Biol.*, vol. 62, no. 9, pp. 3392, 2017. doi: 10.1088/1361-6560/aa5340.

[6] J. Lampe, C. Bassoy, J. Rahmer, J. Weizenecker, H. Voss, B. Gleich, and J. Borgert. Fast reconstruction in magnetic particle imaging. *Phys. Med. Biol.*, vol. 57, no. 4, pp. 1113–1134, 2012. doi: 10.1088/0031-9155/57/4/1113.

[7] T. Knopp and A. Weber. Sparse Reconstruction of the Magnetic Particle Imaging System Matrix. *IEEE Trans. Med. Imag.*, vol. 32, no. 8, pp. 1473–1480, 2013. doi: 10.1109/TMI.2013.2258029.

[8] S. Ilbey, E. U. Saritas, and C.B. Top. Fast Calibration with Compressive Sensing and Image Reconstruction using a Lagrangian Method in Magnetic Particle Imaging. *XXI. National Meeting on Biomedical Engineering*, Istanbul, Turkey, 2017 (Submitted).

[9] S. Ilbey, C. B. Top, T. Çukur, E. U. Saritas, and H. E. Güven. Image Reconstruction for magnetic partical imaging using an augmented Lagrangian method. *International Symposium on Biomedical Imaging*, 2017. doi: 10.1109/ISBI.2017.7950469.

Spatial Resolution in MPI: The Role of Phase

H. Bagheri* and M.E. Hayden

Department of Physics, Simon Fraser University, Burnaby BC, CANADA V5A 1S6
*Corresponding author, email: hbagheri@sfu.ca

I. Introduction

Spatial resolution is a key metric for characterizing any imaging modality. Previous investigations of spatial resolution in Magnetic Particle Imaging (MPI) have focused on the role of particle size, distribution, and susceptibility, magnetic field gradients, drive field amplitude, and harmonic order [1-5]. Here we examine the role of signal phase. This is a somewhat unusual experimental parameter in MPI; it is directly accessible in our work because the scanner we employ is one in which the processes of field free point (FFP) manipulation and particle excitation are intentionally decoupled from one another [6]. Hence, phase-sensitive detection can be – and is – employed in our signal recovery strategy.

We demonstrate significant trends in image quality as acquired signals are projected onto the real axis of a series of coordinate systems that are phase-shifted relative to the excitation field; that is, relative to the applied oscillating magnetic field responsible for harmonic generation. We observe a marked spatial sharpening effect as the phase of the demodulation reference is delayed by up to 90° relative to the phase that yields images with the highest signal-to-noise ratio (SNR). This increase in resolution is accompanied by degradation in contrast or SNR, to the point where reconstructed images effectively vanish when the quadrature component of the demodulated signal is employed. In between the high-contrast/low-resolution and low-contrast/high-resolution limits, images with resolutions of order a few hundred microns or better and signal-to-noise ratios of order 10 dB or more are obtained.

II. Material and Methods

Our imaging experiments are performed using an MPI scanner in which the field free point (FFP) is defined by a 7 MA/m^2 radial (14 MA/m^2 axial) magnetic field gradient. Counter-rotating permanent magnet arrays periodically displace the FFP, causing it to execute a 56-lobe Rose pattern spanning a 1 cm diameter, two-dimensional Field of View (FOV) in the transverse plane. Radial excursions of the FFP occurred at a rate of about 4 s^{-1} during the experiments reported here.

Particle excitation is accomplished by driving current through a solenoid to produce an axially-directed oscillating drive field $\mathbf{H}_{ac}$ at some frequency that is typically in the range 40 to 400 kHz. The emf induced in a second (coaxial) solenoid is then fed to a dual-phase homodyne (phase-sensitive) detector to monitor particle responses at any desired harmonic (or combination of harmonics) of the fundamental. Data reported here were acquired at the third harmonic of a 76 kHz fundamental, employing a fourth-order low pass filter with a 100 Hz demodulation bandwidth. The (complex) discrete-time output of the phase-sensitive detector was then sampled at 450 s^{-1} and mapped onto the instantaneous FFP location inferred from measurements performed at 1000 s^{-1}.

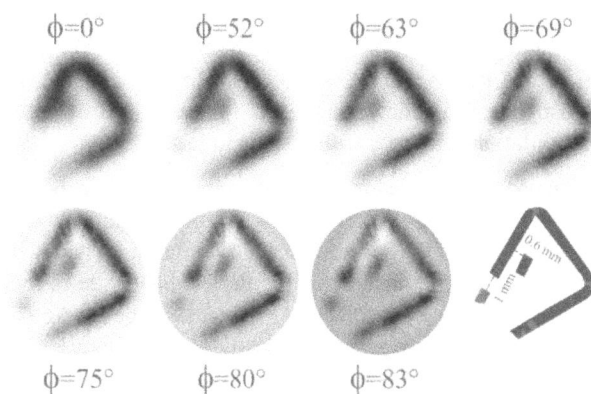

Figure 1: Images reconstructed from the component of the acquired signal that is in-phase with a demodulation reference that is delayed with respect to the excitation field. The lower right-hand panel shows the gross distribution of iron in the phantom, drawn to scale; a few dimensions are also indicated.

The phantom employed in our imaging experiments is a short length of PTFE tube with an inner diameter of 0.56 mm, filled with LodeSpin Labs polyethylene glycol (PEG)-coated superparamagnetic iron oxide (SPIO) particles (product code LS-008; 25 nm core diameter; iron concentration 5.1 mg/ml). The tube is bent into the rectilinear shape suggested by the drawing in the lower right-hand corner of Fig. 1. Voids are present, leading to the appearance of isolated SPIO-filled slugs or droplets in images. The total mass of iron within the FOV is 24 μg.

Complementary Magnetic Particle Spectroscopy (MPS) experiments were also performed, using a purpose-built MPS system that permits arbitrary alignment of the applied static ($\mathbf{H}_{dc}$) and oscillating ($\mathbf{H}_{ac}$) magnetic fields. The MPS data reported here were acquired from MicroMod

Perimag® nanoparticles comprising a 50% (w/w) iron-oxide in a dextran matrix (product code 102-00-132; 130 nm diameter; iron concentration 17 mg/ml).

III. Results

Complex or dual-phase demodulated particle response data, comprising signal amplitude and phase, were acquired for 20 complete scans of the FFP over the FOV. These data were then projected onto the real axis of various reference frames that were phase-shifted with respect to the excitation field $\mathbf{H}_{ac}$. This is equivalent to recording the amplitude of the in-phase component of the phase-sensitive detector output as measured with respect to a reference oscillator locked to $\mathbf{H}_{ac}$, but phase-shifted from it by some fixed angle. Next, an image was generated for each of the 20 scans by mapping the projected signal amplitude onto the instantaneous FFP location, and then interpolating and gridding the result (via triangulation) at 40 μm × 40 μm resolution. Finally the 20 images so obtained were averaged and scaled to a 255 bit depth grayscale. This protocol was then repeated for phase shifts spanning a 360° range; a few representative images are shown in Fig. 1. The indicated phase angle ϕ is defined such that the peak signal amplitude (and hence SNR) is maximum when ϕ = 0° and (effectively) zero when ϕ = 90°. Note that increasing ϕ corresponds to increasing the phase lag of the demodulation reference with respect to $\mathbf{H}_{ac}$.

As the phase employed in the image reconstruction process increases, the spatial blurring that is quite evident in the vicinity of ϕ = 0° diminishes. At ϕ = 52°, the small isolated tracer-filled droplet located on the far left-hand side of the image is first barely resolved. As ϕ increases beyond 69°, the 0.6 mm gap between the centrally-located feature and the main body of the phantom is clearly revealed. Meanwhile, the degradation in contrast or SNR that accompanies the resolution enhancement is apparent. These opposing trends continue as ϕ approaches 90°, at which point images effectively vanish.

Insight into this spatial sharpening effect is provided by the MPS data shown in Fig. 2. Here the sample is driven at 70 kHz with a 4 kA/m (peak) oscillating magnetic field, and the third harmonic component of the acquired signal is projected onto the real axis of three phase-shifted reference frames. The range of static magnetic fields over which a strong particle response is observed narrows considerably as the phase shift increases. This narrowing is accompanied by a decrease in signal amplitude or SNR, which is manifest in Fig. 2 as an apparent increase in noise amplitude as ϕ is increased. Note that the indicated phase is defined in the same manner as in Fig. 1: the maximum signal amplitude is obtained when ϕ = 0°. Direct quantitative comparison of the data in Figs. 1 and 2 should be avoided, since the tracer particles employed in the two experiments are not the same. Nevertheless, the trends in particle responses and image quality as the demodulation phase is changed are clear and consistent.

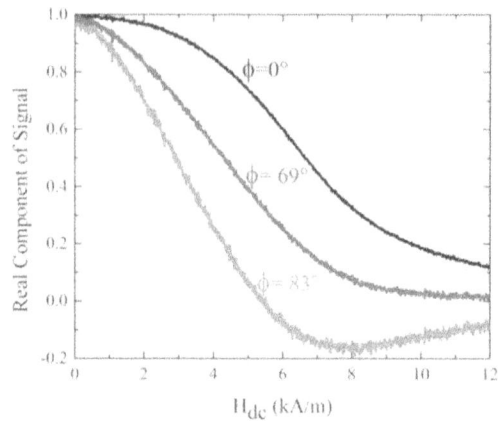

Figure 2*: Normalized MPS amplitude data acquired at the third harmonic of a 70 kHz fundamental, as measured with respect to a reference that is phase-locked to the applied ac field $\mathbf{H}_{ac}$. The uniform static field $\mathbf{H}_{dc}$ is oriented perpendicular to $\mathbf{H}_{ac}$.*

IV. Summary

The data presented here illustrate a powerful MPI signal conditioning protocol that can be employed to achieve significant enhancements in spatial resolution, at the expense of contrast or SNR. This enhancement is accomplished through the judicious use of information that is ultimately linked to the phase-response of tracer particles to applied oscillating magnetic fields.

The methods we have described are ideally-suited to MPI scanners in which the processes of FFP manipulation and particle excitation are decoupled from one another. This permits direct phase-sensitive detection of particle responses. Nonetheless, extensions of the principles employed here may find application in post-processing of MPI data from conventional scanners. A somewhat subtle but essential precondition for implementation is that the applied static and oscillating magnetic fields must be orthogonal to one-another. If they aren't, resolution enhancement is not observed. A full account of these investigations will be given elsewhere.

ACKNOWLEDGEMENTS

This work is funded by the Natural Sciences and Engineering Research Council of Canada. We are grateful to MicroMod Partikeltechnologie Gmbh and Lodespin Labs LLC for providing tracer materials.

REFERENCES

[1] R. M. Ferguson et al., "Optimization of nanoparticle core size for magnetic particle imaging," *J. Magn. Magn. Mater.* **321**, 1548 (2009).

[2] T. Knopp et al., "Prediction of the Spatial Resolution of Magnetic Particle Imaging Using the Modulation Transfer Function of the Imaging Process," *IEEE Trans. Med. Imag.* **30**, 1284 (2011).

[3] P. W. Goodwill and S. M. Conolly, "The X-Space Formulation of the Magnetic Particle Imaging Process: 1-D Signal, Resolution, Bandwidth, SNR, SAR, and Magnetostimulation," *IEEE Trans. Med. Imag.* **29**, 1851 (2010).

[4] L. R. Croft et al., "Low drive field amplitude for improved image resolution in magnetic particle imaging," *Med. Phys.* **43**, 424 (2016).

[5] H. Bagheri and M. E. Hayden, "Spatial Resolution in MPI: The Role of Harmonic Number, in *Proc. 6th IWMPI* (Infinite Science, 2016).

[6] H. Bagheri et al., "A novel scanner architecture for MPI," *Proc. 5th IWMPI*, 63 (2015). doi: 10.1109/IWMPI.2015.7107089

Ghost Correction for Multi-Parameter MPI

Michael Herbst [a*] **and Jochen Franke** [a,b]

[a] *Bruker BioSpin MRI GmbH, Ettlingen;* [b]*Physics of Molecular Imaging Systems, RTWH Aachen, Germany*
[*] *Corresponding author, email: michael.herbst@bruker.com*

I. Introduction

Multi-parameter MPI has been shown to be able to separate signal from N particles with sufficiently different signal properties. To achieve this separation, system matrices $(SM_n|n=1:N)$ from all particles are measured prior to the experiment and are fed to the image reconstruction as introduced in [1]:

$$s(f) = [SM_1 \dots SM_N] \begin{bmatrix} c_1 \\ \dots \\ c_N \end{bmatrix}.$$

A particles signal appears in a subvolume connected to its system matrix. However, since the signals from the particles in the field of view (FOV) might not be fully independent, traces from one particle do not only appear in their own parameter volume but are projected into other subvolumes where they appear as 'ghosts'.

Potential applications of this promising method, like automated catheter tracking, might suffer from these ghosts, due to hindered object identification. In this work, we introduce a method to reduce these unwanted signal intensities.

II. Material and Methods

II.I. Theory

The method is described using the flow chart in Fig. 1. Starting from a multi-parameter dataset with two parameters (N=2) and a combined system matrix (SM) the algorithm consists of six steps, which are executed for each parameter n which removes the ghosts from the image volume(s) m.

1) The state of the art multi-parameter reconstruction. A thin line separates the two subvolumes. Signal from particle one (square) mainly appears in volume one (v1), signal from particle two (circle) in volume two (v2).
In each subvolume, the related particle concentration is depicted in dark gray, the ghost of the other particle is shown in lighter color.
2) After zero-filling $(Z_m | m=2)$, v2 appears white. (In the general case: All subvolumes but v1 are set to zero.)
3) This artificial volume $c_{vn}(r)$ is back-transformed to its signal according to $s_n(f) = SM(r,f) \cdot c(r)$.
4) When this signal is reconstructed, the new image volume not only shows signal in v1 but also in v2, which was set to zero earlier.

- This new concentration contains information of the ghost in v2, which is created by a signal in v1.
- Note that for higher numbers of parameters, the ghost would appear in all other subvolumes.
- Since in our example this signal consists of the signal of particle one as well as the ghost signal from particle two, v2 also contains a ghost of the ghost signal. This 'second order' ghost is shown in the drawing for completeness, but can be expected to have relatively low intensity.
- Signal originating from v1, which now appears in v2 might lower the signal amplitude in v1. Therefore, the extracted ghost might have slightly lower amplitude than the original ghost as well. Assuming that the ghost intensity scales linearly with the intensity of the particle signal, this signal loss can be corrected by adjusting the particle signal of the new image volume to the original.

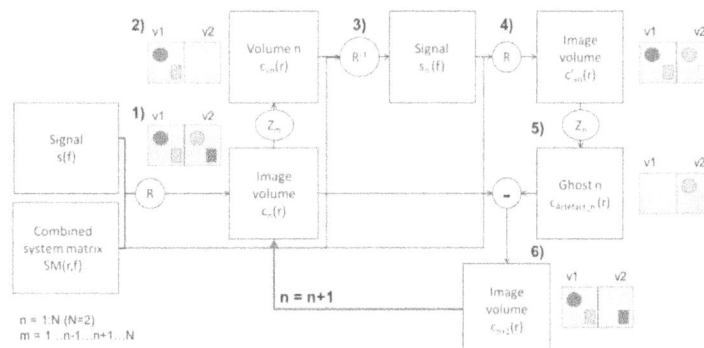

Figure 1*: A multi-parameter ghost correction scheme for two (N=2) materials is shown. R stands for an image reconstruction, R^{-1} for the back-transformation of the image to its signal, and Z for zero-filling of one sub-volume. Each step (1-6) of the ghost correction is described in the theory section.*

5) Now, v1 of this new image volume is set to zero (Z_n).

6) The extracted ghost is subtracted from the original image volume. In the resulting image volume the ghost from particle one disappeared. This new image volume can now be corrected for the ghost of particle two following the same procedure (n = n+1).

II.II. Experiments

Two experiments were performed using a custom-made probe holder. The data were measured using a 3D Lissajous trajectory on a Bruker MPI-Scanner (MPI25/20FF). Imaging parameters: drive fields (x,y,z): 14 mT, selection field: 2.5 T/m. System matrices (26×26×13 voxel) were acquired for all materials.

Exp.1) The phantom was equipped with two probes containing Perimag® and Ferro-Powder respectively.

Exp.2) Two additional probes were placed in the phantom: Resovist® and a magnetic nailpolish.

Data were reconstructed in ParaVision® with the combined system matrices, using the Kaczmarz algorithm. Reconstruction parameters: SNR threshold: 10, Iterations: 3, relative regularization: 10^{-5}.

III. Results

Figure 2 shows one slice of the imaging volume from Exp.1 for one Tracer (Perimag®). In A) the data were reconstructed with the known multi-parameter approach. The red line shows the profile through the ghost artifact, the blue line the profile of the particle signal. After ghost correction, the signal from the ghost was substantially reduced as shown in image B). Note that the blue profile line remains unchanged.

Figure 3 displays the data from Exp.1 in a volumetric view, color-coding the two tracer materials. In A) the standard multi-color approach is shown, ghost artifacts are highlighted by the white arrows. B) shows the same data after ghost correction, which lead to substantially reduced ghosting.

Figure 4 shows images from Exp.2 as reconstructed and displayed in ParaVision® in real-time. To accelerate reconstruction, the processing (reconstruction as well as ghost correction) was performed in the sparse domain. Each image (A, B, and C) displays three projections (X, Y, and Z) of the multi-parameter dataset. In A) the standard multi-parameter reconstruction is shown. In the Y and Z projection, most of the ghosting artifacts are overlaid by the particle signal. In B) the same data are shown after ghost correction. In C) difference images, displaying the artifacts subtracted from the original reconstruction are shown.

IV. Discussion

In all datasets, the presented method for the correction of the well-known multi-parameter artifact shows a clear improvement over the uncorrected data. Additionally, first results on the effect on the 'real' particle signal are promising. However, this needs to be investigated in more detail.

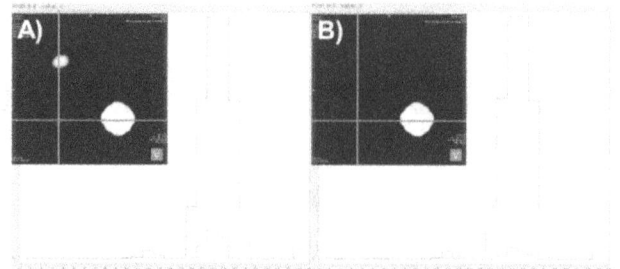

Figure 2: Images and profiles from Exp.1. The profiles are shown for the particle position as well as for the ghost. A) Standard multi-parameter reconstruction, B) results after ghost correction.

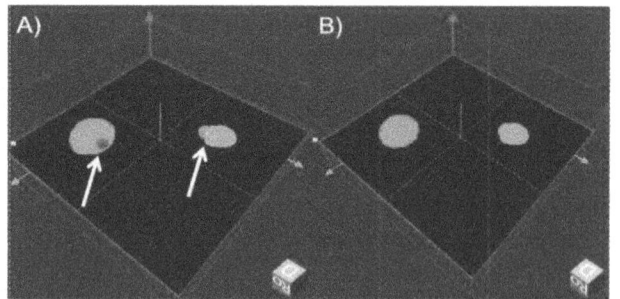

Figure 3: Volumetric view in ParaVision®, color-coding the two parameters (green and red) from Exp.1 A) Multi-parameter reconstruction, ghost artifacts are marked (white arrows) B) results after ghost correction.

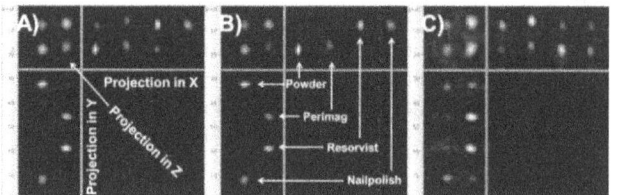

Figure 4: Images from Exp.2 as seen in the ParaVision® real-time display during acquisition. For each dimension, a projection image is shown. The particle volumes are appended in the Z-dimension. A) Multi-parameter reconstruction B) with ghost correction C) difference image.

V. Conclusions

This works shows that image artifacts in multi-parameter MPI can be substantially reduced. The presented ghost correction method uses the similarities in the particles' frequency responses (which lead to the artifacts in the first place) to separate and subtract the erroneous concentrations from the particle distribution. Since this approach can operate in the sparse domain as well as on dense data, this enables real-time correction of multi-parameter MPI data.

ACKNOWLEDGEMENTS

The authors acknowledge the financial support from the German Federal Ministry of Education and Research, FKZ 13GW0069D.

REFERENCES

[1]   J. Rahmer, A. Halkola, B. Gleich, I. Schmale, and J. Borgert, "First experimental evidence of the feasibility of multi-color magnetic particle imaging," *Phys. Med. Biol.*, vol. 60, no. 5, pp. 1775–1791, Mar. 2015

On the Determination of the Sensitivity in Magnetic Particle Imaging

Matthias Graeser[a,b], Patryk Szwargulski[a,b], Thomas Friedrich[c], Anselm von Gladiss [c], Michael Kaul[d], Kannan M Krishnan[e], Harald Ittrich[d], Gerhard Adam[d,] Thorsten M. Buzug[c] , Tobias Knopp[a]

[a] Section for Biomedical Imaging, University Medical Center Hamburg-Eppendorf, Hamburg, Germany.
[b] Institute for Biomedical Imaging, Hamburg University of Technology, Hamburg, Germany.
[c] Institute of Medical Engineering, University of Lübeck, Lübeck, Germany.
[d] Department for Diagnostic and Interventional Radiology and Nuclear Medicine, University Medical Center Hamburg-Eppendorf, Hamburg, Germany.
[e] Department of Materials Science and Department of Physics, University of Washington, Seattle, USA.
* Corresponding author, email: ma.graeser@uke.de

I. Introduction

Magnetic Particle Imaging (MPI) can provide a very high sensitivity at high imaging speed [1]. In recent publications, this sensitivity improved towards its theoretical limits [2-5]. As no central convention is being used to measure the sensitivity, the reported values differ by unit and measurement procedure. Values ranging from 50 µmol/L in one voxel of 0.216 µL [3], over 200 cells [4] to 1 ng [5] have been reported. In addition to the different unit systems, the values were obtained at different encoding schemes, different drive field amplitudes, different time scales and different phantom measurements. To evaluate new imaging concepts, sequences and reconstruction methods, it is, however, crucial to compare sensitivity values across different scanner architectures. The aim of this work is to develop a standardized protocol that allows determining the detection limit across different scanners with their respective technologies and encoding schemes. We evaluate the protocol using two different receive coils of which one is optimized for high sensitivity in a small field of view. This abstract is based on an article published in [2].

II. Material and Methods

II.I. Experiment Design

The sensitivity of an MPI scanner is not a fixed number but depends on various acquisition parameters and also the applied encoding scheme. To still make sensitivity numbers comparable we have developed the following guidelines:

1. Use a dilution series: The SNR of a highly concentrated sample is not suitable for sensitivity determination. Only a sample with a known iron concentration should be used as reference.
2. Use the smallest sample size that is reproducible to reduce the impact of the encoding scheme. Encoding scheme advantages are highly object dependent and in turn should be investigated in a separate step.
3. Use reconstructed data: Raw data may indicate sensitivity limits, but it is not guaranteed that a suitable image can be reconstructed. Background signal might be mixed up with particle signal in the raw data.
4. Move the sample: With lower SNR reconstruction, artifacts could be falsely interpreted as an image. Therefore, a movement of the sample should be performed. A moving object in the image then correctly identifies the phantom.
5. Relate the data to scanning parameters: Several imaging parameters have an additional impact on the sensitivity like drive field strength and frequency, scanning time and bore diameter. These parameters are scanner specific and cannot always be adapted to a unified protocol. However, it is possible to relate the results and therefor make a comparison possible.

These guidelines were taken into account in following protocol. Two different dilution experiments with LS008 [6] were performed. The first sample had a constant volume of 1 µl while the contained iron amount was reduced in each step by a factor of 2 from 5.1 µg to 2.5 ng. In a second experiment, a constant iron content of 10 ng was diluted from 1 µl to a maximum volume of 128 µl. In both experiments the sample was moved by the calibration robot along the bore axis. In addition, a healthy mouse was examined with three subsequent boli of each 10 µl containing 510 ng, 5.1 µg and 51.2 µg iron content. All measurements were performed with 12 mT drive field amplitude. The in vitro measurements were averaged 100 times in maximum leading to 2.14 seconds acquisition time per frame. The in vivo measurements were not averaged to resolve the full dynamic of the heart.

II.II Hardware development

At the UKE a commercial preclinical MPI scanner (Bruker Biospin MRI GmbH, Karlsruhe, Germany) is used for the experiments. To improve the sensitivity of the system a receiver with an optimized coil and receive chain was designed.

The coil is designed as a gradiometer with a length of 34 mm which is a compromise of the optimum for the field of view (FOV) center and the FOV border. The induced signal is filtered by a 4th order resonant filter. Before amplification with a JFET based amplifier it is noise-matched by a ferrite core transformer. A detailed description of the hardware can be found in [2].

III. Results

III.I *In Vitro* Experiments

The *in vitro* experiment with constant volume showed an accurately identifiable sample at a minimum iron content of 160 ng for the preinstalled receive chain and at 5 ng with the gradiometer receive chain.

At the dilution example with constant iron content the moving sample was identifiable until a total volume of 64 µl corresponding to a dilution of 2.8 µmol/L which is

64µl	128µl
156 µg/L	78 µg/L
2.8 µmol/L	1.4 µmol/L

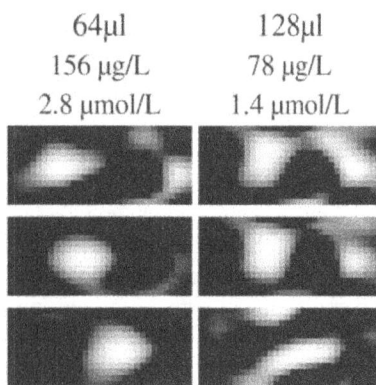

Figure 1: Low concentration imaging. Here the lowest iron concentration of only 2.8 µmol/L could be imaged as a moving dot (Here three different time points are shown). The imaging of the 128 µl failed although the SNR of the raw data suggested otherwise. Image is part of Fig.7 published in [2] with a CC BY licence.

0.514 µg / 10 µl

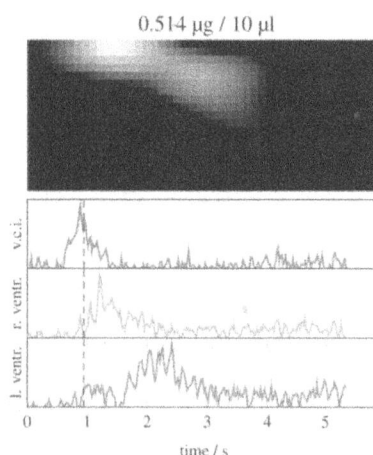

time / s

Figure 2: Reconstructed image at one time point (dashed marker) and intensity over time at the tail vein the right ventricle and the left ventricle. Image is part of Fig. 8 published in [2] with a CC BY licence.

the lowest iron concentration imaged with MPI to date (see Fig 2).

III.II *In Vivo* Experiments

The *in vivo* experiments were able to image in inflow of the bolus from the tail vein in the heard already at the lowest dose of only 510 ng iron content. This is the lowest iron dose, which was imaged by MPI until today.

IV. Discussion

The work showed how complex a unified definition of sensitivity can be and how important a common agreement is. From a hardware perspective, a sensitivity limit in absolute iron content is more suitable than a concentration. As this might differ from a medical point of view, we propose to include both parameters in the experiments. The protocol does not include the reconstruction parameters until now. Since reconstruction parameters, raw data preprocessing, and image processing have an impact on the sensitivity and the spatial resolution, we plan to formalize these parameters in a future sensitivity determination protocol.

V. Conclusions

The improvement of the MPI sensitivity is crucial on the way to clinical use. To be able to compare different receive techniques a unique protocol was presented. Although this protocol is currently not covering all parameters that influence the sensitivity, it introduces a standardized experimental scheme that can be further developed to a sensitivity measurement norm. The developed hardware was able to improve the sensitivity of the preclinical MPI system at the UKE by a factor of 32. With the improved sensitivity the lowest iron concentration and the lowest *in vivo* dose imaged by MPI until today was presented.

ACKNOWLEDGEMENTS

M.G., A.v.G., T.F. and T.M.B. thankfully acknowledge the financial support of the German Research Foundation (DFG) and the Federal Ministry of Education and Research (BMBF) (Grant Numbers BU 1436/10-1 and 13GW0069A). T.K., P.S. thankfully acknowledge the financial support by the German Research Foundation (DFG, grant numbers KN 1108/2-1 and AD 125/5-1). Work at UW was supported by NIH grant R42 EB013520-02A1. K.M.K. also acknowledges the Alexander von Humboldt Foundation for the 2016 Forschungspreis.

REFERENCES

[1] B. Gleich and J. Weizenecker. Tomographic imaging using the nonlinear response of magnetic particles. *Nature*, 435(7046):1217-1217, 2005. doi: 10.1038/nature03808.

[2] Graeser et al. "Towards pictogram detection of superparamagnetic nanoparticles using a gradiometric receive coil", Scientific Reports, 7:6872, 2017, doi: 10.1038/s41598-017-06992-5

[3] Rahmer, J. et al., Nanoparticle encapsulation in red blood cells enables blood-pool magnetic particle imaging hours after injection. *Physics.in Medicine and Biology* 58, 3965–3977, 2013. doi:10.1088/0031-9155/58/12/3965.

[4] Zheng, B. et al. Magnetic particle imaging tracks the long-term fate of in vivo neural cell implants with high image contrast. Sci. Rep.5: 14055,2015, doi:10.1038/srep14055.

[5] Jeff Gaudet et al., Micrometer Resolution, High Linearity, and Picogram Sensitivity in a Field-Free Line Magnetic Particle Imaging Scanner, EMIM, PS 02 /5, 2017

[6] Khandhar, A. P. et al. Evaluation of peg-coated iron oxide nanoparticles as blood pool tracers for preclinical magnetic particle imaging. *Nanoscale* 9, 1299–1306, 2017, doi:10.1039/C6NR08468K.

Session 05 - Talks

Instrumentation I

Improved Receive Hardware Unit for Magnetic Particle Imaging

Hendrik Paysen [a,*], James Wells [a], Olaf Kosch [a], Jochen Franke [b], Lutz Trahms [a], Tobias Schaeffter [a], Frank Wiekhorst [a]

[a] *Physikalisch-Technische Bundesanstalt, Abbestrasse 2-12, 10587 Berlin, Germany*
[b] *Bruker BioSpin MRI GmbH, Rudolf-Plank-Str. 23, 76276 Ettlingen, Germany*
[*] *Corresponding author, email: hendrik.paysen@ptb.de*

I. Introduction

Magnetic particle imaging (MPI) is capable of determining the spatial distribution of magnetic nanoparticles (MNP) in a biomedical environment [1]. An oscillating magnetic field is used to generate a time-dependent magnetization response of the MNP, which can be detected using inductive receive coils. The simultaneous presence of the rather strong excitation field during the measurement hampers the clear identification of the weak signal generated by the MNP. Notch-filters are used to strongly suppress the signal feed-through at the excitation frequency. Higher harmonic frequency components caused by the non-linear magnetic susceptibility of the MNP are measured and used for the MPI image reconstruction. However, non-linear hardware elements in the transmission- and receive-chain also generate background signals at multiples of the excitation frequency.

To further minimize the influence of the excitation fields for higher harmonic frequency components, one can use a combination of two coils in a gradiometric arrangement placed inside the excitation field coil [2]–[6]. By this, the excitation signals are cancelled in a broad bandwidth, while the particle signal remains. Here, we present initial measurement results acquired with a prototype gradiometric receive coil, designed and manufactured for the Berlin preclinical MPI scanner (Bruker BioSpin, Germany), depicting the improvement of the limits-of-detection compared to the conventional built-in MPI transmit-receive coil hardware setup.

II. Material and Methods

II.I. Gradiometric Receive Coil

The prototype receive coil consists of an inner pick-up coil (radius R=36 mm) and an outer cancelation coil (R=52 mm) with opposite winding direction (Fig. 1). The positioning of both coils is chosen to minimize the mutual induction with the excitation coil. The choice of different coil diameters for the pick-up and the cancelation coil lead to a homogenous sensitivity around the center (deviation

between maximum and minimum sensitivity in a 6x3x3 cm³ cuboid around the center of <16%).

The installed prototype was oriented with its axis parallel to the scanner bore (x-direction) of our preclinical MPI scanner and was connected to the same hardware elements as used for the conventional coil in the receive chain (also x-direction). This allows for simultaneous measurements and a fair comparison of both coil geometries.

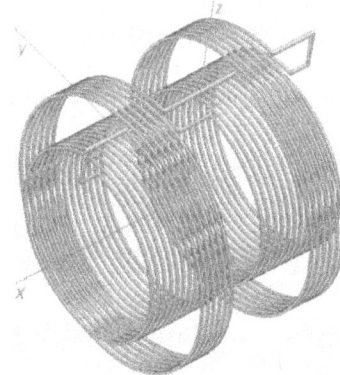

Figure 1: *Model of the prototype gradiometric receive coil designed to suppress the signal components generated by the excitation field.*

II.II. Serial Dilution Measurements

Samples containing 1 µL of Ferucarbotran (Meito Sangyo, Japan) at different iron concentrations ranging from 7.9 mmol/mL to 90 nmol/mL (diluted by water, resulting iron amounts of 440 ng-5 ng) were measured using drive field amplitudes of 12 mT and a gradient strength of 2.5 T/m in z-direction, and 1.25 T/m in x- and y-direction. 100 measurement repetitions were averaged resulting in a total acquisition time of 2 s. All samples were measured at three locations inside the field-of-view (FOV) to avoid misinterpretations due to image artefacts as it was proposed in [5]. Image reconstructions were performed using a measured system function (SF) acquired with the same receive concept as for the object measurement over a FOV of 25x25x13 mm³ with a 1 µL sample of Ferucarbotran at full concentration (0.935 mol/L). The Kaczmarz algorithm with Tikhonov regularization was used for the reconstruction process. The data acquired with the conventional and the prototype receive coil (both sensitive in x-direction) were used separately to calculate individual images. Truncation of the used frequency components were done based on the signal-to-noise ratio (SNR) derived from the SF. Measurements of an empty scanner were subtracted from the object measurement and the SF to remove background signal contributions. For all reconstructions, a single Kaczmarz iteration, a SNR-threshold of 200/300 (for the conventional/prototype coil) and a regularization of $1 \cdot \lambda_0$ [7] were chosen.

III. Results

The 1 µL sample was reconstructed successfully at all three positions for iron masses of 130 ng for the conventional and 20 ng for the prototype receive coil. Fig. 2 displays the reconstruction results of both coils at one location. Since the measured signals for this iron masses are extremely small, a high SNR-threshold and a high regularization are used for the reconstruction, which leads to image blurring. The samples containing larger amounts of iron can be reconstructed using a smaller SNR-threshold and less regularization. For comparison, we have chosen the same parameter set for all measurements with the respective coil. Although a higher SNR threshold was chosen for the prototype coil, more frequency components were used in the reconstruction process (38 for the conventional, 157 for the prototype coil) based on a higher sensitivity and therefore higher SNR-values of the prototype coil.

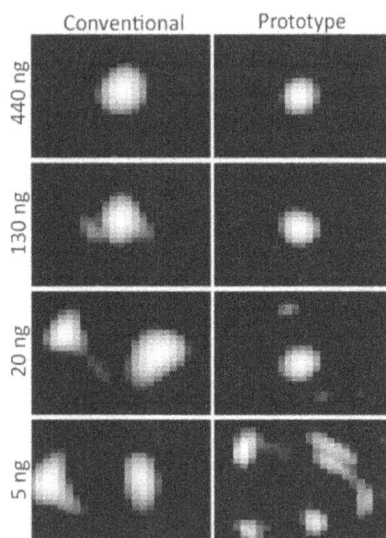

Figure 2: Maximum intensity projections of the reconstruction results using the conventional (left column) and the prototype receive coils (right column). The brightness was scaled to the individual maximum intensities of each image. The displayed masses represent the iron mass contained in the measured samples.

IV. Discussion and Conclusion

A new gradiometric receive coil was successfully implemented in our MPI system allowing for an about 7-fold lower detection limit compared to the built-in conventional transmit-receive coil, allowing for the detection of MNP samples containing iron down to 20 ng.

These improvements were made based on a smaller coil diameter and a gradiometric design, which lead to a higher sensitivity and a better suppression of background signals generated by the excitation field.

In a previous publication a detection limit of 5 ng was reached with a similar approach of a gradiometric receive coil. In this publication, the same coil diameters were chosen for the pick-up and the cancelation coil, which lead to zero-crossings of the sensitivity along the central x-axis. The presented approach of different coil diameters yields a homogenous sensitivity over a large imaging volume. This is crucial for future applications such as full body mice imaging, in which a large FOV is needed.

A more in-depth analysis of the characterization and the improvements gained by the prototype receive coil will be presented at the conference.

ACKNOWLEDGEMENTS

This project was supported by the DFG research grants "AMPI: Magnetic particle imaging: Development and evaluation of novel methodology for the assessment of the aorta in vivo in a small animal model of aortic aneurysms" SHA 1506/2-1, "quantMPI" 1 FKZ TR 408/9-1, and by the European Commission FP7 project "NanoMag", grant agreement no 604448.

References

[1]   B. Gleich and J. Weizenecker, "Tomographic imaging using the nonlinear response of magnetic particles," *Nature*, vol. 435, no. 7046, pp. 1214–1217, 2005. doi: 10.1038/nature03808

[2]   P. B. Roemer, W. A. Edelstein, C. E. Hayes, S. P. Souza, and O. M. Mueller, "The NMR phased array," *Magn. Reson. Med.*, vol. 16, no. 2, pp. 192–225, Nov. 1990. doi: 10.1002/mrm.1910160203

[3]   V. Schulz, M. Straub, M. Mahlke, S. Hubertus, T. Lammers, and F. Kiessling, "A Field Cancelation Signal Extraction Method For Magnetic Particle Imaging .," *IEEE Trans. Magn.*, vol. 51, no. 2 Pt 1, Feb. 2015. doi: 10.1109/TMAG.2014.2325852

[4]   M. Graeser, T. Knopp, M. Grüttner, T. F. Sattel, and T. M. Buzug, "Analog receive signal processing for magnetic particle imaging," *Med. Phys.*, vol. 40, no. 4, 2013. doi: 10.1118/1.4794482

[5]   M. Graeser *et al.*, "Towards Picogram Detection of Superparamagnetic Iron-Oxide Particles Using a Gradiometric Receive Coil," *Sci. Rep.*, vol. 7, no. 1, pp. 1–13, 2017. doi: 10.1038/s41598-017-06992-5

[6]   J. Wells *et al.*, "Characterizing a preclinical magnetic particle imaging system with separate pick-up coil," *IEEE Trans. Magn.*, pp. 1–1, 2017. doi: 10.1109/TMAG.2017.2708419

[7]   J. Weizenecker, J. Borgert, and B. Gleich, "A simulation study on the resolution and sensitivity of magnetic particle imaging.," *Phys. Med. Biol.*, vol. 52, no. 21, pp. 6363–6374, 2007. doi: 10.1088/0031-9155/52/21/001

Adaptive Hardware lens for Traveling Wave MPI

Martin A. Rückert [a,*], Patrick Vogel [a,b], Thomas Kampf [a,c], Stefan Herz [b], Thorsten A. Bley [b], Volker C. Behr [a]

[a] Department of Experimental Physics 5 (Biophysics), University of Würzburg, 97074 Würzburg, Germany
[b] Department of Diagnostic and Interventional Radiology, University Hospital Würzburg, 97080 Würzburg, Germany
[c] Department of Diagnostic and Interventional Neuroradiology, University Hospital Würzburg, 97080 Würzburg, Germany
* Corresponding author, email: Martin.Rueckert@physik.uni-wuerzburg.de

I. Introduction

Traveling Wave Magnetic Particle Imaging (TWMPI) uses a dynamic linear gradient array (dLGA) for the generation and movement of a strong magnetic field gradient represented by a field-free point (FFP) in one direction [1, 2]. The linear movement along the main axis as well as the specific hardware configuration offer a flexible and versatile system providing large FOVs. Additional saddle-coil pairs orientated perpendicularly to the dLGA give the possibility to move the FFP on arbitrary trajectories through the field of view (FOV) covering a sample in 2D [3, 4] or 3D [5]. In all cases the sequence controlling the dLGA is identical.

In this manuscript a novel approach is presented to manipulate the FFP trajectory modifying the control of the dLGA. In the result a zoom effect can be achieved, which increase the resolution by up to 30 % within a specific area.

II. Material and Methods

The dynamic linear gradient array (dLGA) consists of several electro magnets, which can be driven separately with the same sinusoidal current (frequency f_1) but with a phase difference $\Delta\varphi$ between adjacent elements generating a sinusoidal magnetic field traveling in one direction through the dLGA (Traveling Wave approach) [1]. In Fig. 1 (a) a simplified dLGA system is sketched, which can be driven with two channels [2]. The sequence to control a dLGA-4 is given as follows:

$$\text{Ch1: } A_1 \sin(2\pi f_1 + \varphi_1)$$
$$\text{Ch2: } A_2 \sin(2\pi f_1 + \varphi_2)$$

(1)

with the phases $\varphi_1 = 0°$ and $\varphi_2 = 90°$. Running one saddle-coil at a frequency $f_2 \gg f_1$ provides a trajectory scanning the center slice of the FOV (see Fig. 1 (a)). By adaption of the difference between φ_1 and φ_2 the dynamics of the magnetic field generated by the dLGA are changed. Using the saddle-coil as before the trajectory is strongly modified. Fig. 1 (b) shows the simulated trajectories in dependence of the phase difference [6]. The simulation of an imaging experiment (here several lines) shows in the result a zoom effect (adaptive lens).

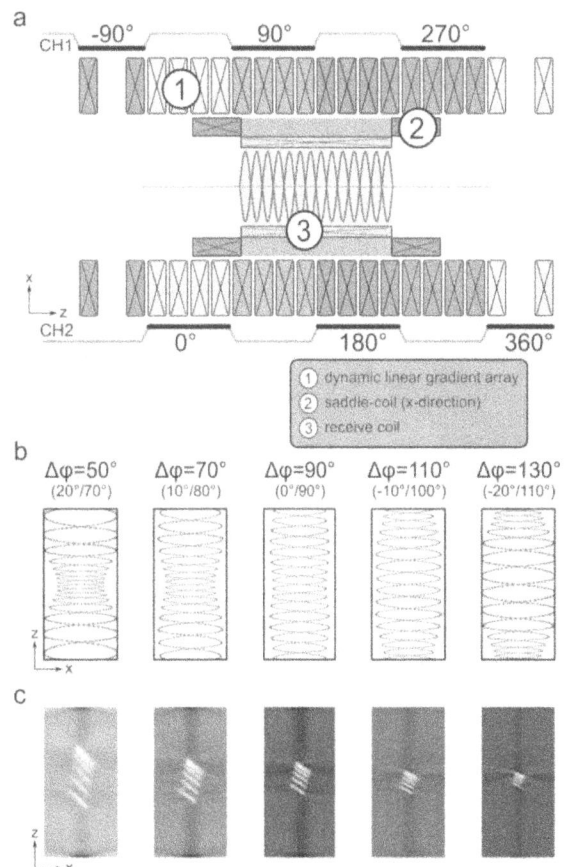

Figure 1: (a) Sketch of a TWMPI system consisting of a dLGA-4 system (1), a saddle-coil pair (2) and a receive coil (3). The dLGA can be driven with two amplifiers running the same frequency f_1 but with a phase shift of $\Delta\varphi=90°$. By driving the saddle-coil pair with the frequency f_2 the FFP travels along a sinusoidal trajectory through the FOV. (b) By changing the phase difference $\Delta\varphi$ between the dLGA channels, the trajectory is modified. (c) The result for imaging is a zoom-effect (adaptive lens).

III. Results

For initial testing of the zoom effect a common TWMPI scanner is used [1] applying the frequencies f_1=723.57 Hz for the dLGA and f_2=16823 Hz for the saddle-coil and a gradient strength of approx. G_z=2.55 T/m. For reconstructing the raw-data, an image-based system matrix approach is used (system matrix size: 2059×6480) [7].

In Fig. 2 (a) the change of the magnetic field gradient strength in the center of the TWMPI scanner is shown. By changing the phase difference e.g. from 90° to 70° an increase of about 17 % can be measured.

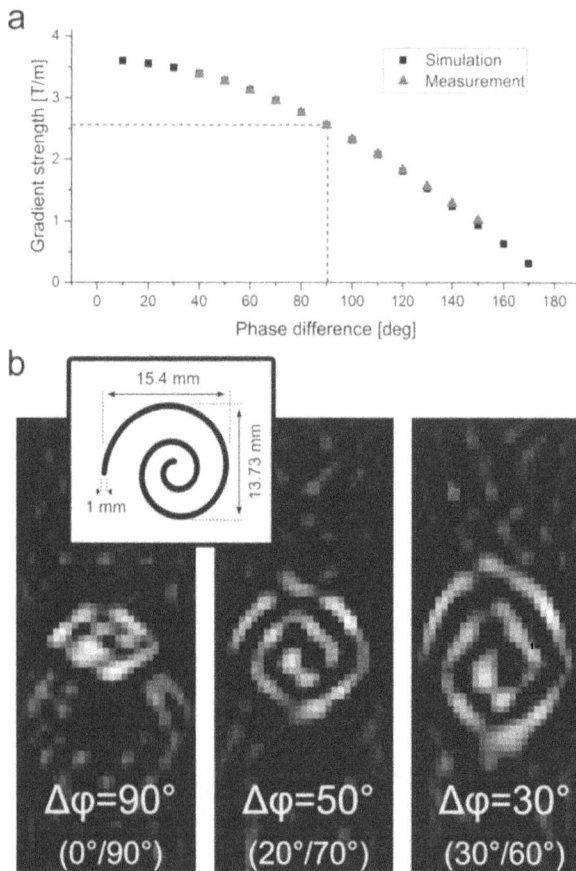

IV. Discussion

The zoom effect is the result of the change of the superimposed magnetic fields generated by each individual element of the dLGA resulting in a spatial change of the gradient strength over the length of the system [2]. This result in a higher resolution ether in the center of the FOV (see Fig. 1 $\Delta\phi$=50°) or at the edges (Fig. 1 $\Delta\phi$=130°).

For implementation of this new feature, no changes in hardware are required, which makes it easy accessible.

V. Conclusions

In this abstract, a novel feature for Traveling Wave MPI scanners have been demonstrated, the adaptive hardware lens (zoom effect). Modifying the phase of the main gradient system (dLGA) provides a change of the gradient strength and resolution. By applying this feature, it is possible to increase gradient strength from 2.55 T/m to about 3 T/m without changing any hardware components. As result, samples, which cannot be resolved in standard operation, can be visualized with a high accuracy.

Acknowledgements

We thank Tobias Knopp and Patryk Szwargulski for providing the 3D printed spiral sample.

References

[1] P. Vogel, et al., Traveling Wave Magnetic Particle Imaging, *IEEE TMI*, vol. 33(2), pp. 400-7, 2014. Doi:10.1109/TMI.2013.2285472.

[2] P. Vogel & P. Klauer, et al., Dynamic Linear Gradient Array for Traveling Wave Magnetic Particle Imaging, *IEEE Trans. Magn.*, (in press). Doi: 10.1109/TMAG.2017.2764440

[3] P. Vogel, et al., Real-time 3D Dynamic Rotating Slice-Scanning Mode for Traveling Wave MPI, *Int. Journal on MPI*, vol. 3(2):1706001, 2017. Doi:10.18416/ijmpi.2017.1706001

[4] S. Herz, et al., Selective Signal Suppression in Traveling Wave MPI: Focusing on Areas with low Concentration of Magnetic Particles, *Int. Journal on MPI*, vol. 3(2):1709001, 2017. Doi: 10.18416/ijmpi.2017.1709001

[5] P. Vogel, et al., Rotating slice-scanning mode for Traveling Wave MPI, *IEEE Trans. Magn.*, vol. 51(2):6501503, 2015. Doi: 10.1109/TMAG.2014.2335255

[6] P. Vogel, et al., 3D-GUI Simulation Environment for Magnetic Particle Imaging, Proc. on IWMPI (Lübeck), p.95, 2016.

[7] P. Vogel, et al., Flexible and Dynamic Patch Reconstruction for Traveling Wave MPI, *IJMPI*, vol. 2(2):1611001, 2017. Doi: 10.18416/ijmpi.2016.1611001

Figure 2: (a) Results of the determination of the gradient strength in the center of the dLGA. (b) Measurements of a spiral sample demonstrating the zoom effect: with a phase difference of 90° the sample cannot be resolved, where with decreased phase difference (adaptive lens) the structure can be reconstructed.

In Fig. 2 (b) the reconstructed images from an imaging experiment with a 3D printed spiral sample filled with PeriMag (MicroMod, Germany, 2.8 mg (Fe)/ml) is shown. The experiment using a standard sequence (0°/90°) with a gradient of about 2.55 T/m is not able to resolve the structure of the spiral sample. Applying the adaptive hardware lens (zoom feature), which increases the gradient to about 3.5 T/m, it is possible to reconstruct the structure.

The entire acquisition time was 2 s with 100 averages.

An Approach for Actively Cancelling Direct Feedthrough

Jonas Beuke[a,*], Thomas Friedrich[a], Matthias Gräser[bc], Thorsten M. Buzug[a], Philipp Rostalski[d]

[a] Institute of Medical Engineering, Universität zu Lübeck, Lübeck, Germany
[b] Institute for Biomedical Imaging, Technische Universität Hamburg, Hamburg, Germany
[c] Section of Biomedical Imaging, University Medical Center Hamburg Eppendorf, Hamburg, Germany
[d] Institute for Electrical Engineering in Medicine, Universität zu Lübeck, Lübeck, Germany
* Corresponding author, email: beuke@imt.uni-luebeck.de

I. Introduction

In magnetic particle imaging (MPI), an oscillating magnetic field is used to excite magnetic nanoparticles. The common way of measuring the magnetization of the nanoparticles is to use a receive coil in which the particles induce a signal [1]. This signal is superimposed by the excitation signal, which couples into the receive chain and is usually several orders of magnitude higher. Due to the limited dynamic range of available analogue-to-digital converters (ADC) it is a challenge to distinguish the particle signal from the system background [2].

One common solution to this problem are analogue highpass filters removing the strong signal at the fundamental frequency. Another approach are gradiometer setups cancelling the excitation signal with a second coil of an opposing polarity which only detects the excitation signal [2]. However, both solutions have intrinsic issues. Highpass filters do not only remove the excitation signal but also reduce the first harmonic of the particle signal. This presents a problem in the reconstruction [3]. Gradiometer coils on the other hand must be tuned very precisely to minimize the residual excitation. Both methods are subject to temperature dependencies in their components [2]. Here, we introduce an alternative solution to the problem by actively creating an inverse signal which can be used to cancel the interfering signal and extend the dynamic range of the particle signal. A related approach has been used by Zheng et al. for the cancellation of power amplifier harmonics on the sending side [4].

II. Material and Methods

II.I. Converters

ADCs and their counterparts, digital-to-analogue converters (DAC), are limited in their dynamic range. The dynamic range is closely linked to the sampling rate, which must be high enough to resolve the particle signal harmonics without aliasing. Since the excitation signal has a limited bandwidth, the creation of the active cancellation signal can be performed with a high signal-to-noise ratio

(SNR) by a DAC. This is necessary to avoid undesired noise to the system. If the SNR of the DAC is higher than necessary, the bandwidth of the DAC can be increased, allowing for the cancellation of more harmonics. Fig. 1 shows this idea for a specific combination of DAC and ADC. Since the output of the DAC is known, the canceled particle response can be recovered. With an empty measurement, the remaining excitation signal can be removed digitally and the overall dynamic range is improved.

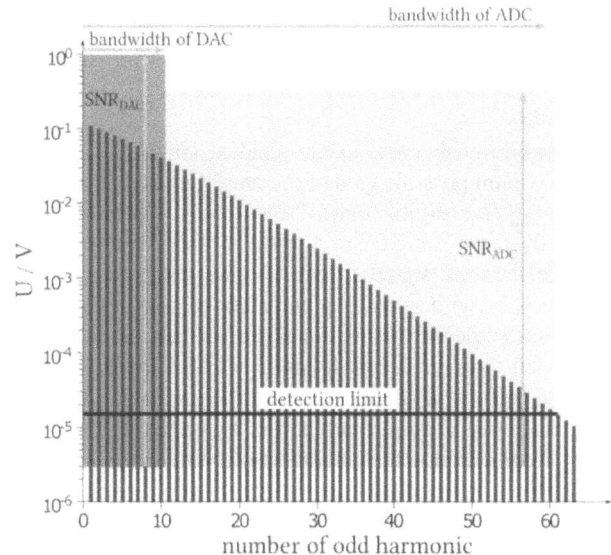

Figure 1: Exemplary combination of a 16-bit ADC with a sampling rate of 10 MHz and an 18-bit DAC with a sampling rate of 1 MHz. Due to the limited bandwidth of the DAC its SNR is better than the SNR of the ADC. This allows for the cancellation of higher harmonics resulting in a higher overall SNR.

II.II. Setup

The setup for a first prototype consists of a custom transformer, a commercial low noise amplifier (LNA; SR560, Stanford Research Systems, Inc., California) with an integrated lowpass filter with a cut-off frequency of

1 MHz and an embedded signal generation and acquisition board (Red Pitaya; RP). The transformer is used to match the maximum amplitude of the RP's DAC to the maximum amplitude of the measured signal via its turn ratio. The focus of this study was the cancellation of the strong lower harmonics allowing a higher amplification of the remaining harmonics. To assess the principle feasibility of the proposed compensation strategy without a full implementation in an MPI scanner, a simulated particle signal from a field free point MPI scanner (FFP) based on the Langevin theory was calculated (see [5,6]) and programmed in an arbitrary wave form generator.

II.III. Algorithm

The real-time cancellation of the measured signal requires feedback and therefore creates a control loop. The phase shifts of the electronics combined with the periodicity of the signal prevent the use of simple control algorithms. However, the periodicity of the signal can be taken into account for which different approaches are known from control theory. The selected algorithm for this study is Adaptive Feedforward Control (AFC) which allows for a memory efficient implementation in the Field Programmable Gate Array (FPGA) of the RP. It mainly consists of a gradient descent for the phase and amplitude of the different harmonics and a Fourier synthesis of the cancellation signal [7]. The implementation of the algorithm was made for cancelling 10 odd harmonics of the measured signal with the first harmonic being at 25 kHz. The whole algorithm could be implemented within the limited resources of the RP's FPGA Xilinx Zynq 7010.

III. Results

The peak-to-peak value of the residual signal determines the maximum possible gain of the amplifier that allows for a clipping-free digitization of the signal. Therefore, we define the dampening factor Δ as the ratio of the undamped and the damped signal's peak-to-peak value. For a fair comparison with the implementation, the maximum possible dampening factor for a perfect cancellation was calculated for the 10 first harmonics and a lowpass filter with a cut-off at 1 MHz. This maximum is $\Delta = 4.6$. Simulations of the algorithm reveal a dampening factor of $\Delta = 4.0$ compared to the measurements with $\Delta = 2.7 \pm 0.3$. Simulations show, that a steady state can be reached within two periods of the measured signal.

IV. Discussion

The dampening factor of the implemented algorithm shows, that the real-time generation of a sufficiently accurate cancellation signal is feasible with limited computational resources. The simulation of the algorithm almost reaches the same dampening factor as the ideal one where the first 10 harmonics are set to zero. Due to limiting factors like noise and inaccuracies in the system function measurements the realized setup does not completely reach the simulated dampening factor. Further simulations show, that including an internal model with more harmonics increases the dampening factor and reduces resulting stable periodic oscillations in steady state which occur due to the gradient descent not being able to completely cancel the residual signal with a limited number of harmonics. Because of the limited resources of the board, it was not possible to add a refined internal model to the implementation. Since the steady state is reached quickly, the algorithm is suitable for the purpose of dampening even the possibly changing particle signal to a certain extend if the SNR allows for this. Combining this method with the gradiometer approach would allow for a more flexible receive chain since no filters tuned for a specific frequency would be needed.

V. Conclusions

The study shows, that an active cancellation can be realized not only for the excitation frequency but also for the harmonics of the resulting particle signal. Depending on the dynamic range of both ADC and DAC a combination of the presented method with a cancellation unit as in [2] is favorable. This would not only allow for the suppression of the excitation signal but even going beyond. Partly cancelling the comparably slowly changing particle signal allows for a higher amplification and leads to a higher spatial resolution. The next step will be the integration into an MPI scanner or into a spectrometer. For this purpose, the algorithm has to be extended to cancel not only a single period but also a complete trajectory. Multidimensional excitation utilizes two or three different frequencies, which leads to a dense spectrum of mixing frequencies and thus significantly increases the computational effort. Today's advances in FPGA technology allow for exactly this.

ACKNOWLEDGEMENTS

This research was partially supported by the Federal Ministry of Education and Research, Germany (BMBF) in the project SAMBA-PATI (13GW0069A).

REFERENCES

[1] B. Gleich and J. Weizenecker. *Tomographic imaging using the nonlinear response of magnetic particles.* Nature, 435(7046):1217-1217, 2005. doi: 10.1038/nature03808.
[2] M. Gräser, T. Knopp, M. Grüttner, T. F. Sattel and T. M. Buzug. *Analog receive signal processing for magnetic particle imaging.* Medical Physics 40.4 (2013), S. 042303. doi: 10.1118/1.4794482.
[3] P. W. Goodwill and S. M. Conolly. *Multidimensional X-Space Magnetic Particle Imaging.* IEEE Transactions on Medical Imaging 30.9 (Sep. 2011), S. 1581–1590. doi: 10.1109/tmi.2011.2125982.
[4] B. Zheng, W. Yang, T. Massey, P. W. Goodwill and S. M. Conolly. *High-power active interference suppression in magnetic particle imaging.* 2013 International Workshop on Magnetic Particle Imaging (IWMPI). Institute of Electrical and Electronics Engineers (IEEE), March 2013. doi: 10.1109/iwmpi.2013.6528381.
[5] S. Blundell. *Magnetism in Condesed Matter.* Oxford University Press, U.S.A., 2001
[6] H. Landolt and R. Börnstein, editors. *Numerical Data and Functional Relationships in Science and Technology,* B. III/4b Magnetic Oxides and Related Compounds. Springer, Berlin/Heidelberg, 1977.
[7] C.-H. Chung and M.-S. Chen. *A robust adaptive feedforward control in repetitive control design for linear systems.* Automatica 48.1 (2012), S. 183–190. doi: 10.1016/j.automatica.2011.09.034.

MPI Meets CT: First Hybrid Scanner Design

Jonathan Markert [a,b,*], Patrick Vogel [b,c], Martin A. Rückert [b], Fabian Piekarek [b], Benedikt Kessler [a], Thorsten A. Bley [c], Simon Zabler [d], Thorsten M. Buzug [e], Volker C. Behr [b], Walter H. Kullmann [a]

[a] Institute of Medical Engineering, University of Applied Sciences Würzburg-Schweinfurt, 97421 Schweinfurt, Germany
[b] Department of Experimental Physics 5 (Biophysics), University of Würzburg, 97074 Würzburg, Germany
[c] Department of Diagnostic and Interventional Radiology, University Hospital Würzburg, 97080 Würzburg, Germany
[d] Department of Experimental Physics (X-Ray Microscopy), University of Würzburg, 97074 Würzburg, Germany
[e] Institute of Medical Engineering, University of Lübeck, 23562 Lübeck, Germany
* Corresponding author, email: Jonathan.Markert@physik.uni-wuerzburg.de

I. Introduction

Magnetic Particle Imaging (MPI) is a tomographic technique that directly detects the distribution of superparamagnetic iron-oxide nanoparticles (SPIONs) in a volume without acquiring signal from the surrounding tissue [1]. For a more precise diagnostic statement, MPI has to be combined with another tomographic technique to fill this gap of information. Previous projects showed that a combination of MPI with Magnetic Resonance Imaging (MRI) is possible [2]. Both are non-invasive techniques with a minimum of burden for the patient with MRI requiring higher hardware efforts and longer measuring times. The next step is the combination of MPI and Computed Tomography (CT), both being fast tomographic techniques.

CT is a method which uses projections of the measuring object in the FOV. To acquire a complete CT image, a rotation of the system of at least 180 degrees is required. For an MPI-CT hybrid system, the hardware requirements of the MPI side are moderate. Using a field free line (FFL) concept [3], MPI offers the acquisition of projections as well. Since the CT hardware (gantry) will be rotated mechanically, for the FFL generation a static concept can use the same mechanism. Previous research also showed that an FFL-MPI-scanner can provide the same resolution by using a tenth of the ferro-fluid compared to an FFP-scanner [3]. A preliminary concept of a hybrid MPI-CT system is presented in this abstract.

II. Material and Methods

To create the FFL, two Halbach ring arrays are used. A Halbach array is a special arrangement of permanent magnets that focusses the magnetic flux on one side, while vanishing it on the other side [5]. A special form of Halbach arrays is the Halbach ring, where the individual magnets

are arranged in ring shape and oriented at a constant angle φ with respect to each other (see Fig. 1).

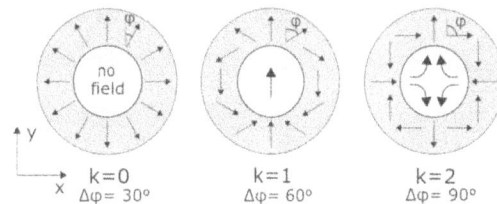

Figure 1: Halbach rings with different orientation φ of the permanent magnets and the resulting magnetic field in the center of the Halbach rings.

The angle $\varphi=(k+1)*360°/N$ determines the number of magnetization directions k inside the Halbach ring depending on the amount of magnets N [4]. For the FFL-scanner two Halbach rings with $k=1$ configuration are used.

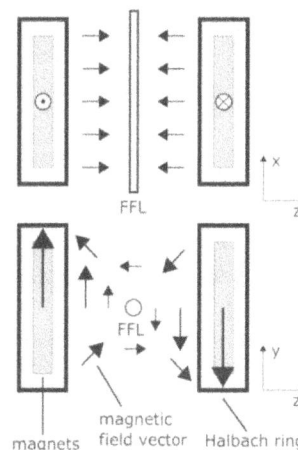

Figure 2: Generation of the FFL in the x-z and y-z plane by using Halbch rings with k=1 configuration.

They are placed facing each other with opposing magnetization vectors thereby creating an FFL in the center *(see Fig. 2)*. An external driving coil (solenoid in *z*-direction) generates a magnetic field of $\pm$ 100 mT with which the FFL can be shifted in the *x-y* plane through the FOV. Figure 3 shows a first concept of a combined system between MPI and CT. Both systems are assembled on a common gantry and can be rotated mechanically around the sample volume (*z*-axis).

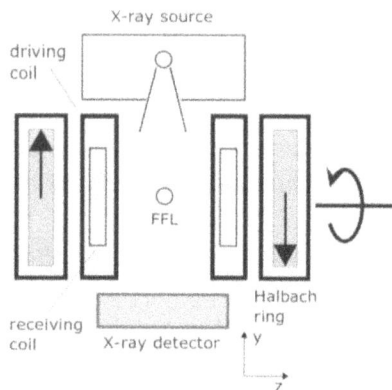

Figure 3: Sketch of the hybrid MPI-CT system consisting of two Halbach rings, driving coil and receiving coil, X-ray source and detector. The system is assembled on a gantry and can be rotated mechanically around the z-axis.

III. Results

To create the Halbach ring, 12 cubic neodymium magnets (NIB-N-52) with a side length of 10 mm are used. They are arranged in a $k=1$ configuration and generate a homogeneous magnetic field of about 90 mT in the center of the ring (Fig. 4). The distance between the two rings is set to 4 cm generating a magnetic field gradient of about 4.5 T/m.

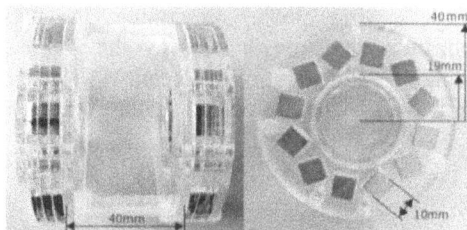

Figure 4: Assembled Halbach rings with k=1 configuration and dimensions

In a first experiment with the FFL-system a sample carrier with two samples of ferro-fluid (Resovist®, Bayer, Germany) (Fig. 5) was placed in the center between the Halbach rings. Six projections were acquired with a sample carrier rotation of 30° per measurement. The acquired data were processed (correction of receive-chain distortion) and digitally filtered.

IV. Discussion

Figure 5 shows the reconstruction of the six acquired projections. The two samples are clearly visible in which the oblong smearing is a result of the low amount of projections. The distance between the samples is 17 mm and the scanner achieves a round FOV with a diameter of 32 mm.

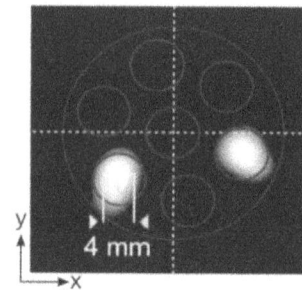

Figure 5: Reconstruction of six acquired projections with the FFL-system. A sample carrier (grey) with two ferro-fluid samples was placed in the center between the Halbach rings. Six projections were acquired with a rotation of the sample carrier of 30°.

By using permanent magnets instead of electromagnets the system consumes less power and the cabling effort is reduced, especially regarding to the system rotation.

V. Conclusions and Outlook

A novel concept of a hybrid design between MPI and CT is presented, which combines information about the SPION distribution and the surrounding tissue. This concept allows more precise diagnostic statement than MPI on its own. In a next generation, the Halbach arrangement is realized on three concentric rings around the measuring field (see Fig. 6). In this way, it is possible to generate a field gradient of 5 T/m in a measuring field with a diameter of 80 mm (FOV approx. 50 mm).

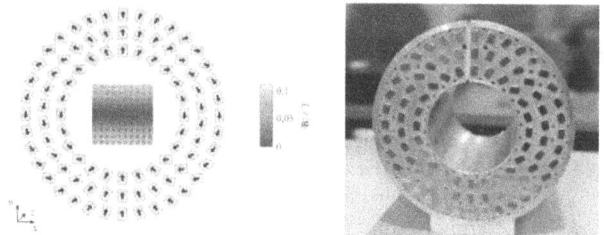

Figure 6: Halbach arrangement with an inner diameter of 80 mm and an outer diameter of 180 mm [6,7].

References

[1] B. Gleich and J. Weizenecker. Tomographic imaging using the nonlinear response of magnetic particles. *Nature*, 435(7046):1217-1217, 2005. doi: 10.1038/nature03808.

[2] P.Vogel, S. Lother, M. A. Rückert, W. H. Kullmann, P. M. Jakob, F. Fidler and V. C. Behr. MRI Meets MPI: A Bimodal MPI-MRI Tomograph, *IEEE TMI*, Vol. 33: 1954-1959, 2014

[3] J. Weizenecker, B. Gleich and J. Borgert, Magnetic particle imaging using a field free line, *J. Phys. D: Appl Phys.*, 41 (105009) : 3pp, 2008. doi:10.1088/0022-3727/41/10/105009

[4] H. Raich and P. Blümler, Design and construction of a dipolar Halbach array with a homogeneous field from identical bar magnets: *NMR Mandhalas. Concepts in Magnetic Resonance Part B:Magnetic Resonance Engineering*, 23B(1): 16–25, 2004. doi: 10.1002/cmr.b.20018.

[5] K. Halbach, "Design of permanent multipole magnets with oriented rare earth cobalt material", *Nucl. Instr. Meth. Phys. Res*, 169: 1-10, 1980. doi:10.1016/0029-554X(80)90094-4

[6] M. Weber, T. M. Buzug, *Magnetic Field-Generating Device for Magnetic Particle Imaging*, 2017, PCT, WO 2017/050789 A1

[7] M. Weber, Magnetic Particle Imaging, Neuartige Bildgebungskonzepte mit einer feldfreien Linie, *Research Series of the Institute of Medical Engineering, Volume 6*, Infinite Science Publishing, Lübeck, 2017, ISBN 978-3-945954-42-3.

A Receive Coil Topology Based on Oppositely Tilted Solenoids for a Predefined Drive Field

Jan Stelzner [a,*], Matthias Weber [a], Thorsten M. Buzug [a]

[a] Institute of Medical Engineering, Universität zu Lübeck, Lübeck, Germany
[*] Corresponding author, email: stelzner@imt.uni-luebeck.de

I. Introduction

The proper design of drive-field generating coil topologies and receive coils in Magnetic Particle Imaging (MPI) is a decisive element within the construction of the signal chain. Most commonly, the desired properties of such coils or coil assemblies are high efficiency, low power loss and high homogeneity [1]. In this work, a receive coil topology that is based on tilted solenoids is proposed. Caspi et al. presented a similar concept which is based on magnetic dipoles and features an exceptionally high field quality perpendicular to the bore axis [2]. The proposed application of the tilted solenoids from the original work lies in the area of magnetic accelerators and employed high temperature superconductors.

In this work, an analogous approach is investigated which utilizes tilted solenoids for an MPI system that applies a field-free line (FFL) for spatial encoding [3]. Furthermore, an augmented setup is simulated that is expanded by means of further coils. This gradiometric approach [4] is tailored for a magnetic field of a particular existing MPI setup [5].

II. Material and Methods

II.I. Functional Principle of the Topology Based on Tilted Solenoids

Most two-dimensional MPI systems, independent of field-free point or FFL technology, feature a cylindrical bore and require a drive field or a receive-coil sensitivity that is perpendicular to the bore axis Likewise, the magnetic field or sensitivity profile within the measurement scope should be as homogeneous as possible considering the direction of the magnetic flux density and its magnitude as well [6].

While a regular cylindrical coil generates a magnetic field pointing mainly in the axial direction, the field direction can by skewed by tilting the solenoid. By superimposing the emerged field by a similar one which is mirrored at the center plain perpendicular to the bore axis, a magnetic field that is orthogonal to the bore of the coil can be obtained (see Fig. 1).

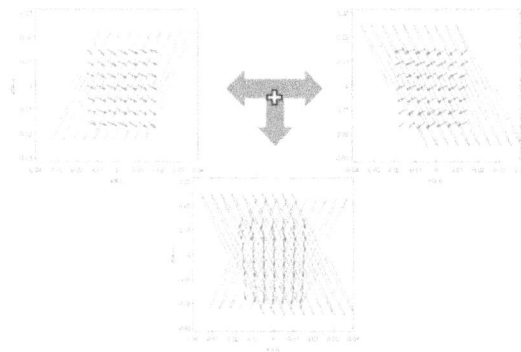

Figure 1: Basic principle of the tilted-solenoid topology.

The magnetic flux density can be approximated by the following equation

$$B_{\text{Dipole}} = 2B_{\text{Solenoid}} \sin \alpha \qquad (1)$$

with α being the tilt angle and B_{Dipole} and B_{Solenoid} representing the magnitude of the magnetic flux densities of the partial and the whole structure, respectively. Regarding the coordinate system in Fig. 1, B_{Dipole} is aligned with the z-axis.

II.II. Construction and Measurement of a Simplified Test Object

To validate simulated values and examine the construction process of such structures, a simplified prototype was designed and measured. Table 1 lists its geometric parameters.

Table 1: Geometric parameters of the prototype

Inner diameter (bore) d_{inner}	50 mm
Number of Windings n_1, n_2	10 per solenoid
Winding thread	5 mm
Tilt angle α	30°

A winding support has been constructed by a 3D printer (Ultimaker 2) for each of the solenoids, subsequently wound with enameled copper wire of 0.4 mm thickness, assembled and finally sealed with epoxy resin (see Fig. 2).

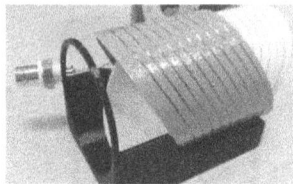

Figure 2: Simplified test object

The magnetic field, respectively the coil sensitivity profile, was measured utilizing a DC-source (1 A). Therefore, a multi-axis hall probe recorded the magnetic field data at various points being precisely moved by a 3-axis Cartesian robot.

II.III. Simulation of an Enhanced Setup for a Predefined Drive Field

Using the magnetic field produced by a drive-field component of an existing MPI-FFL field generator [5], an enhanced topology is designed and simulated. The dimensioning of the topology was optimized for the purpose of cancelling out the sum of all partial voltages that are induced by the drive field into the tilted solenoids. In turn, this facilitates a solely sensitivity of the designed topology regarding spatial field distortions inside the measurement scope e.g. by a particle sample when the tilted-solenoid topology is used as a receiver.

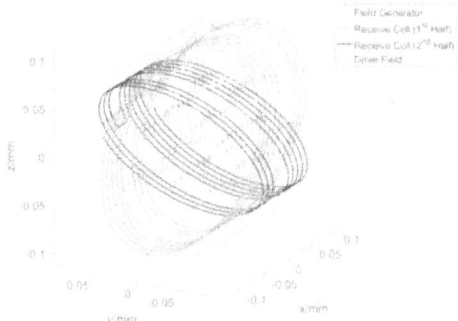

Figure 3: Enhanced simulation model

Fig. 3 shows a design, where the induced voltage is computed via Faraday's law of induction

$$U_{\text{ind}} = 2\pi f \sum_A |B(r) \times dA| \qquad (2)$$

with $B(r)$ describing the magnetic field generated by the drive-field coil and computed by (3). A is the effective area spanned by the wire of the tilted solenoids. For the drive-field computation, ds represents elements of the discretized wire path and r' the location of each wire part.

$$B(r) = \frac{\mu_0}{4\pi} I \sum_V ds \times \frac{r-r'}{|r-r'|^3} \qquad (3)$$

III. Results

III.I. Magnetic Field of the Prototype

The measurement results of the magnetic field of the simplified test object is depicted in Fig. 4. As expected, the magnetic field points mainly in vertical direction ($B_{\text{vertical}}/|B|_{\text{mean}} > 99\%$) and is highly homogeneous ($\sigma_B/|B|_{\text{mean}} < 3\%$). The maximum deviation of B_{vertical} within the measurement field amounts to 15 μT, which is

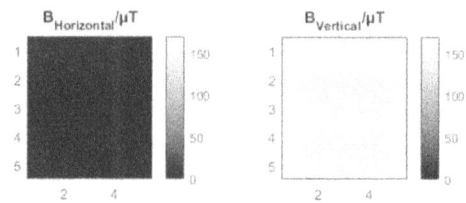

Figure 4: Magnetic field in the center plane perpendicular to the bore axis of the magnetic dipole fed with 1 A_{DC}. The distance between two measurement points is 5 mm.

less than 10% of its mean value. As a comparison, the drive-field coil would provide 17% if it was down-scaled to the size of the investigated prototype.

III.II. Results for the Enhanced Setup

After various geometrical parameters have been tested within the simulation environment, Table 2 lists a combination of parameters that leads to an induced voltage of the existing drive-field coil of effectively zero.

Table 2: Geometric parameters of the simulated enhanced coil

Inner diameter (bore) / outer diameter	17 cm / 17.2 cm
Number of windings	50 per solenoid
Additional windings in opposite direction	40 per solenoid
Thread	1 mm
Tilt angle α	40°

IV. Conclusion and Outlook

The feasibility of manufacturing a magnetic dipole based on tilted solenoids and its homogeneous magnetic sensitivity profile has been shown. A reasonable design for a receive-coil topology for an existing MPI-FFL scanner setup has been successfully simulated that is capable of cancelling out empty measurements.

A further enhancement will enable the acquisition of two-dimensional signals. Accordingly, subsequent simulations and tests are already planned.

REFERENCES

[1] M. Weber, K. Bente, M. Graeser, T. F. Sattel, T. M. Buzug, Implementation of a High-Precision 2-D Receiving Coil Set for Magnetic Particle Imaging. *IEEE Transactions on Magnetics*, 51(2): 6502404, 2015, doi: 10.1109/TMAG.2014.2331987

[2] S. Caspi, D. R. Dietderich, P. Ferracin, N. R. Finney, M. J. Fuery, S. A. Gourlay, and A. R. Hafalia. Design, Fabrication, and Test of a superconducting Dipole Magnet Based on Tilted Solenoids. *IEEE Transactions on Applied Superconductivity*, 17(2):2266-2269, 2007. doi: 10.1109/TASC.2007.899243.

[3] J. Weizenecker, B. Gleich, J. Borgert. Magnetic Particle Imaging Using a Field Free Line. *Journal of Physics D: Applied Physics*, 41(10):105009, 2008. doi: 10.1088/0022-3727/41/10/105009

[4] V. Schulz, M. Straub, et al. A Field Cancelation Signal Extraction Method for Magnetic Particle Imaging, *IEEE Transactions on Magnetics*, 51(2 Pt 1):6501804. doi: 10.1109/TMAG.2014.2325852

[5] J. Stelzner, T. M. Buzug. Magnetic-Field Measurement and Simulation of a Field-Free Line Magnetic-Particle Scanner, *Current Directions in Biomedical Engineering*, 3(2):837-840, 2017, doi: https://doi.org/10.1515/cdbme-2017-0191.

[6] P. W. Goodwill, S. M. Conolly. The X-space formulation of the magnetic particle imaging process: 1-D signal, resolution, bandwidth, SNR, SAR, and magnetostimulation. *IEEE Trans Med Imaging*, 29(11):1851-1859, 2010, doi: 10.1109/TMI.2010.2052284

MPI Scanner with Rotating Permanent Magnets

Ismail Harbi[a], Waldemar Schneider[a], Dieter Gann[a], Jochen Franke[b], Ulrich Heinen[a],[*]

[a] Fakultät für Technik, Hochschule Pforzheim, Tiefenbronner Straße 65, 75175 Pforzheim
[b] Bruker BioSpin MRI GmbH, Rudolf-Plank-Str. 23, 76275 Ettlingen
[*] Corresponding author, email: ulrich.heinen@hs-pforzheim.de

I. Introduction

Magnetic Particle Imaging (MPI) is a novel imaging technique that utilizes the magnetization signal of tracer materials containing superparamagnetic nanoparticles (MNPs).

Since the inception of MPI [1], a number of different scanner designs have been realized [2]. Most scanner designs feature three major components. First, a Selection Field (SF) is required that is provided either by permanent magnets or by a set of coils and determines the spatial resolution. The SF is a gradient field with a zero crossing that can take the shape of a point (field free point, FFP) or a line (field free line, FFL) which in this contribution will be dubbed Field Free Region (FFR). Secondly, a Drive Field (DF) excites the MNPs and provides the spatial encoding by moving the FFR over the region of interest. Finally, a set of detection coils records the magnetization signal of the MNPs. The detected signal is dominated by the DF excitation signal and must therefore be filtered to recover the particle signal. Thus, most scanners employ strictly monochromatic excitation signals. Without further shift coils, the achievable field-of-view (FOV) volume is limited by

$$V_{FOV} = \prod_{i=x,y,z} \frac{2B_{DF,i}}{G_{SF,i}}$$

where $B_{DF,i}$ and $G_{SF,i}$ are the amplitude of the Drive Field and the field gradient provided by the Selection Field along direction i. Thus, for a large FOV either a small Selection Field is required, sacrificing spatial resolution, or a higher Drive Field amplitude must provide a larger FFR shift. The DF's power consumption rises with the square of the amplitude; and simultaneously the effort to ensure monochromatic excitation increases with DF power. Likewise, for SFs realized by coils, there is a substantial increase in power when a higher spatial resolution is required. Shift coils have been employed to realize larger FOVs at the expense of temporal resolution.

High DF amplitudes mandate the use of resonant circuits. Together with the required signal filtering this implies that current scanners are restricted to fixed excitation frequencies.

Some of these restrictions of conventional scanners have been solved in the TWMPI scanner design [3, 4] where the FFP generation and movement is realized by a linear arrangement of coils, which however are still driven by sinusoidal currents. The same authors have also demonstrated the use of permanent magnets for generations of ultra-high gradient fields [5].

In this contribution, these ideas are combined into a feasible scanner design that is no longer restricted to fixed excitation frequencies.

II. Signal excitation by moving magnets

The high-power DF setup could be avoided if it were possible to oscillate the Selection Field generator mechanically with a sufficiently high frequency to generate a tracer signal. However, a large distance SF magnet oscillation is not feasible due to the involved high moments of inertia. As an alternative, multiple adjacent pairs of permanent magnets with different lateral offsets and alternating polarity can be pulled past the FOV at high speed to generate an FFR movement. Such a movement is most easily achieved by mounting the magnet pairs on the perimeter of a cylindrical wheel. Each magnet pair generates an FFP, which is moved through the FOV to perform a line scan. Due to their lateral offsets, each magnet pair generates a distinct line scan. One rotation of the wheel completes scan of an entire image plane. If the FOV is small compared to the wheel diameter, an almost flat image plane results. Owing to the rotating magnets, the term RotoMPI is proposed for the novel setup [6].

The resulting field layout closely resembles the TWMPI except that the moving encoding field is generated by pairs of permanent magnets rather than a dynamic linear gradient array.

A critical factor of all MPI scanners is the elimination of the background signal generated in the detection coils by the Drive Field. Typically, gradiometer setups are used in combination with frequency-domain filtering. As the RotoMPI does not provide strict sinusoidal excitation signals, this approach is not applicable here. Instead, the magnet pairs in opposite positions of the rotating wheel are mounted with identical lateral offsets but opposite shift directions, so that an overall inversion symmetry of the wheel results. With two identical sets of detection coils at

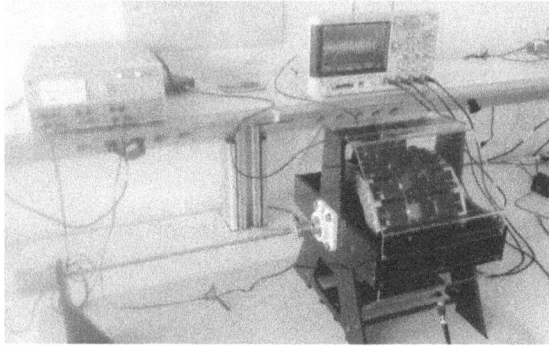

Figure 1: Setup of the RotoMPI prototype. The rotating wheel carries 16 magnet pairs. Two sets of detection coils are mounted on the front and rear side bar. Trigger circuits for measuring the speed of rotation and for providing a unique reference position are mounted at the rear end of the principal axis.

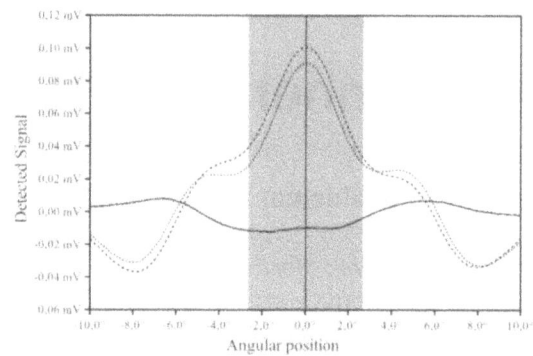

Figure 2: Detection signals. Dashed line: Signal induced by encoding magnets in detection coil pair at measuring volume. Dotted line: Signal induced by opposite pair of encoding magnets in compensation coil pair. Solid line: residual signal after (digital) subtraction. The gray area marks the FFP passage between the detection coil pair. FFP speed was 4.5 m/s. Magnet gap and positions were not yet optimized during this measurement.

opposite sides around the rotating drum, identical magnet signals are obtained on both sides and an excellent first order signal cancellation can be achieved.

II. Material and Methods

II.I. Scanner prototype

A prototype of the proposed scanner design was realized in the workshop of Pforzheim University. The current setup provides a nearly planar detection area of 8×8mm which is scanned by 16 magnet pairs with a scan line spacing of 0.5 mm. Volume imaging is possible by moving the object forward through the imaging plane. Each magnet pair consists of two NbFeB permanent magnets sized $20 \times 20x \times 5$mm (Q-20-20-5N, Webcraft GmbH, Germany) mounted with a 20mm pole gap on a rotating cylinder with the magnet center located at r=153mm from the axis. The magnet pairs provide a maximum field gradient of 18 T/m at the FFP perpendicular to the direction of motion. With an alternative magnet type ($20 \times 20 \times 10$mm) an even higher field gradient of 32 T/m has been observed. The cylinder is driven by a small motor (Hosiden R4801) with up to 7 rps, resulting in a field change of ~60 T/s. Besides the motor and a small home-built trigger circuit, no further electrical power is required for field and signal generation. Initial signal detection has been realized by a conventional oscilloscope (Keysight InfiniiVision MSOX3054). The scanner is operated by a custom-written software package. The entire setup is shown in figure 1.

II.II. Scanner adjustment

The positions of the detection coils and the lateral position of each magnet pair were adjusted to optimize magnet signal cancellation during FFP passage through the FOV. For calibration, the signals of both coil pairs are recorded individually, and both coil positions and magnet positions are modified, until optimum signal cancellation is obtained. Usually, a reduction of up to a factor of 10 is readily achievable, further reduction are possible but will require finer adjustment mechanisms. An example signal is shown in figure 2.

III. Results

Although no image has been recorded yet, a signal change upon sample insertion was already noticeable without further signal amplification or background correction even at this small encoding speed. This suggests that the RotoMPI concept is principally sound.

IV. Discussion

The proposed scanner setup realizes strong selection field gradients in a very inexpensive setup. Although the design is not scalable to a human scanner, a FOV enlargement sufficient for mouse imaging appears feasible, while the current prototype could be considered an MPI microscope. As the speed of rotation can be chosen freely, the novel setup will permit imaging studies with a wide range of encoding speeds, allowing exploration of the tracer material's relaxation kinetics in a convenient way. It is estimated that the ultimate encoding speed can approach that of conventional scanners.

V. Outlook

Planned further work on the present prototype aims at increasing the speed of rotation, improving the calibration procedure for finer adjustment of the signal compensation, implementation of a full residual background compensation, and an optimization of the magnet pair placement. These steps will allow further assessment of the concept's feasibility. With the experience in prototype optimization, the key design parameters of a RotoMPI scanner suitable for mouse imaging can be determined.

REFERENCES
[1]   B. Gleich, J. Weizenecker, *Nature* **2005**, *435*, 1214.
[2]   N. Panagiotopoulos, R. L. Duschka, M. Ahlborg, G. Bringout, C. Debbeler, M. Graeser, C. Kaethner, K. Lüdtke-Buzug, H. Medimagh, J. Stelzner et al., *International journal of nanomedicine* **2015**, *10*, 3097.
[3]   P. Vogel, M. A. Ruckert, P. Klauer, W. H. Kullmann, P. M. Jakob, V. C. Behr, *IEEE transactions on medical imaging* **2014**, *33*, 400.
[4]   P. Vogel, M. A. Ruckert, P. M. Jakob, V. C. Behr, *IEEE Trans. Magn.* **2015**, *51*, 1.
[5]   U. Heinen, J. Franke, EP 3048452 A1, **2015**.

Session 06 - Posters

Applications I

Effect of Agarose gel pore size on SPIO MPI Signal Strength

Matthias Stoeckmann[a]*, Jan Sedlacik[b], Svenja Zapf[c], Florian Thieben[d], Jens Fiehler[e]

[a]*University Medical Center Hamburg-Eppendorf*
[b]*Center for Radiology and Endoscopy, Department of Neuroradiological diagnostics and intervention, University Medical Center Hamburg-Eppendorf*
[c]*Head and Neurocenter, Department of Neurosurgery, University Medical Center Hamburg-Eppendorf*
[d]*Department of experimental Biomedical Imaging, University Medical Center Hamburg-Eppendorf and Technical University of Hamburg-Harburg*
[e]*Center for Radiology and Endoscopy, Department of Neuroradiological diagnostics and intervention, University Medical Center Hamburg-Eppendorf*
**Corresponding author, email:* Matthias.stoeckmann@stud.uke.uni-hamburg.de

I. Introduction

Rotational freedom of Superparamagnetic Iron Oxide Nanoparticles (SPIOs) dissolved in agarose is influenced by the agarose concentration. Relaxation time and MPI as well as MPS signal strength are measures of the SPIOs' rotational freedom [1]. Agarose concentration has an effect on pore size. One can notice a steep decrease in pore size between 0,5% and 1% agarose concentration [2]. When dissolved in agarose, SPIOs are thought to be located inside the pore mesh. The hypothesis investigated by the authors was that the aforementioned abrupt decrease in gel pore size leads to an equally strong reduction in MPI and MPS signal strength generated by the SPIOs.

II. Material and Methods

A serial dilution of SPIOs mixed with distilled water was established. This suspension was then used to produce agarose gels showing different amounts of SPIO (1:10, 1:50 and 1:100 of Perimag plain SPIO solutions, respectably) and different agarose concentrations, namely 0.5%, 0.75%, 1%, and 1.5%. Two other series of samples served as zero tests. One only contained agarose and distilled water without SPIOs, verifying the reliability of the MPS measuring. The other was a likewise concentrated solution of distilled water and Perimag, but free from agarose. In such a solution, the SPIOs' Brownian motion and rotational freedom are thought to be less restricted than in agarose, allowing more accurate statements about the kinetic changes caused by the agarose pore mesh. To estimate the effect of pore size and agarose concentration on the SPIOs' rotational freedom, the MPS signal of in total 20 samples was measured. Thereafter, we plotted the

amplitudes, i.e. the absolute values of the spectra, for each measured sample.

To illustrate the results of the MPS measuring, we chose the series a, containing a SPIO dilution of 1:10 and an agarose concentration ranging from 0.5% (a1) to 1.5% (a4), see Figure 1. To emphasize the differences between the harmonics, we multiplied the spectra by the same number to even out the third harmonic.

III. Results

Part of the MPS measuring results are shown in Figure 1 below. One can notice that there is a more abrupt decrease between the third and the fifth respectably seventh harmonic in the 1.5% agarose sample than there is in the 0.5% agarose sample. This difference can be seen when comparing the harmonics one to another. The absolute values measured seem to be highly dispersed, forbidding a conclusive comparison.

The measuring of the d series, distilled water with agarose and free from SPIO, showed no measurable MPS signal in these four samples. This proves our MPS measuring technique to be reliable.

The other zero test, distilled water with similar Perimag concentrations as in series a to c but without agarose, showed a linear correlation between the amount of SPIOs and the signal strength. The maximum frequencies measured, serving as an indicator for the SPIOs concentration, were 800 kHz, 700 kHz, and 500 kHz, respectively. The relative signal ratio at the fifth uneven harmonic (225 kHz), another indicator for the SPIO concentration, was 1, 0.1875 and 0.1. These measurements show that the MPS signal decreases in direct proportion to reduced amounts of SPIOs. No abrupt decline in signal strength was seen, unlike series a to c.

REFERENCES

[1] J. B. Weaver and E. Kuehlert. Measurement of magnetic nanoparticle relaxation time. American Association of Physicisists in Medicine 39 (5), May 2012, 2765-2770. doi: 10.1118/1.3701775

[2] J. Narayanan, J.Y. Xiong and X.-Y. Liu. Determination of agarose gel pore size: Absorbance measurements vis a vis other techniques. Journal of Physics: Conference Series 28 (2006), 83-86. doi: 10.1088/1742-6596/28/1/017

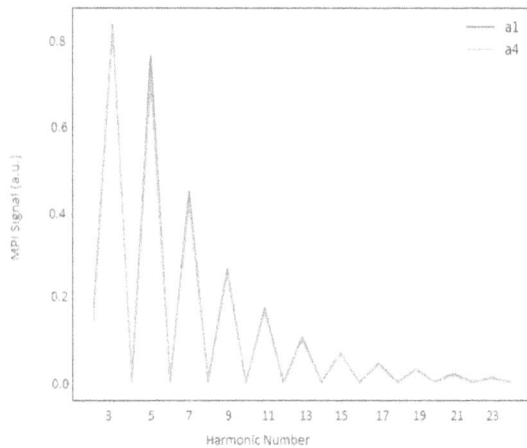

Figure 1 shows the MPI signal (a.u.) in dependence on the harmonic number. The a1 sample (darker shade) contains 1:10 SPIO dilution and 0.5% agarose, the a4 sample (lighter shade) contains the same amount of SPIOs but 1.5% agarose.

IV. Discussion

The results of our experiment show that the agarose concentration and gel pore size influence the MPS signal measured. The fact that the fifth and seventh harmonics show a stronger decrease than the third harmonic in the 1.5% agarose gel compared to the 0.5% agarose gel indicate that the narrower pore mesh limits the SPIOs' Brownian motion and rotational freedom, thus changing their measured relaxation time. The observed dispersion of the absolute values suggests that the amount of SPIO Perimag solution used in three of the series differed too much. This represents an improvement opportunity for further experiments.

Apart from the zero agarose sample series, the lowest agarose concentration we used in this experiment was 0.5%. One can wonder whether this is the critical concentration that accounts for the sudden limitation of SPIO rotational freedom, or an even lower concentration: less than 0.5% but unequal to zero.

V. Conclusions

Relaxation time, being a function of the SPIOs' rotational freedom, is very sensitive to changes in pore size, caused by varying agarose concentrations. Our experiment showed that there is a critical agarose concentration along with a certain pore size that leads to an abrupt decrease in the SPIOs' rotational freedom and decrease in their relaxation time, both measurable by the means of MPI and MPS. Further experiments are needed in order to confirm the exact critical agarose concentration and permit an exact comparison of the absolute values measured, thanks to absolutely equal SPIO concentrations in each series of samples.

MPI Arthrography – Proof of Concept in a Phantom Study

Stefan Herz [a],*, Patrick Vogel [a,b], Thomas Kampf [b], Martin A. Rückert [b], Volker C. Behr [b], Thorsten A. Bley [a]

[a] *Department of Diagnostic and Interventional Radiology, University Hospital Würzburg, Germany*
[b] *Department of Experimental Physics 5 (Biophysics), University of Würzburg, Germany*
[c] *Department of Diagnostic and Interventional Neuroradiology, University Hospital Würzburg, Germany*
 * *Corresponding author, email: Herz@ukw.de*

I. Introduction

Arthrography is an important technique in musculoskeletal radiology for the detailed assessment of structures of joints, such as shoulder, knee or hip [1]. In direct arthrography a thin needle is used to inject contrast agent into a joint [2] prior to standard imaging methods such as X-rays, ultrasound, computed tomography (CT) or magnetic resonance imaging (MRI). The injected contrast agent leads to joint distention, separates intraarticular structures and thus facilitates the detection of pathological findings. It may be applied if standard joint imaging methods do not show the needed detail of joint structure and function.

Magnetic Particle Imaging (MPI) visualizes the distribution of superparamagnetic iron-oxide nanoparticles (SPIOs) background-free [3]. This new tomographic imaging modality is now on its way from proof of principle to preclinical applications especially in vascular and targeted imaging [4]. An additional possible application for MPI in musculoskeletal imaging could be direct arthrography. The direct visualization of anatomical structures is not possible with MPI. However, joint structures could be visualized indirectly via the generation of a negative image based on intra-articular injected contrast agent.

Here, initial results of a first MPI arthrography proof-of-concept experiment are presented.

II. Materials and Methods

II.I. MPI Scanner and Software

A simulation study was performed using a tailored simulation environment to optimize MPI scanner settings for imaging of joints [5]. Experiments were conducted on a Traveling Wave MPI Scanner (TWMPI) [6] featuring an in-plane resolution of ~1.5 mm and a field of view of 65 x 29 x 29 mm^3. 3D datasets were collected using a rotating slice scanning mode, which acquired 36 'quasi'-projections through the sample under different angles [6,7].

II.I. Phantoms and Measurements

A simple plastic joint phantom was constructed consisting of a tube (Diameter 16 mm) containing two convexly shaped hemispheres that were oppositely arranged to each other (Fig. 1, left). The tube represented the joint capsule and the hemispheres the articulating bones. The resulting articular space was filled with diluted Ferucarbotran (10 mmol (Fe)/l). Each measurement (acquisition time: 20 ms per image) was averaged 10 times to increase image definition.

III. Results

MPI visualized the intraarticular space of the joint phantom in a 2D setting (Fig. 1, right). The negative image of the contrast filled volume outlined the basic articular structure. In the peripheral and central edge regions the exact anatomy was slightly blurred. Furthermore, accentuated in the center of the phantom geometric distortions were visible.

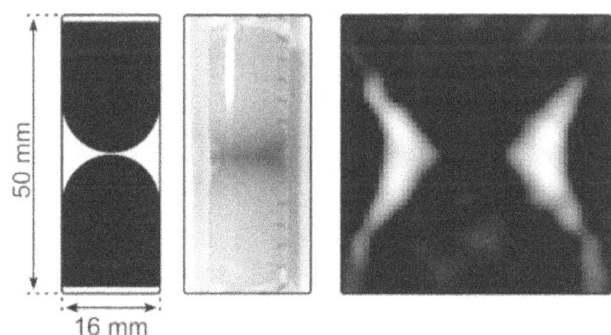

Figure 1: *Left: Sketch and photo of the simple joint phantom consisting of a tube and two convexly shaped hemisspheres. Right: 2D MPI reconstruction of the joint phantom visualizing the intraarticular space.*

IV. Discussion

MPI arthrography of joint phantoms is principally feasible. As a drawback in contrast to established musculoskeletal imaging techniques such as MRI intra-articular structures can only be visualized indirectly. The visualization of edge regions in joints using TWMPI, however, remains challenging due to issues such as the dynamic range of the MPI scanner [8]. This can lead to blurring of the image in edge regions and underestimation of the extent of small findings. Geometric distortions could be reduced using an optimized reconstruction matrix. Further research is necessary to address these issues.

V. Conclusions

Arthrography of a simple joint phantom using MPI is feasible. Further research is necessary to improve the 2D visualization capabilities and the dynamic range of the TWMPI scanner.

ACKNOWLEDGEMENTS

This work was partially funded by the DFG (BE-5293/1- 1).

REFERENCES

[1] L.S. Steinbach et al., Special focus session: MR arthrography, *Radiographics*, vol. 22 (5), pp. 1223–1246, 2002. Doi: 10.1148/radiographics.22.5.g02se301223

[2] A.K. Rastogi et al., Fundamentals of Joint Injection, *American Journal of Roentgenology*, vol. 207, pp. 484-494, 2016. Doi: 10.2214/AJR.16.16243

[3] B. Gleich and J. Weizenecker, Tomographic Imaging using the nonlinear response of magnetic particles, *Nature*, vol. 435, pp. 1214-7, 2005. Doi: 10.1038/nature03808

[4] T. Knopp, et al., Magnetic Particle Imaging: from proof of principle to preclinical applications, *Phys. Med. Biol.*, vol. 62(14), pp. R124-R178, 2017. Doi: 10.1088/1361-6560/aa6c99

[5] P. Vogel, et al., 3D-GUI Simulation Environment for MPI, *Proc. IWMPI*, p. 95, Lübeck, 2016.

[6] P. Vogel, et al., Traveling Wave Magnetic Particle Imaging, *IEEE TMI*, vol. 33(2), pp. 400-7, 2014. Doi:10.1109/TMI.2013.2285472.

[7] P. Vogel, et al., Rotating Slice-Scanning Mode for Traveling Wave Magnetic Particle Imaging, *IEEE Trans Magn.*, vol. 51(2):6501503, 2015. Doi: 10.1109/TMAG.2014.2335255

[8] S. Herz, et al., Selective Signal Suppression in Traveling Wave MPI: Focusing on Areas with Low Concentration of Magnetic Particles, *Int. Journal on MPI*, vol. 3 (2), 1709001, 2017. Doi: 10.18416/ijmpi.2017.1709001

MPI Based 4D flow Estimation – a Simulation Study

Jochen Franke [a,b,*], Romain Lacroix [(a)], Heinrich Lehr [a], Volkmar Schulz [b]

[a] *Bruker BioSpin MRI GmbH, Ettlingen, Germany*
[b] *Physics of Molecular Imaging Systems, University RWTH Aachen, Germany*
[*] *Corresponding author, email: Jochen.Franke@Bruker.com*

I. Introduction

Flow estimation is a common tool in the field of cardiology to screen for or to evaluate and stage cardiovascular diseases. Magnetic Particle Imaging (MPI) features a 4D capability with fast repetition rates of approx. 46 Hz [1] and thus is a promising candidate for 4D velocity vector field estimation. By analyzing pulsed tracer information, an MPI based flow analysis has been proposed by means of Optical flow techniques [2,3].

II. Material and Methods

II.I. Optical flow based 4D flow analysis algorithm

A Flow Analysis Toolbox (Bruker BioSpin MRI GmbH, Germany) described in [3] uses time as well as frequency signal processing approaches to extract from reconstructed MPI datasets the velocity information from time-intensity-curves. In this approach, only signal components within narrow bands around the tracer pulse frequency and its harmonics are used for analysis. Quantitative velocity vector fields are estimated by calculating local propagations from the spatial gradient vectors of the pulsatile tracer distribution by means of an Optical Flow algorithm [4]. The scope of this simulation study is the verification of the quantitative validity of the proposed Flow Analysis Toolbox.

II.II. Simulation Study

Synthetic 4D image datasets of constant, laminar max. fluid velocities of 5, 10, 50, 200, 500 and 800 mm/s within Poiseuille tubes were generated in MATLAB®. The simulation was set up for pulsatile tracer concentrations with a tracer modulation frequency of 6 Hz, a tracer concentration modulation depth of 1 [a.u.], volume rate of approx. 46 Hz, isotropic spatial resolution of 1 mm³ and a field of view of 31×31×15 mm³. For each velocity setting, the Poiseuille tube with radius of 7 mm was oriented in z-direction (i.e. short field of view axis).

Setup I: 200 consecutive volumes of each synthetic 4D image data with fluid velocity of 5...800 mm/s were fed into the MPI Flow Analysis Toolbox described in [3]. For the flow field reconstruction, an noise level (2 %) was added to the input data and a Tikhonov optical flow regularizer ($\lambda=3e^{-12}$) was used. From each dataset, 15 adjacent 3D velocity vector (with TR = 21 ms) were estimated and analyzed in terms of $|\vec{v}|$ at the center of the tube.

Table 1: Simulated flow velocities and the resulting tracer wave length and wave front propagation per repetition for volume rates of approx. 46 Hz and tracer modulation frequency of 6 Hz.

V [mm/s]	5	10	50	100	200	500	800
Tracer wave length [mm]	0.8	1.7	8.3	16.7	33.3	83.3	133.3
Capture range [mm]	0.4	0.8	4.2	8.3	16.7	41.7	66.7
Propagation [mm]	0.1	0.2	1.1	2.2	4.3	10.8	17.2

Setup II: To investigate the noise dependency, one synthetic data set of flow rate 500 mm/s was fed with different noise levels [0.5...15 %] into the MPI Flow Analysis Toolbox, while the optical flow regularizer was kept constant ($\lambda=3e^{-12}$).

Setup III: To investigate the Tikhonov optical flow regularizer dependency, one synthetic data set of flow rate 500 mm/s was fed with different λ [$1e^{-20}$...1] into the MPI Flow Analysis Toolbox, while the noise level of the input data was kept constant (2 %).

III. Results

Resulting pulsatile tracer wave length and wave front propagations for the different synthetic 4D data are summarized in Table 1. Fig. 1 shows exemplarily two adjacent time points of the 500 mm/s synthetic 4D dataset dataset, which serves as input for the flow analysis. Here, a wave front propagation in the centerline of the tube can be deduced to approx. 11 mm in z-direction. In Fig. 2, a 3D representation of the reconstructed velocity vector field can be seen, depicting a parabolic velocity profile as expected for laminar flows in Poiseuille tubes. Velocity estimation results over a wide range of velocities are presented in Fig.

3. Results of setup II are shown in Fig. 4. The influence of the Tikhonov optical flow regularizer for a given noise level input data is shown in Fig. 5.

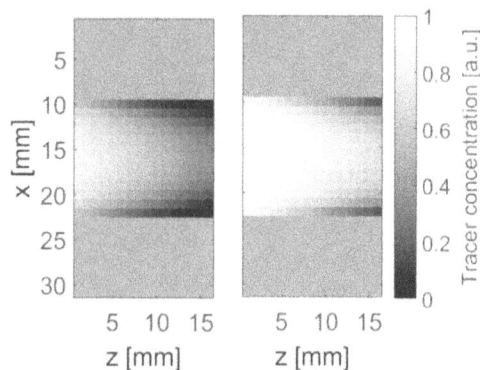

Figure 1: Central slice of the simulated synthetic 4D data of a constant laminar fluid velocity of 500 mm/s in a Poiseuille tube. Two adjacent time points are presented to illustrate the tracer wave front propagation in the z-direction.

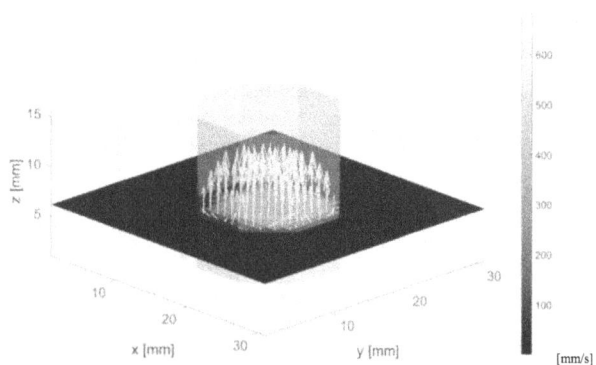

Figure 2: One time point of the reconstructed 4D velocity vector field in a Quiver-representation of the 500 mm/s constant laminar flow dataset. The color-code displays the reconstructed $|\vec{v}|$ in mm/s.

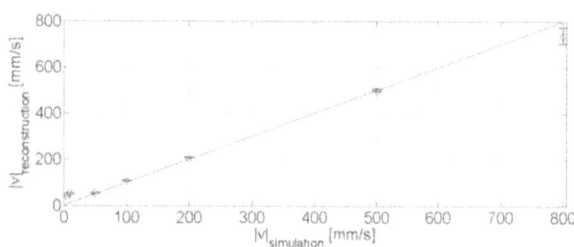

Figure 3: $|\vec{v}|$ mean and standard deviation values extracted from the central part of the Poiseuille tube, reconstructed for different simulated constant laminar fluid velocity datasets.

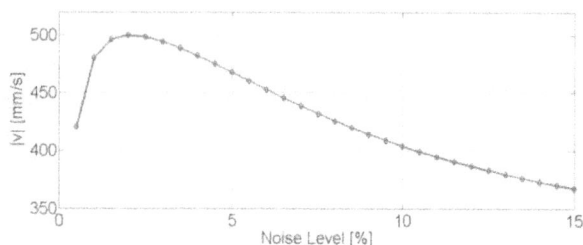

Figure 4: Reconstruction result of the 500 mm/s constant laminar flow dataset for a constant Tikhonov optical flow regularizer and variable noise level.

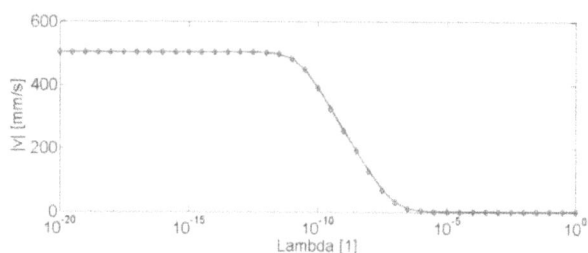

Figure 5: Reconstruction result of the 500 mm/s constant laminar flow dataset for a constant noise level and variable Tikhonov optical flow regularizer, lambda.

IV. Discussion

It was observed that both, the Tikhonov optical flow regularization as well as the noise level have a significant influence onto the reconstructed velocity results. Thus the Tikhonov optical flow regularizer, which stabilizes the Optical Flow solution, has to be adapted carefully for a given noise level of the input image data to not underestimate the velocities. The simulated fluid velocities in the range of 50…500 mm/s were reconstructed precisely with a preserved flow profile of a Poiseuille tube. As prerequisites for the Optical Flow analysis, the tracer pulsatile information has to meet the Nyquist criterions with respect to the spatial as well as the temporal sampling rate of the image data. Furthermore, the wave front propagation has to be significant smaller compared to the capture range as well as smaller than the field of view to prevent folding artifacts in form of reversed flux directions. To reconstruct velocities outside the above stated limits, either the tracer modulation frequency, the spatial and or temporal sampling rate and the field of view has to be adapted.

V Conclusion

This simulation study has proven the quantitative output validity of the proposed Flow Analysis Toolbox [3] with a reconstructed time resolution of 21 ms. The simulated fluid velocities in the range of 50…500 mm/s were reconstructed precisely with a preserved flow profile of a Poiseuille tube. The reconstructed velocity vectors at the tube boundary were aligned parallel and diminish to zero, preserving the no-slip condition at solid interfaces in fluid mechanics. To prevent artifacts, the velocities under investigation have to meet the spatial and temporal limits of the respective Nyquist criterions. MPI signal alteration, induced by particle motion, was not addressed in this contribution.

REFERENCES

[1] B. Gleich and J. Weizenecker. Tomographic imaging using the nonlinear response of magnetic particles. *Nature*, 435(7046):1217-1217, 2005. doi: 10.1038/nature03808.

[2] R. Lacroix "3D Optical flow analysis of a pulsed contrast agent in the bloodstream. Application to virtual angiography and Magnetic Particle Imaging" HAL Id: tel-01298049

[3] J. Franke et Al. „MPI Flow Analysis Toolbox exploiting pulsed tracer information–an aneurysm phantom proof", International Journal on Magnetic Particle Imaging, 3(1).

[4] B.D. Lucas, and T. Kanade. "An iterative image registration technique with an application to stereo vision." Imaging, 130(x):674-679.

Incorporation of Superparamagnetic Iron Oxide Nanoparticles into Erythrocytes for MPI

Kristin Müller [a], Kerstin Lüdtke-Buzug [a,*]

[a] Institute of Medical Engineering, University of Lübeck, Lübeck, Germany
[*] Corresponding author, email: luedtke-buzug@imt.uni-luebeck.de

I. Introduction

Magnetic Particle Imaging (MPI) is an imaging modality introduced by Gleich and Weizenecker in 2005 [1]. By using superparamagnetic iron oxide nanoparticles (SPIONs) as tracer material, MPI can measure their spatial distribution and concentration within the body. Its high temporal and spatial resolution offers real-time functional imaging of e.g. the blood flow in patients with occluded blood vessels [2].

However, SPIONs have a limited blood circulation duration. The reticuloendothelial system (RES) recognizes SPIONs as a foreign object and initiates degradation of the SPIONs. In angiography for observation, a prolonged circulation time in the blood from 4-6 hours [3] up to several days [2] is desirable. Fortunately, the RES does not recognize particles that embark to red blood cells (RBCs), which leads to a prolonged circulation time.

Antonelli et al. [2] reported a method to encapsulate SPIONs into erythrocytes using carboxydextran coated Resovist® (hydrodynamic diameter approx. 60 nm) and silica coated SPIONs (hydrodynamic diameter 40-140 nm). Resovist® has been fully taken up, whereas the silca coated particles were attached to the cell membrane only.

To investigate the feasibility of using this method to incorporate different magnetic nanoparticles into RBCs, on-site synthesized SPIONs (UL-D) with a dextran coating and hydrodynamic diameter of approx. 100 nm were used.

II. Material and Methods

II.I. Incorporation procedure

The loading procedure of RBCs with SPIONs was carried out as described by Antonelli [2]. The UL-D are added to porcine erythrocytes for hypotonic dialysis.

During dialysis, the swelling RBCs become permeable to the SPIONs that enter the cells. Afterwards, a regenerating PIGPA-solution brings the erythrocytes down to their original size by means of isotonic resealing before incubation. Multiple washing with HEPES buffer removes any unentrapped SPIONs so that only loaded erythrocytes remain. To determine the outcome of the incorporation, the remaining, loaded RBCs and supernatant fluids from washing are analyzed by Magnetic Particle Spectroscopy (MPS) and Transmission Electron Microscopy (TEM).

II.I. Magnetic Particle Spectroscopy

To analyze how well the RBCs incorporated the SPIONs, MPS is used. MPS gives information on the magneti-zation characteristics of SPIONs in the sample. An alternating magnetic field magnetizes the particles and the resulting magnetization is determined indirectly by a voltage in the receiver coil. Chosen measurement parameters are: 25 mT field strength, 5 s measurement time, 12500 repetitions, 25 kHz frequency, whereas each measurement was repeated three times. The standard procedure is to put a 10 µl sample into the sample holder.

When there are magnetic nanoparticles in the SPIONs-erythrocytes-sample, a specific signal is obtained. However, it is not possible to decide whether the particles are in the cells or only adhere to the cell membrane. If, in addition, there are no nanoparticles in the supernatant fluid from the latest washing step, it can be assumed that the RBCs are loaded with SPIONs.

III. Results

After the last washing process, the supernatant fluids of the first and last washing step were measured in the MPS as well as the loaded erythrocytes. The MPS results are shown in Fig. 1 that plots the spectral magnetic moment m as a function of the odd harmonics. A high amplitude and even decay of m reveals the presence of SPIONs. The absence of SPIONs is assumed at a spectral magnetic moment from the third harmonic less than 10^{-10} Am^2/Hz. The supernatant fluid of the first washing contains particles. However, the fluid of the latest washing shows none, whereas the erythrocytes sample contains magnetic nanoparticles. This means that all unentrapped particles have been removed and the RBCs are loaded with SPIONs.

To confirm this result, TEM images of the loaded erythrocytes were acquired and are shown in Fig. 2. The black spots in the images are most likely the iron oxide cores and not the whole particle. The majority of the SPIONs are located within the RBCs, whereas some particles appear to be on or partially in the cell membrane. The nanoparticle distribution is not homogenous as there are several condensed clusters of SPIONs. The RBCs have changed into echinocytes, deformed erythrocytes.

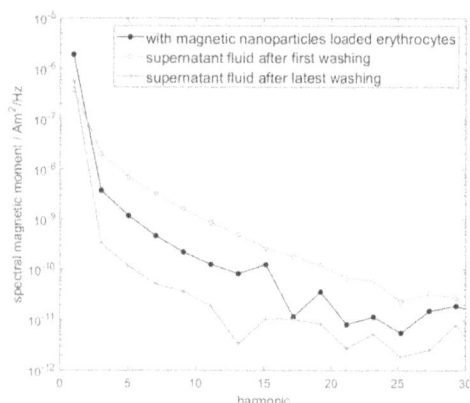

Figure 1: *MPS result in the amplitude spectrum over the odd harmonics.*

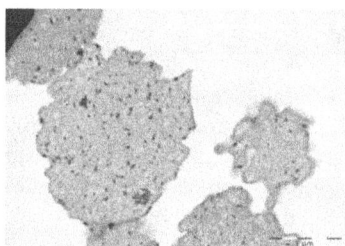

Figure 2: *TEM image of porcine red blood cells loaded with SPIONs. The particles' iron oxide cores (black spots) are unevenly distributed, forming agglomeration clusters.*

IV. Discussion

The MPS results show that all unentrapped magnetic nanoparticles have been removed and the RBCs are loaded with SPIONs. The TEM images as a counter-check confirm the successful incorporation of the nanoparticles into the erythrocytes.

However, the red blood cells have shrinked and deformed into echinocytes. The reason could be an intracellular water loss due to buffer hyperosmolarity. The quality of SPION incorporation strongly depends on osmolarity. Antonelli et al. [2] took into account the osmolarity during the loading procedure, reporting a dialysis buffer osmolarity of 64 mOsm for human RBCs. A specific osmolarity value has not been considered during the experiments reported here. If the osmolarity is too low, the cell membrane can be damaged irreversibly. If the osmolarity is too high, the poration can be limited [4]. Takeuchi et al. [5] recommend 120 mOsm for human RBCs for shape preservation and highest *m* when adding 0,2 ml Resovist® for loading. In addition, the method of [2] is adjusted to human RBCs. Antonelli et al. [6] used an 88 mOsm dialysis buffer for murine erythrocytes. This suggests the need for different parameters for ideal SPION encapsulation when using porcine RBCs.

Within the cells, the SPIONs are not distributed homogeneously, some appear to be in the cell membrane. The black spots in the TEM image are most likely the iron oxide cores and not the whole particle, based on their size. Magnetic nanoparticles on or partially in the cell membrane would mean that the RES can recognize the particles and induce phagocytosis. The condensed clusters suggest that the dextran coating has been damaged at some point during the encapsulation which resulted in an agglomeration of the particles or iron oxide core, respec-tively. As the dextran coating does not give contrast to the image, a damaged coating cannot be identified by the TEM images. The use of SPIONs with a fluorescent dyed dextran coating and a fluorescence microscope could be used to examine the coating after encapsulation.

V. Conclusions

We presented the use of an approved method of Antonelli et al. [2] to incorporate on-site synthesized SPIONs into porcine erythrocytes for prolonged vascular circulation time. We showed that RBCs can be loaded with dextran coated nanoparticles with a hydrodynamic diameter of approximately 100 nm.

The result was evaluated by MPS and TEM. Both showed successfully incorporated UL-D-SPIONs. However, the cells dehydrated due to intracellular water loss and some SPIONs were attached to the cell membrane. It is not clear if the dextran coating was still intact after entering the RBCs. Further research should focus on buffer osmolarities and comparison to non-loaded erythrocytes as well as different particle sizes and the use of human RBCs. In addition, investigating vascular circulation efficiency should be aimed for.

ACKNOWLEDGEMENTS
The authors thank Prof. Matthias Klinger and Kerstin Fiebelkorn, Institute of Anatomy, University of Lübeck, for their realization of the TEM images.

REFERENCES
[1] B. Gleich and J. Weizenecker. Tomographic imaging using the nonlinear response of magnetic particles. *Nature*, 435:1214-1217, 2005. doi: 10.1038/nature03808.
[2] A. Antonelli et al. New Biomimetic Constructs for Improved In Vivo Circulation of Superparamagnetic Nanoparticles. *Journal of Nanoscience and Nanotechnology 8*, 5:1-9, 2008. doi: 10.1166/jnn.2008.190.
[3] K. Lüdtke-Buzug et al. Preparation and Characterization of Dextran-Covered Fe₃O₄ Nanoparticles for Magnetic Particle Imaging. *Springer IFMBE Series 22*, 2343-2346, 2008. doi: 10.1007/978-3-540-89208-3_562.
[4] D. E. Markov et al. Human erythrocytes as nanoparticle carriers for magnetic particle imaging. *Phys. Med. Biol. 55*, 6161-6473, 2010. doi: 10.1088/0031-9155/55/21/008.
[5] Y. Takeuchi et al. Encapsulation of Iron Oxide Nanoparticles into Red Blood Cells as a Potential Contrast Agent for Magnetic Particle Imaging. *Advanced Biomedical Engineering 4*, 37-43, 2014. doi: 10.14326/abe.3.37.
[6] A. Antonelli et al. New Strategies to Prolong the In Vivo Life Span of Iron-Based Contrast Agents for MRI. *PloS ONE 8*, 10:e78542, 2013. doi: 10.1371/journal.pone.0078542.

Fluorescence Labeled MPI Tracer as a Visualization Tool for Different Cell Types

Kerstin Lüdtke-Buzug[b,*], Ralph Pries[a,*], Ann-Kathrin Steuer[b], Thorsten M. Buzug[b], Barbara Wollenberg[a]

[a]Department of Otorhinolaryngology, University Hospital of Schleswig-Holstein, Campus Luebeck, Luebeck, Germany
[b] Institute of Medical Engineering, University of Luebeck, Luebeck, Germany
* Corresponding authors, email: luedtke-buzug@imt.uni-luebeck.de, rallepries@yahoo.de

I. Introduction

I.I. Subsection

Recent investigations have indicated that MPI tracers based on superparamagnetic iron oxide nanoparticles (SPIONs) have highly biocompatible characteristics [1] and thus are very promising for cell labeling. In this contribution, the cellular uptake of magnetic particles and its biological impact was analyzed using head and neck squamous cancer cells (HNSCCs). Particles that meet specific MPI requirements have been synthesized as tracers (UL-D) and subsequently, the cellular uptake was analyzed using different methods such as magnetic particle spectroscopy (MPS). The biological impact of the synthesized SPIONs was investigated with respect to various molecular and cellular characteristics. The results suggest that UL-D SPIONs are a promising tracer material for use in innovative analysis of different cell types in MPI. Labeled tracers coupled to fluorophores are introduced, which are suitable for MPI. With these modified tracers the particle cell upload can be monitored with fluorescence microscopy.

II. Material and Methods

Unlabeled tracers have been manufactured by alkaline co-precipitation. The iron (II) and iron (III) salts are precipitated with a base, like sodium hydroxide or ammonia, in the presence of the coating material and converted into magnetite (Fe_3O_4) under heating.

In the presence of dextran the reactions

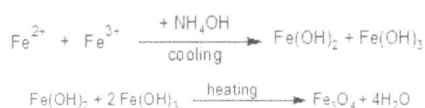

$$Fe^{2+} + Fe^{3+} \xrightarrow[\text{cooling}]{+ NH_4OH} Fe(OH)_2 + Fe(OH)_3$$

$$Fe(OH)_2 + 2 Fe(OH)_3 \xrightarrow{\text{heating}} Fe_3O_4 + 4 H_2O$$

take place.

For the synthesis of with fluorophores labeled SPIONs two different methods have been used.

In the first method, SPIONs were produced as described above and in a consecutive step the corresponding dyes were coupled to the SPIONs. In the second method, dextran, which is used as the coating material, was first coupled with the fluorescent dyes. Then this labeled dextran was used for the synthesis of the SPIONs. The synthesis process is the same as described for unlabeled SPIONs.

For the labeling, we used different dyes. The best results have been achieved with fluorescein and Rose Bengal (see Fig. 1.)

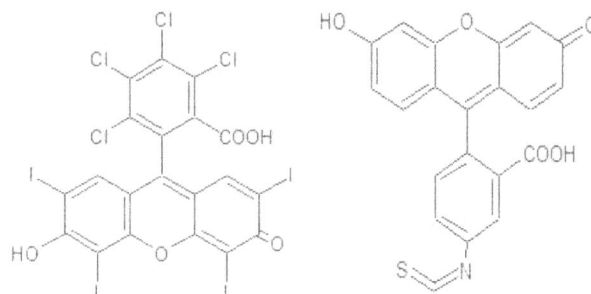

Figure 1: Structure of Rose Bengal and Isothiocyanatofluorescein for labeling of the SPIONs

For the labeling of the dextran (MW 70.000) with Isothiocyanatofluoresccein the dextran has to be dissolved in methyl sulphoxide. The reaction is catalyzed by dibutyltin dilaurate. The result (Fig. 2) is a stable thiocarbamoyl linkage. The labeling procedure does not lead to any depolymerisation of the dextran [2].

For the labeling of the dextran with Rose Bengal the steglich esterification, which is a mild reaction, and which allows the conversion of sterically demanding and acid labile substrates [3] was used. The ester preparation is catalyzed by 4-(N,N-dimethylamino)pyridine (DMAP).

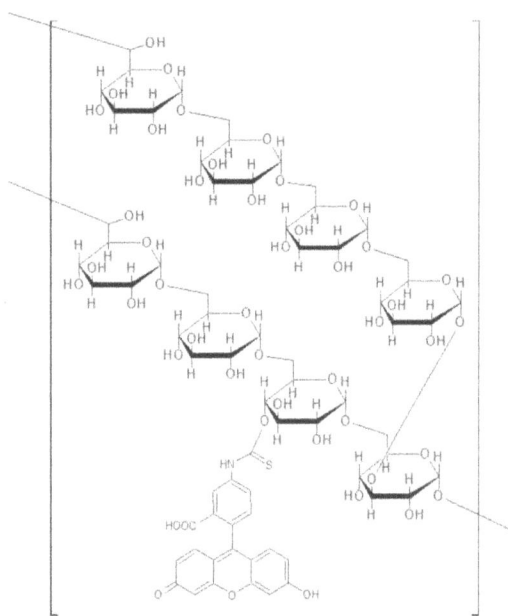

Figure 2: *Labeled dextrane with Isothiocyanofluorescein*

maximum field strength: 25 mT, measurement period: 5 s, number of repetitions: 12500, frequency 25 kHz. Each measurement was repeated 3 times. The MPS standard procedure is to put a 10 µL sample into the sample holder. As demonstrated in Fig. 4, the decay of the harmonics is independent of the coating.

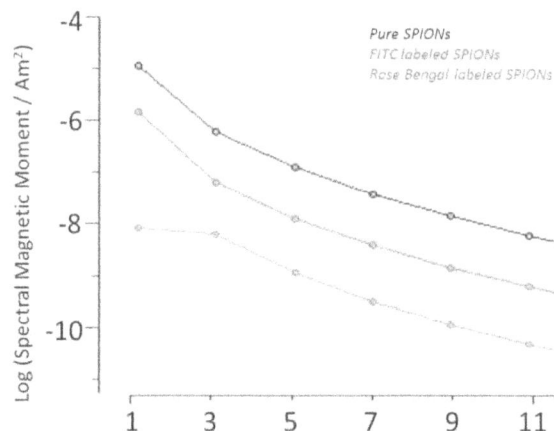

Figure 4: *MPS measurements of pure and labeled SPIONs*

III. Results and Discussion

Dose and time dependent effects of SPIO labeling on cell viability, proliferation, migration as well as on inflammatory and oxidative stress responses were evaluated. UL-D SPIONs that were taken up *in vitro* by human head and neck cancer cells showed good labeling efficiencies.

IV. Conclusions

The aims of this study are the optimization of the SPION synthesis process and the development of different kinds of specific labels. The visualization of different cell types *in vitro* and *in vivo* has been studied. The results of the experiments presented here suggest that UL-D SPIONs are a promising tracer material for use in analysis of different cell types in MPI.

ACKNOWLEDGEMENTS

The authors are grateful to Birgit Hüsing for technical support in several parts of this work. This work was supported by grants of the following funding bodies to B.W.: the Monika Kutzner Stiftung, the Werner and Klara Kreitz Stiftung and the Rudolf Bartling Stiftung.

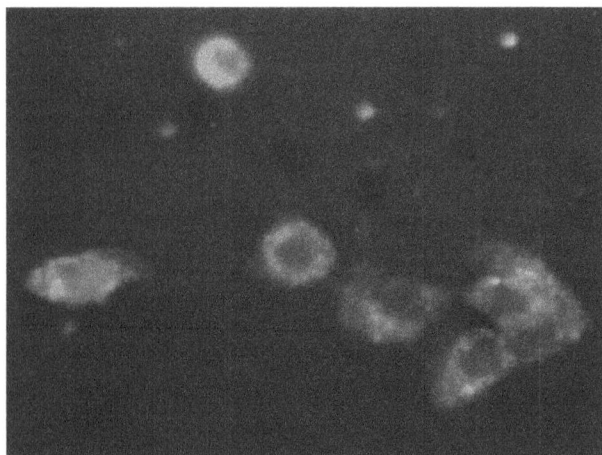

Figure 3: *Uptake of FITC labeled SPIONs.*

Flow cytometry analysis demonstrated that the cell viability of UL-D SPION labeled cells was not influenced. We observed decreased cell proliferation in response to increased SPIO concentrations. The cellular migration and the intracellular production of reactive oxygen species (ROS) were not impaired. Tumor necrosis factor alpha (TNF-α) and the interleukins -6 (IL-6) -8 (IL-8) and -1 beta (IL-1ß) were measured indicating inflammatory responses. Our data suggest UL-D SPIONs as a promising agent for innovative tumor cell analytics.

For the characterization of labeled SPIONs a magnetic particle spectrometer (MPS, Fork Labs) was used [4,5]. The following measurement parameters have been chosen:

REFERENCES

[1] A. Lindemann, K. Lüdtke-Buzug, B.M. Fraederich, K. Gräfe, R. Pries, and B. Wollenberg, *Biological impact of superparamagnetic iron oxide nanoparticles for magnetic particle imaging of head and neck cancer cells*, International Journal of Nanomedicine, 9, 5025–5040, 2014. DOI: 10.2147/ijn.s63873.

[2] A.N. de Belder and K. Granath. *Preparation and properties of fuorescein labelled dextrans.* Carbohydr. Res. 1973; 30:375-378

[3] B. Neises, W. Steglich, *Simple Method for the Esterification of Carboxylic Acids,*. Angew. Chem. Int. Ed., 17 (7), 522–524, 1978. DOI: 10.1002/anie.197805221

[4] S. Biederer. *Magnet-Partikel-Spektrometer Entwicklung eines Spektrometers zur Analyse superparamagnetischer Eisenoxid-Nanopartikel für Magnetic Particle Imaging.* Springer Vieweg, Berlin, 2012.

[5] S. Biederer, T. Sattel, T. Knopp, K. Lüdtke-Buzug, B. Gleich, J. Weizenecker, J. Borgert, T. M. Buzug, *Magnetization response spectroscopy of superparamagnetic nanoparticles for magnetic particle imaging*, Journal of Physics D: Applied Physics, 42 (20), 205007, 2009. DOI: 10.1088/0022-3727/42/20/205007.

Adaption of a System Function for *in-vivo* Media

Olaf Kosch [a,*], Harald Kratz [b], Patricia Radon [a], Azadeh Mohtashamdolatshahi [b], Jörg Schnorr [b], Matthias Taupitz [b], Lutz Trahms [a], Frank Wiekhorst [a]

[a] *Department 8.2 Biosignals, Physikalisch-Technische Bundesanstalt, Berlin, Germany*
[b] *Institute of Radiology, Charité – Universitätsmedizin Berlin, Berlin, Germany*
* *Corresponding author, email: olaf.kosch@ptb.de*

I. Introduction

Magnetic particle imaging (MPI) is an emerging tomographic imaging technique capable of quantitatively determining the 3D distribution of a magnetic nanoparticle (MNP) based tracer material. Besides, this technique shows a high specificity to the magnetic properties of the MNPs utilized in multi-color MPI [1]. However, the magnetic behavior of these particles may be already changed by opsonization [2], different ionic strength and other influences of biological fluids as already shown by magnetic particle spectroscopy in [3]. Here, we analyze MPI measurements of two magnetic MPI tracers in biological media, with an emphasis on blood. In [4] the case of an adapted system function (SF) of MNPs distributed among stem cells was published first time. In contrast, we study the case of MNPs distributed in blood, where rotation of the MNPs is not blocked. We analyze the temporal changes of the MNPs' MPI performance in the media; to ascertain the potential impact during SF measurements. To include the influence of the biological fluids into the SF based reconstruction, a suitable reference sample of MNP dispersed in the target media is required.

II. Material and Methods

II.I. MPI spectrum

MPI measurements were performed using a preclinical MPI system (Bruker MPI 25/20 FF) installed at Charité University Hospital Berlin, equipped with an additional separate receiving coil [5] to increase sensitivity. The spectra were measured with orthogonal drive fields, with frequencies of 2.5 MHz divided by 102/96/99 in x-/y-/z-direction and amplitudes of 12 mT without applying a selection field gradient. At the beginning of each measurement, we recorded the background signal and then the sample was moved robotically to the center of the field of view (FoV). The background was removed from the recorded spectra. Additionally, we removed the transfer function of the MPI signal chain. We analysed two magnetic MPI tracers MCP 2-2 [6] and Resovist with a concentration of 145.5 mmol/L. The tracers were measured in blood, fetal valve serum (FCS), bovine serum albumin (BSA), NaCl solution and distilled water (used as reference).

II.II. SF and phantom measurement

The imaging measurements were performed using a drive field of 12 mT and a selection gradient field of 2.5 T/m in the z-direction (1.25 T/m in x- and y-directions). Three SF were measured with MCP 2-2 applying the original concentration diluted 1:2 by water, FCS or blood. The size (x*y*z) of the reference sample applied in the SF was $2*2*1$ mm^3. The SFs have a geometrical size of $26.4*26.4*13.2$ mm^3 with a grid of 33*33*33 resulting in a voxel size of $0.8*0.8*0.4$ mm^3. A PCR tube (s. Fig 2 a, inner diameter max. 5 mm) with 10 μL MCP 2-2 at original concentration diluted by 90 μl blood was used in the phantom measurement. The same background cleaning was used like in the spectrum measurements before. The Kaczmarz algorithm with 5 iterations and a regularization factor of 10^{-2} was used for reconstruction. 2535 frequency components were selected for use in the reconstruction of the phantom measurements.

II.III. Rat measurement and reconstruction

A bolus of MCP 2-2 with administered doses 100 μmol Fe/kg of bodyweight was injected into the tail vein. The rat was placed in the FoV of the MPI scanner with the abdominal section of the vena cava, distal aorta and kidney to image the passage through the renal artery. A moving average of 5 was applied to the measurement data of the animal experiment and the regularization factor was increased to 0.2. By SNR-thresholds, 2355 frequency component were selected for reconstructions employing either the SF recorded with MCP 2-2 in water or MCP 2-2 in blood.

III. Results

The amplitudes in the spectra were reduced in all biological fluids compared to MNP in water. As an example, this comparison is shown for MCP 2-2 in blood Fig. 1. Remarkably, the spectra were time invariant for 48 hours window starting from a few seconds after mixing. The temporal stability is therefore sufficient for the recording of detailed SFs. A similar reduction pattern was exhibited by the particles in FCS. This behavior is contrary to Resovist and blood, where the spectra in blood is time-dependent, especially for higher concentrations of Resovist. The spectra of Resovist together with the different media will be presented at the conference.

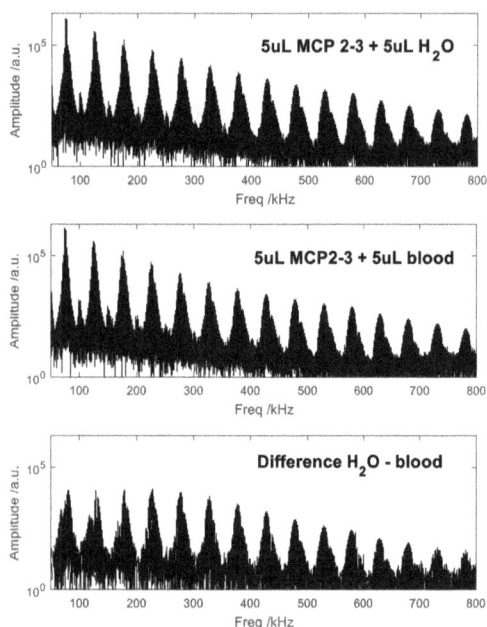

Figure 1: *Spectra of MCP 2-2 (top): in water, (middle) in blood and (bottom): the difference (H₂O – blood).*

By employing the SF of MNP dispersed in water, the reconstruction of the described phantom extends the nominal volume of the phantom (s. Fig 2 b, c), and the whole image contains more noise. This qualitative impression is supported by a quantitative analysis, that was performed by integrating the iron content over all voxels inside and outside of the real phantom volume (s. Table 1).

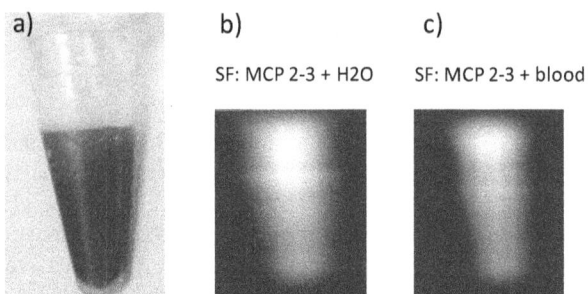

Figure 2: *a) Phantom with 10 µL MCP 2-2 + 90 µL blood and the reconstructions applying SF from sample b) MCP 2-2 + H₂O and c) MCP 23 + blood*

Table 1: *Iron content (without hemoglobin) of the phantom.*

Iron content	Original	SF sample MCP 2-2 + H₂O	SF sample MCP 2-2 + blood
inside phantom in µmol in µg	1.455 81.25	0.876 48.95	1.414 78.94
outside phantom in µmol in µg	0 0	1.884 105.21	0.786 43.92

Surprisingly, the reconstructed image indicated a huge iron content outside the phantom volume, even for the SF in blood.

From the rat experiment data, we reconstructed images with higher noise in a similar way. Here, the image of the

vessel appeared to be partially bloated or broken if the SF was taken from water, while the image appeared more realistic for the SF in blood (s. Fig 3).

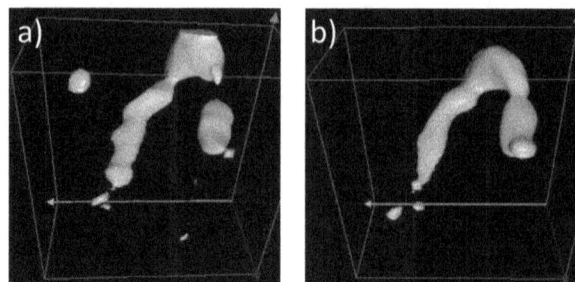

Figure 3: *Reconstruction of the renal passage applying the SF of MCP 2-2 dispersed in a) H₂O and b) blood*

IV. Discussion

Interestingly, the tracer MCP 2-2 exhibits a time invariant behavior, even in a complex medium like blood, and enables the recording of SF for non-aqueous media, e.g. blood. Applying SFs recorded in media other than those physiologically required for *in-vivo* imaging can result in a mismatch between calibration and measurement data sets, and reduce the MPI reconstruction quality in animal and human models. The increased magnetic mobility of the MNP in water during the SF recording is not relevant if the mismatch to the target medium is considered.

V. Conclusions

By adaption of the SF using MNP dispersed in the target medium, we have achieved an essential increase in quantitative MPI reconstruction. Especially, for lower tracer concentrations, or after the injected bolus has distributed over the whole blood circle, the imaging result is improved by using a SF measured in a matching media to the imaging measurement.

ACKNOWLEDGEMENTS

This work was supported by the DFG research program (quantMPI, grant TR408/9-1).

REFERENCES

[1]   J. Rahmer, A. Halkola, B. Gleich, I. Schmale, and J. Borgert, "First experimental evidence of the feasibility of multi-color magnetic particle imaging," *Phys. Med. Biol.*, vol. 60, no. 5, pp. 1775–1791, 2015.

[2]   C. Gräfe *et al.*, "Intentional formation of a protein corona on nanoparticles: Serum concentration affects protein corona mass, surface charge, and nanoparticle-cell interaction," *Int. J. Biochem. Cell Biol.*, vol. 75, pp. 196–202, 2016.

[3]   N. L??wa, M. Seidel, P. Radon, and F. Wiekhorst, "Magnetic nanoparticles in different biological environments analyzed by magnetic particle spectroscopy," *J. Magn. Magn. Mater.*, vol. 427, pp. 133–138, 2017.

[4]   K. Them *et al.*, "Increasing the sensitivity for stem cell monitoring in system-function based magnetic particle imaging," *Phys. Med. Biol.*, vol. 61, no. 9, pp. 3279–3290, 2016.

[5]   J. Wells *et al.*, "Characterizing a preclinical magnetic particle imaging system with separate pick-up coil," *IEEE Trans. Magn.*, pp. 1–1, 2017.

[6]   H. Kratz *et al.*, "Novel magnetic multicore nanoparticles designed for MPI and other biomedical applications : From synthesis to first in vivo studies," pp. 1–22, 2018.

Lateral Movement of a Helical Swimmer Induced by Rotating Focus Fields in a Preclinical MPI Scanner

Anna Bakenecker [a,*], Thomas Friedrich [a], Anselm von Gladiss [a], and Thorsten M. Buzug [a]

[a] Institute of Medical Engineering, Universität zu Lübeck, Lübeck, Germany
* Corresponding author, email: {bakenecker, buzug}@imt.uni-luebeck.de

I. Introduction

The magnetic fields of a magnetic particle imaging (MPI) scanner system cannot only be used to image the distribution of magnetic nanoparticles [1], but also to manipulate magnetic devices [2, 3, 4]. The manipulation of a 3D printed helical swimmer, made of magnetic printing material, is presented in this work. Rotating magnetic fields of an MPI scanner induce a force on the swimmer. Furthermore, the suitability of the printing material for MPI was investigated by magnetic particle spectrometry (MPS).

I.I. Motivation in Context of Clinical Applications

In a clinical application scenario, one may think of the manipulation of macroscopic devices, such as catheters, video capsules or screws, which can be directed towards the region of interest. A commercially available manipulation system consisting of permanent magnets is already available (Stereotaxis Niobe). In combination with MPI the devices need to be coated with magnetic nanoparticles for simultaneous imaging [5]. This application has the potential to maintain minimal invasive surgery techniques. Also, magnetic capsules filled with therapeutics are of potential interest, since drugs can be administered to the region of interest and for certain therapies the systemic treatment can be reduced. However, the tomographic in vivo monitoring of the manipulation process remains an open task, and therefore the combination of magnetic manipulation with MPI is of great interest [6].

I.II. Generation of Forces in an MPI Scanner

MPI scanner systems typically feature three magnetic field topologies: First, a drive field, which excites the magnetic nanoparticles. Second, a selection field, which features either a field free point or a field free line. Only particles nearby the field free region contribute to the particle signal. Third, a focus field, which is a homogeneous offset field enabling to enlarge the field of view [7].

There are two ways to apply a magnetic force. One is to utilize the selection field. A force is induced in the direction of the field gradient pointing towards the highest magnetic field strength. The other way is to apply an oscillating current to the focus field coils and therefore, to induce a magnetic torque to the object inside the scanner. The torque τ depends on the externally applied magnetic field strength B, the magnetic moment of the device μ and the angle between these two:

$$\tau = \mu \times B \qquad (1)$$

Since the direction of B is circularly moving and μ has a certain relaxation time, there is always an angle between B and μ inducing a torque.

In order to move screws or other helical structures around their long axis pointing in e.g. x-direction, an alternating current needs to be applied to the focus field coils in y- and z-direction with a 90° phase shift, respectively. This induces a rotation of the object in the y-z plane.

II. Material and Methods

The macroscopic swimmers are 3D printed with magnetic iron PLA, which consists of PLA and micrometer sized iron particles (Proto Pasta, Vancouver, USA). The swimmer has a diameter of 5 mm, a total length of 17.5 mm and weights 0.28 g. The swimmer has been put in a water filled silicon tube at room temperature with a diameter of 7 mm. The swimmer can be seen in Fig. 1. The tube has been positioned in the middle of the MPI scanner along the bore axis (x-direction). The experiments were performed with a preclinical MPI system (Bruker, Ettlingen, Germany). A maximum focus field strength of 18 mT and a maximal focus field frequency of 10 Hz can be applied. Focus fields were applied in y- and z-direction. The movement has been observed with a small camera positioned inside the scanner bore below the phantom.

In a second step, the suitability of the printing material for the use in MPI was investigated with a spectrometer, featuring a 2D excitation of about 25 kHz [8]. 0.12 g of printing material have been used. The receive signal has been compared to a measurement of 1:1 diluted Resovist (see Fig. 2).

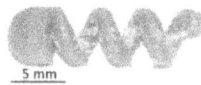

Figure 1: A picture of the helical swimmer, which is 3D printed with magnetic iron PLA. It has a diameter of 5 mm and a length of 17.5 mm.

III. Results

The macroscopic swimmer could be laterally moved through the water filled tubes by rotating the focus fields. The swimmer was moved because of its continuous rotation along its long axis. The helical shape induces a propulsion. The swimmer could only be moved by applying the maximal field strength of 18 mT. A rotation frequency of 1 Hz results in a continuous rotation of the helical swimmer and a forward movement. However, the lateral movement was only a few mm when the swimmer was rotated twenty times. Smaller field strength, larger and smaller frequencies did not lead to a full rotation of the helical swimmer and therefore, no lateral movement was observed.

In Fig. 2 the amplitude spectrum of the 3D printing material can be seen in comparison to Resovist and an empty measurement. The amplitudes of the printing material are smaller compared to Resovist, but mixing frequencies up to the approximately thirteen harmonic can be seen for the 3D printing material.

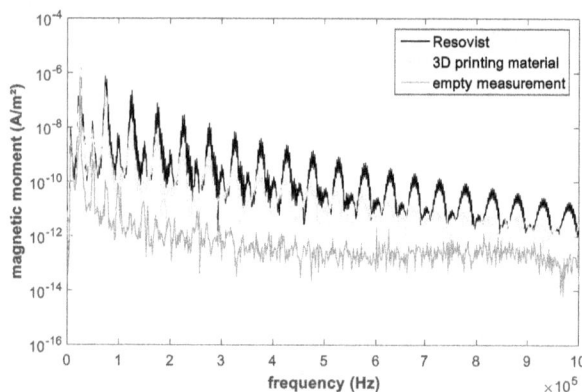

Figure 2: Amplitude spectrum of 3D printing material (magnetic iron PLA) in comparison to Resovist (10 μl, dilution 1:1) and an empty measurement. The measurement was performed with an MPS featuring 2D excitation.

IV. Discussion

The fluid dynamic properties of the helical swimmer are not yet optimized. Most probably, a larger lateral movement may be achieved by optimizing the shape of the swimmer.

It has been observed that lower as well as higher frequencies than 1 Hz did not result in a continuous rotation of the swimmer. That is because at lower frequencies the angle between the magnetic moment of the swimmer and the magnetic field is very small and therefore only a small

torque is induced (see eq. 1). At higher frequencies the magnetic moment of the swimmer cannot follow the magnetic field anymore, because of its relaxation time.

Since the iron concentration of the printing material is not known, it is not possible to compare the amplitude spectra of Resovist and the printing material quantitatively. However, a comparable amount of printing material has been used and since multiple frequency components show an MPI signal (see Fig. 2), the precondition for image acquisition with an MPI scanner is fulfilled.

V. Conclusions

It has been qualitatively shown that a lateral movement of a magnetic helically shaped swimmer can be carried out by rotating the focus fields of an MPI scanner system. The amplitude spectrum (see Fig. 2) shows, that image acquisition of the 3D printed helical swimmer is possible with an MPI scanner.

Further steps would be the additional use of the selection field with which it is possible to selectively move swimmers positioned in different tubes. Then, more sophisticated phantoms containing more tubes of different directions could be used. Different shapes of the swimmer, which produce more propulsion, are of future investigation. Last, the combination of the manipulation of the used swimmer with MPI is of future interest.

ACKNOWLEDGEMENTS
Funding by the Federal Ministry of Education and Research, Germany (BMBF) under grant number 13GW0069A is gratefully acknowledged.

REFERENCES
[1] B. Gleich and J. Weizenecker. Tomographic imaging using the nonlinear response of magnetic particles. Nature, 435(7046):1217-1217, 2005. DOI: 10.1038/nature03808.
[2] N. Nothnagel, J. Rahmer, B. Gleich, A. Halkola, T. M. Buzug and J. Borgert: Steering of Magnetic Devices With a Magnetic Particle Imaging System. IEEE Transactions on Biomedical Engineering, 63(11): 2286-2293, 2016, DOI: 10.1109/TBME.2016.2524070.
[3] J. Rahmer, C. Stehning, and B. Gleich: Spatially selective remote magnetic actuation of identical helical micromachines, Science Robotics, 2(3), 2017, DOI: 10.1126/scirobotics.aal2845.
[4] A. Mahmood, M. Dadkhah, M. Ok Kim, J. Yoon: A Novel Design of an MPI-Based Guidance System for Simultaneous Actuation and Monitoring of Magnetic Nanoparticles. IEEE Transactions on Magnetics, 51(2), 2015, DOI: 10.1109/TMAG.2014.2358252.
[5] J. Rahmer, D. Wirtz, C. Bontus, J. Borgert, B. Gleich: Interactive Magnetic Catheter Steering with 3D Real-Time Feedback Using Multi-Color Magnetic Particle Imaging. IEEE Transactions on Medical Imaging, 2017, DOI: 10.1109/TMI.2017.2679099.
[6] T. Kuboyabu, A. Ohki, N. Banura, and K. Murase: Usefulness of Magnetic Particle Imaging for Monitoring the Effect of Magnetic Targeting. Open Journal of Medical Imaging, 6: 33-41, 2016, DOI: 10.4236/ojmi.2016.62004.
[7] T. Knopp and T. M. Buzug. Magnetic Particle Imaging: An Introduction to Imaging Principles and Scanner Instrumentation. Springer, Berlin/Heidelberg, 2012. DOI: 10.1007/978-3-642-04199-0.
[8] M. Graeser, A. von Gladiss, M. Weber and T. M. Buzug: Two dimensional magnetic particle spectrometry, Physics in Medicine and Biology, 62(9), 3378-3391, 2017, DOI: 10.1088/1361-6560/aa5bcd.

Towards the Visualization of Biohybrid Implants with MPI: SPION Infused PCL

Henning Nilius [a,*], Robert Siepmann [a], Merle Orth [b], Marcel Straub [a], Seyed Mohammadali Dadfar [c], Milita Darguzyt [c], Volkmar Schulz [a]

[a] *Physics of Molecular Imaging Systems, RWTH Aachen University, Aachen, Germany*
[b] *Institut für Textiltechnik, RWTH Aachen University, Aachen, Germany*
[c] *Experimental Molecular Imaging, RWTH Aachen University, Aachen, Germany*
[*] *Corresponding author, email: henning.nilius@pmi.rwth-aachen.de*

I. Introduction

Vascular diseases such as coronary artery syndrome, myocardial infarction and stroke are among the most common death causes in the western world. Many of these diseases are caused by hemodynamic critical stenoses or thrombosis of feeding arteries of the respective organ. One common treatment is stent implantation using angiography. Most frequently used stents are either bare metal stents (BMS) or metal ones eluting a cytostatic drug to prevent restenosis, called drug eluting stent (DES). Those have the disadvantages that they can lead to late stent thrombosis and a loss of vessel function such as adaptive vasodilatation at higher oxygen consumption of the organ [1], [2]. Bioresorbable scaffolds might overcome these disadvantages by stenting the artery during the healing phase in the first three to six months and then later being dissolved by the body. However recent trials with drug eluting bioresorbable scaffolds for coronary intervention have shown that they are associated with a higher rate of thrombosis compared to DES [3]. Long-term in vivo monitoring will help to better understand why this happens and to find a solution for this problem. As a non-invasive imaging method with high sensitivity and no ionizing radiation magnetic particle imaging (MPI) might be suitable to observe the implanted scaffolds over a long period without doing harm to the patient.

Our work approaches this idea by infusing the bioresorbable polyester polycaprolactone (PCL) with super paramagnetic ironoxide nanoparticles (SPIONs). In this work, we outline the process of creation and confirm visibility in the MPI.

II. Material and Methods

PCL granulate (PCL Capa 6506, Perstorp, Malmo, Sweden) was mixed with 0,1,2,5 and 7 weight percent (wt%) of a SPION powder, obtained by air drying C2 particles that were synthesized in our institute [4]. The mixtures were then given into a micro extruder (MC15, Xplore Instruments BV, Sittard, Netherlands) one after another, starting with the lowest concentration. The extruder was set to 75°C and 5-6 RPM resulting in a maximum extrusion force of 700N. A filament was produced by winding the melt on a spool using a winder unit (Winder unit, Xplore Instruments BV, Sittard, Netherlands) set to a speed of 50 m/min. The filament with 5 wt% SPIONs can be seen in Fig 1. After each mixture, the extruder was cleaned with pure PCL until the melt showed no visible contamination. Resulting filaments were sewed onto a chip forming a small loop structure.

All phantoms were measured using our preclinical MPI [5]. The drive field amplitude was (18, 18, 8) mT in the (X, Y, Z)-direction and the gradient field was set to (3.4, 3.4, 1.7) T/m in (X, Y, Z)-direction. For image reconstruction, an established Kaczmarz algorithm with non-negative constraints was applied. We used MIPAV (Center for Information Technology, National Institutes of Health, Bethesda, United States of America) to create a maximum intensity projection (MIP) of the resulting image volumes and the windowing was set to the same parameters for every imaging phantom.

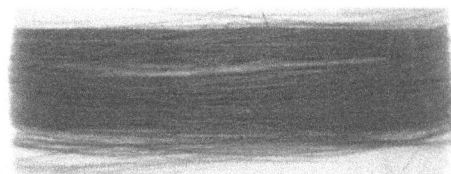

Figure 1: PCL-filament infused with 5 wt% of SPIONs. The filament is tenuous and becomes darker the more SPIONs is added to the PCL.

III. Results

We successfully produced thin filaments that could be processed for all the mixtures. The filaments were not homogenous in thickness and at 7 wt% fresh filaments attached to each other.

Pure PCL was not visible in the MPI but the filaments infused with SPIONs showed a signal which increased with the wt% of added SPIONs. The resulting MIP of the 7 wt% phantom can be seen in Fig. 2. Furthermore, the frequency response in the MPI showed mostly lower harmonics as presented in Fig. 3 and the signal strength was below the expected strength of SPIONs in water at similar concentrations.

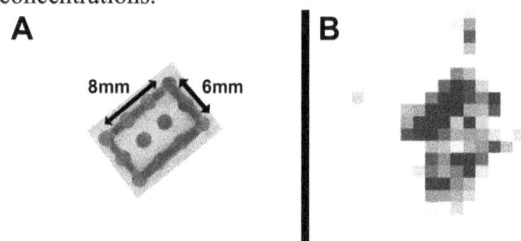

Figure 2: A: Filaments were sewed onto plastic probe holders. The long stroke was 8mm long and the short stroke 6mm. B: MIP of the 7 wt% imaging phantom. Each pixel has an edge length of 1mm.

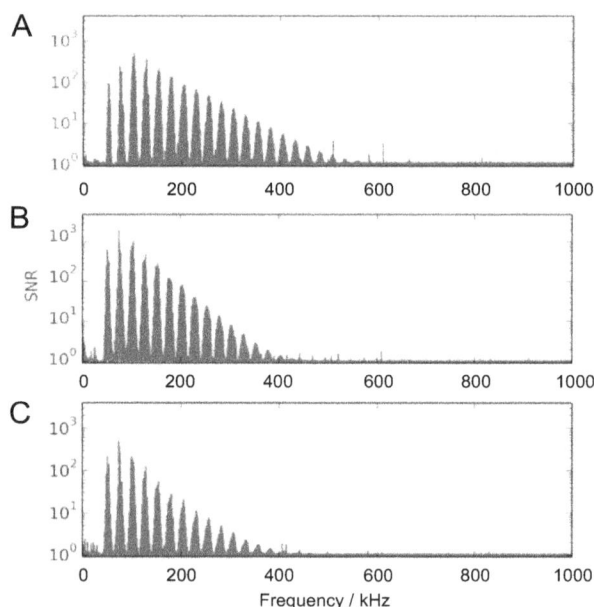

Figure 3: Frequency spectrum of the y-channel of A: SPIONs in water, B: air-dried SPIONs, C: SPION infused PCL at similar iron concentrations. For the SPION infused PCL the higher harmonics and the signal strength are reduced compared to SPIONs in water.

IV. Discussion

The filaments we produced in this work were processable and showed a signal in the MPI indicating that infusing PCL with SPIONs is a feasible way to create a MPI-visible polyester. The inhomogenities in the filament are most likely not due to the added SPIONs but due to the production process, which operated without a pump, since they were also present in pure PCL. A bigger extruder equipped with a melt pump will produce more homogenous filaments. Furthermore, with the current extruder set-up adding more SPION wt% to the PCL will result in more attachments of the filaments. This will impede the unwinding from the spool and therefore further processability.

In accordance with findings of past experiments, the MPI signal is dependent on the concentration of SPIONs and the filament with 7 wt% added SPIONs produced the strongest

signal. However, the frequency spectrum of the filaments shows that higher harmonics, which we expected from experiments with SPIONs in water at similar concentrations, were not present. A possible explanation for this finding is that the Brownian relaxation is impaired due to the incorporation of the SPIONs into the polymer. This also the reason why the signal strength is weaker. A comparison to SPIONs in solution indicates the option to differentiate the filament from circulating SPIONs via multi-color MPI [6] or new methods such as Magnetic Particle Spectroscopy Imaging (MPSI).

V. Conclusions

While the idea of bioresorbable scaffolds is intriguing, we have only limited resources to monitor them from the outside. MPI might be a solution to this problem. In this work, we showed that it is possible to infuse PCL with SPIONs. The polyester that we created generated a concentration dependent signal and could be further processed. As next steps, we plan to investigate if the signal declines when the polymer degrades and the effect of degradation on the surrounding tissue.

ACKNOWLEDGEMENTS

We thank our colleagues from the department of "Physics of Molecular Imaging Systems" who provided knowledge and expertise that greatly assisted the research. Also, we like to thank the "Institute für Textiltechnik" for providing the equipment and expertise to create the filaments.

REFERENCES

[1] Palmerini, T., Benedetto, U., Biondi-Zoccai, G., Della Riva, D., Bacchi-Reggiani, L., Smits, P. C., … Stone, G. W. (2015). Long-term safety of drug-eluting and bare-metal stents: Evidence from comprehensive network meta-analysis. Journal of the American College of Cardiology, 65(23), 2496–2507. https://doi.org/10.1016/j.jacc.2015.04.017

[2] Wiebe, J., Nef, H. M., & Hamm, C. W. (2014). Current status of bioresorbable scaffolds in the treatment of coronary artery disease. Journal of the American College of Cardiology, 64(23), 2541–2551. https://doi.org/10.1016/j.jacc.2014.09.041

[3] Katsikis, A., & Serruys, P. W. (2017). Bioresorbable scaffolds versus metallic stents in routine PCI: The plot thickens. Journal of Thoracic Disease, 9(8), 2296–2300. https://doi.org/10.21037/jtd.2017.07.72

[4] S. M. Ali Dadfar, M. Darguzyte, D. Camozzi, J. Metselaar, S. Banala, N. Güvener, I. Slabu, U. Engelmann, M. Straub, V. Schulz, F. Kiessling and T. Lammers (Ongoing): Maximizing superparamagnetic iron oxide nanoparticles performance for MRI, MPI, and hyperthermia applications.

[5] Weizenecker, J., Gleich, B., Rahmer, J., Dahnke, H., & Borgert, J. (2009). Three-dimensional real-time in vivo magnetic particle imaging. Physics in Medicine and Biology, 54(5), L1–L10. http://doi.org/10.1088/0031-9155/54/5/L01

[6] Rahmer, J., Halkola, A., Gleich, B., Schmale, I., & Borgert, J. (2015). First experimental evidence of the feasibility of multi-color magnetic particle imaging. Physics in Medicine and Biology, 60(5), 1775–1791. https://doi.org/10.1088/0031-9155/60/5/1775

Towards Flow Characterization of Fluids using Magnetic Particle Imaging

Robert Siepmann [a,*], Henning Nilius [a], Marcel Straub [a], Seyed Mohammadali Dadfar [b],
Milita Darguzyte [b], Volkmar Schulz [a]

[a] *Physics of Molecular Imaging Systems, RWTH Aachen University, Aachen, Germany*
[b] *Experimental Molecular Imaging, RWTH Aachen University, Aachen, Germany*
[*] *Corresponding author, email: robert.siepmann@pmi.rwth-aachen.de*

I. Introduction

Cardiovascular diseases (CVD) are widespread and one of the leading causes of death worldwide. Consequently, the importance of cardiovascular diagnostics and therapies has increased rapidly during the last decades. However, clinically established methods have serious drawbacks such as high radiation exposure, toxicity of the commonly used contrast agents or a limit in penetration depth. Magnetic particle imaging (MPI) might have the potential to overcome these disadvantages due to its high spatial and temporal resolution [1] in the absence of radiation. For these reasons, lots of research concerning cardiovascular imaging with MPI has already been done. Several in vivo studies, e.g. a lung perfusion study by Zhou et al. [2] and the visualization of a beating mouse heart using an alternative scanner concept by Vogel et al. [3], support the assumption of MPI's feasibility for this kind of application. Also flow quantifications have already been investigated, most of them focussing on aneurysms. Franke et al. [4] presented a MPI toolbox, which was able to provide flow parameters such as the velocity. Another approach using aneurysm phantoms was done by Sedlacik et al. [5], comparing MPI to DSA and MRI regarding flow estimation.

The aim of this study is to transfer this approach to less complex geometries to understand the flow visualization with MPI at the most basic level. We therefore aim at exploring its limits, artefacts and consequently, possible misinterpretations. This is of great interest, as diagnostics and treatment of many illnesses such as renal artery stenosis or valvular diseases of the heart require a quantification of the blood flow. In this initial study, we visualized boluses in straight glass tubes using MPI in order to assess flow patterns under laminar conditions.

II. Material and Methods

Five glass tubes with diameters ranging from 5 mm to 9 mm were used as imaging phantoms. A diaphragm pump was used to establish a water flow with velocities from 0.08 m/s to 0.22 m/s depending on the diameter of the glass tubes. Velocities and length of glass tubes were chosen in such manner that a laminar flow inside the field of view (FOV) was highly probable. For every tube size, five 1 ml of inhouse developed SPION-boluses (C2, [6]) with an iron content of 67 mmol(Fe)/l were injected into the flow system and visualized by a preclinical MPI-scanner [1].

1 mm isotropic 3D MPI data sets with a temporal resolution of 21.5 ms were generated using selection field gradient of (1.7,1.7,3.4) T/m in (x,y,z)-direction. Drive field amplitudes of ±9 mT in x-,y-direction and ±4 mT in z-direction were used. This leads to a DF-FOV of 10x10x2 mm³ and to a SM-FOV of 23x17x13 mm³. Image reconstruction was done by using the established Kaczmarz algorithm with a non-negativity constraint [7]. Prior to reconstruction, the measurement data was corrected for the background signal. Reconstruction was done with 10 iterations and a L2 regularization of 10^{-1}.

As laminar flow is characterized by a specific velocity distribution we can use this flow system as an initial validation. Under such ideal conditions, plotting the average velocities of a bolus as a function of the location in the cross section of a straight tube will result in a rotationally symmetric parabola as shown in Fig. 1A. This means that the bolus has its maximum speed at the rotational axis of the tube and decelerates to zero towards the inside walls.

When transferring this to MPI, it is important to consider the effect of the temporal resolution of our current setup. If the velocity of the SPION bolus exceeds a particular value, which results from the temporal resolution and the length of the FOV, the MPI scanner is not able to allocate the signal of the bolus to a single location. This causes a motion artefact, which appears as blurred strokes in flow direction in the images. Furthermore, a loss in brightness is to be expected at the beginning and the end of the boluses, as the concentration is averaged over one acquisition frame.

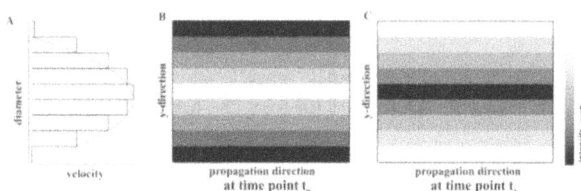

Figure 1: A shows the velocity distribution along the cross section under idealized laminar flow conditions and the discrediting of the voxels in diameter direction when using MPI. B/C show the expected MPI images at two different time points considering the limit of MPI's temporal resolution.

Taking this into consideration, we expect the reconstructed images to look like this: When the bolus enters the FOV (time point t_0), the highest signal intensity should be located in the center of the tube represented as a stroke, shifting to lower values in the tube margins (see Fig. 1B). Supposing that the bolus is short, moments later (time point t_1), the maximum intensity shifts centrifugally to the inside wall while the central signal slowly fades (see Fig. 1C).

III. Results

All boluses were clearly identifiable in the reconstructed MPI images. As an example, Fig. 2 shows the inflow of a SPION bolus in a glass tube of 9 mm inner diameter at an average velocity of 0.08 m/s. At the time the bolus reached the FOV (time point t_0=0s), a central signal saturation in flow direction is observed due to the fact, that the velocity of the bolus in the central line should theoretically be twice as high as the average velocity under laminar flow conditions. Subsequently, in this case approximately 1.8s later, the maximum intensity moves both to the edges of the FOV while a washout in the middle is clearly visible, which is defined as time point t_1. This is consistent with our expectation as outlined above and shows, that MPI is able to visualize laminar flow patterns in simple geometries.

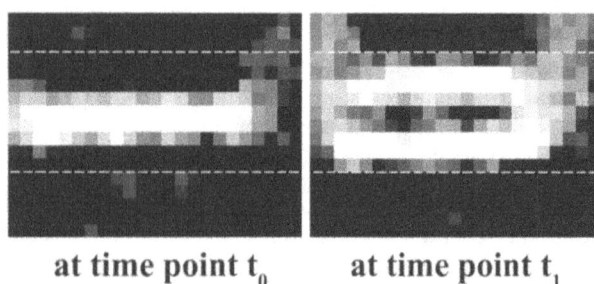

at time point t_0 at time point t_1

Figure 2: Inflow of a SPION bolus in a straight glass tube with 9 mm inner diameter at two different time points. Flow direction is from left to right. The supposed location of the tube is depicted as dashed lines. At first, only a central saturation can be observed. After a short time, the maximum signal intensity shifts centrifugally to both the inside walls of the glass tube.

IV. Discussion

This study dealt with the qualitative approach of flow pattern analysis under laminar conditions using MPI. Other studies have already shown, that MPI might be a useful modality for vascular imaging. Most of them focused on the depiction of organs rather than analysis of the SPION flow itself, for example velocity distributions or bolus shape description. When it comes to diagnostics of CVD, a

dependable characterization of the flow is of great interest. However, there are still some challenges to be dealt with in the future. One of them is the detected decrease in signal intensity at the beginning and the end of fast moving boluses caused by averaging during one Lissajous cycle. Understanding and solving these problems will greatly improve the validity of future perfusion studies.

The next step, which we are currently working on, is to move forward to a full quantification of flow patterns using MPI. This includes a reliable computation of the average velocity, which counts to the most sensitive parameters in detecting pathologic hemodynamics.

V. Conclusions

MPI represents a promising modality for cardiovascular imaging. The chance to depict vessels in high resolution in addition to flow pattern analysis without using radiation could make MPI a strong alternative to clinically established methods. Though, it still remains unclear to what extent MPI is feasible of making its contribution. An important step is to evaluate its limits in flow visualization and consequent possible misinterpretations. This will help assessing MPI's capabilities of clinical use in the future. Further studies should deal with a full quantification of dynamic bolus measurements in more complex geometries and ultimately in vivo.

ACKNOWLEDGEMENTS
We thank our colleagues from the department of "Physics of Molecular Imaging Systems" who provided knowledge and expertise that greatly assisted the research.

REFERENCES
[1] Weizenecker J, Gleich B, Rahmer J, Dahnke H, Borgert J. Three-dimensional real-time in vivo magnetic particle imaging. Phys Med Biol 2009; 54:L1–L10. doi: 10.1088/0031-9155/54/5/L01
[2] Xinyi Y. Zhou, Kenneth E. Jeffris, Elaine Y. Yu, Bo Zheng, Patrick W. Goodwill, Payam Nahid, and Steven M. Conolly. First in vivo magnetic particle imaging of lung perfusion in rats. Physics in medicineandbiology,62(9):3510–3522,2017. ISSN 0031-9155. doi:10.1088/1361-6560/aa616c.
[3] P. Vogel, M. A. Rückert, P. Klauer, W. H. Kullmann, P. M. Jakob, and V. C. Behr. First in vivo traveling wave magnetic particle imaging of a beating mouse heart. Physicsinmedicineandbiology,61(18):6620– 6634, 2016. ISSN 0031-9155. doi:10.1088/00319155/61/18/6620.
[4] Franke, J., Lacroix, R., Lehr, H., & Heinen, U. (2017). MPI Flow Analysis Toolbox exploiting pulsed tracer information - an aneurysm phantom proof, 3(1), 1–5.
[5] Jan Sedlacik, Andreas Frölich, Johanna Spallek, Nils D. Forkert, Tobias D. Faizy, Franziska Werner, Tobias Knopp, Dieter Krause, Jens Fiehler, and Jan Hendrik Buhk. Magnetic particle imaging for high temporal resolution assessment of aneurysm hemodynamics. PloS one, 11(8):e0160097, 2016. ISSN 1932-6203. doi:10.1371/journal.pone.0160097.
[6] S. M. Ali Dadfar, M. Darguzyte, D. Camozzi, J. Metselaar, S. Banala, N. Güvener, I. Slabu, U. Engelmann, M. Straub, V. Schulz, F. Kiessling and T. Lammers (Ongoing): Maximizing superparamagnetic iron oxide nanoparticles performance for MRI, MPI, and hyperthermia applications.
[7] Achiya Dax. On row relaxation methods for large constrained least squares problems. SIAM Journal on Scientific Computing,14(3):570–584,1993. ISSN 1064-8275. doi:10.1137/0914036.

Long-Term Stable Ferrogels for Magnetic Particle Imaging Phantoms

Lucas Wöckel [a], Frank Wiekhorst [b], Olaf Kosch [b], James Wells [b], Volker C. Behr [c], Patrick Vogel [c], Stefan Lyer [d], Christoph Alexiou [d], Cordula Grüttner [e], Silvio Dutz [a,*]

[a]Institute of Biomedical Engineering and Informatics, TU Ilmenau, Ilmenau, Germany
[b]Physikalisch-Technische Bundesanstalt Berlin, Berlin, Germany
[c]Department of Experimental Physics 5 (Biophysics), University of Würzburg, Würzburg, Germany
[d]Department of Otorhinolaryngology,Head and Neck Surgery, Section for Experimental Oncology & Nanomedicine, University Hospital Erlangen, Erlangen, Germany
[e]micromod Partikeltechnologie GmbH, Rostock, Germany
*Corresponding author, email: silvio.dutz@tu-ilmenau.de

I. Introduction

Since the first publications of MPI in 2005 [1], a large amount of experimental and preclinical MPI scanners has been built at various locations all over the world [2]. Due to the rapid development of this new technology, Bruker Biospin launched the first commercially available MPI scanners in 2014. These scanners enable the measurement of the spatial and temporal distribution of magnetic nanoparticles (MNP) within biological tissue, which plays an important role for numerous applications of MNP in biomedicine.

To facilitate investigating the imaging capabilities of this novel modality, detection limits and image resolutions of present MPI scanners have been examined as substantial performance determining parameters. For this reason, appropriate and precisely defined comparable magnetic structures are required to perform comparative studies between different MPI systems. Presently, each group of researchers use their own manufactured phantoms [3, 4]. In most cases, these phantoms consist of MNP-fluids at a certain concentration filled into containers of different volume. Such phantoms often exhibit no long-term stability, and thus do not allow intercomparitive studies between different labs and scanners. Therefore, here we report on our development and evaluation of long-term stable materials for the preparation of MPI phantoms.

II. Material and Methods

First, we aimed to determine suitable combinations of MNPs and matrix materials for the preparation of such phantoms. The main requirements for these material blends are good imaging properties of the tracer particles used, and a homogeneous and agglomeration-free distribution of these particles within the selected matrix. At best, this matrix is long-term stable and guarantees a constant image quality of the phantoms over a long period of at least several months. For our studies, the following MNP types were used:

- Ferucarbotran (Meito Sangyo Co., Nagoya)
- fluidMag-D50 (chemicell, Berlin)
- perimag® (micromod Partikeltechnologie, Rostock)
- SEON[LA-BSA] (SEON-group, Erlangen)

For the phantom matrix, the synthetic polymer (ELASTO-SIL® RT 604 A/B, Wacker Chemie AG) was tested for its suitability in preparing the measurement objects. The group of synthetic polymers seemed to be very suitable for the preparation of such phantoms due to their long-term stability.

The obtained combinations were checked for their mechanical stability by means of mechanical load tests (shore-A). The homogeneity of MNP distribution within the matrix was determined by optical investigation of the samples with a microscope. The influence of embedding the aqueous MNP in a polymer matrix on the MPI performance of the particles was tested by means of Magnetic Particle Spectroscopy (MPS). MPS is a fast and direct method to specifically detect the dynamics of MNP influenced by their environment. For the measurements we used a commercial MPS spectrometer (MPS-3, Bruker) operating at 25 kHz drive frequency and a 25 mT excitation field amplitude. We analyzed changes in the amplitudes of the first odd harmonics between stock MNP and after matrix embedding of the MNP.

The most promising MNP-matrix combination was chosen to manufacture measurement objects of different shape (cubes, cylinders), size, and concentrations. The resulting phantoms were evaluated for their suitability to simulate

MNP loaded areas and the needed MNP concentration for sufficient imaging by means of MPI at PTB (Bruker BioSpin preclinical MPI-scanner) and at University of Würzburg (Traveling-Wave MPI) [5].

III. Results

The transfer of MNP from aqueous suspensions into the synthetic matrix was a challenging part of the phantom preparation. We established a procedure by using ethanol for this transfer, resulting in no alteration of the mechanical properties (shore-A) of the used polymer. Optical investigations showed a low agglomeration behavior of the embedded MNP.

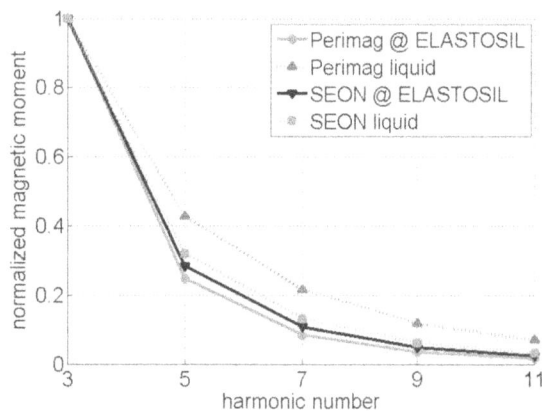

Figure 1: MPS measurements of liquid and immobilized perimag®- and SEON^{LA-BSA} -particles.

The MPS measurements revealed a decrease of the higher harmonics after embedding the MNP into the polymer (see Fig. 1). In repeated MPS measurements, no changes of the magnetic properties were found for all particle types immobilized in the synthetic polymer, and thus they show a long-term stable behavior for up to one year now.

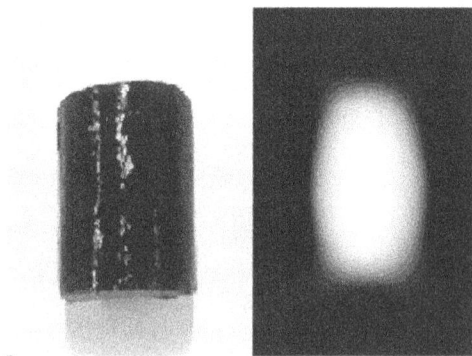

Figure 2: Left: A cylindrical phantom with diameter = height = 13 mm and an iron concentration of 20 mmol/l. Right: The reconstructed MPI-image of the phantom (slice of phantom center).

Of all tested materials, the combination perimag®/ethanol/ELASTOSIL® was the most promising regarding long-term stability and signal performance and was used for the preparation of the phantoms. The imaging of the prepared phantoms with an acceptable spatial resolution was successful (see Fig. 2) down to iron-concentration of c(Fe) = 20mmol/l.

IV. Discussion

With the establishment of an ethanol transfer procedure to embed the MNP into a synthetic polymer matrix, we achieved a way to provide long-term stable MNP phantoms for MPI imaging applications.

We have determined the magnetic properties of phantom materials by means of MPS. Several effects cause the decrease of the higher odd harmonics in the MPS-spectra. The most influencing factor is the immobilization of the MNP in the synthetic matrix, whereby the Brownian rotation of the particles is suppressed. For smaller particles (SEON^{LA-BSA}, fluidMag-D50), which show a smaller proportion of Brownian contribution, this decrease is less pronounced.

The MPI-measurements are influenced by the above-mentioned immobilization effect, too. Due to the lower MPI performance of the immobilized particles, the cylindrical shapes of the phantoms are not reconstructed correctly and appear more elliptical.

V. Conclusions

Here we present suitable combinations of commercial MNP and a polymer for the manufacture of magnetically and physically long-term stable MPI phantoms. The phantoms possess constant magnetic and mechanical properties for at least one year and are capable for MPI. Continuing work will be focused on the provision of defined, more structured MPI measurement objects with a homogeneous particle distribution.

ACKNOWLEDGEMENTS

This work was supported by Deutsche Forschungsgemeinschaft (DFG) (FKZ: AL 552/8-1, DU 1293/6-1 and TR408/9-1).

REFERENCES

[1] B. Gleich and J. Weizenecker. Tomographic imaging using the nonlinear response of magnetic particles. Nature, 435(7046):1217-1217, 2005. doi: 10.1038/nature03808.

[2] N. Panagiotopoulos, R. L. Duschka, M. Ahlborg et al., Magnetic particle imaging: current developments and future directions, International journal of nanomedicine, vol. 10, pp. 3097-114, 2015, doi: https://doi.org/10.2147/IJN.S70488

[3] T. Knopp and T. M. Buzug. Magnetic Particle Imaging: An Introduction to Imaging Principles and Scanner Instrumentation. Springer, Berlin/Heidelberg, 2012. doi: 10.1007/978-3-642-04199-0.

[4] J. J. Konkle, P. W. Goodwill, O. M. Carrasco-Zevallos et al., Projection reconstruction magnetic particle imaging, IEEE Transactions on Medical Imaging, vol. 32, no. 2, pp. 338-347, Feb, 2013. doi: 10.1109/TMI.2012.2227121

[5] P. Vogel et al. Traveling wave Magnetic Particle Imaging, IEEE TMI, 33(2), 400-7, 2014. doi: 10.1109/TMI.2013.2285472

Towards Standardized MPI Measurements

P. Szwargulski [a,b,*], P. Vogel [c,d], M.A. Rückert [c], M. Straub [e], M. Graeser [a,b], T. Knopp [a,b], V. Schulz [e], V.C. Behr [c]

[a] Section for Biomedical Imaging, University Medical Center Hamburg-Eppendorf, Hamburg, Germany
[b] Institute for Biomedical Imaging, Hamburg University of Technology, Hamburg, Germany
[c] Department of Experimental Physics 5 (Biophysics), University of Würzburg, Würzburg, Germany
[d] Dep. of Diagnostic and Interventional Radiology, University Hospital Würzburg, Würzburg, Germany
[e] Department of Physics of Molecular Imaging Systems, RWTH Aachen University, Aachen, Germany
[*] Corresponding author, email: p.szwargulski@uke.de

I. Introduction

Magnetic particle imaging (MPI) is a tomographic imaging method that utilizes the non-linear magnetization response of super-paramagnetic iron oxide nanoparticles to oscillating magnetic fields [1]. MPI provides a positive contrast and is capable of sensitive imaging with a high spatial and temporal resolution. The concrete imaging performance depends on a variety of parameters. The spatial resolution is mainly influenced by the applied gradient, the particle system [2] and on the signal to noise ratio (SNR) of the measurement data. The temporal resolution depends on the applied imaging sequence but also on the desired spatial resolution. The physical detection limit of an MPI system is given by the receive chain dominated by thermal noise.

Worldwide more than 20 MPI scanners have been developed of which each has a unique innovation over previous systems [3]. In addition, several different image reconstruction approaches are available making it almost impossible to compare the results of the different MPI systems. In this work we measure the same phantom in three different MPI scanners and report on the challenges in making comparative MPI measurements and phantoms [4].

II. Material and Methods

II.I. Phantom

To compare the different systems of Würzburg, Aachen, and Hamburg a standardized 3D phantom has been designed and manufactured (3D printer Form 2, Formlabs). The phantom consists of a spiral in the horizontal plane and has a size of about 14 mm × 15.5 mm × 1 mm. The spiral has a lead of 3.2 mm and is built out of 2.5 turns resulting in an arc length of 65.3 mm. The cutout is a circle with a diameter of 1 mm. A schematic view of the phantom is shown in Fig. 1 (right). Each phantom was filled with undiluted Perimag (MicroMod, Germany, conc. 2.8 mg/ml, Lot: 03216102-1). The size of the spiral was matched to fit into the field of view (FoV) of each scanner and the outer dimensions of the phantom were chosen such that the phantom fits into each imaging bore.

II.II. Würzburg

The Traveling Wave MPI (TWMPI) scanner uses a dynamic linear gradient array for the generation and linear movement of several field-free points (FFPs) through the system (dynamic selection field) [5]. With additional saddle-coil pairs (drive field) several trajectories are realizable to cover the FoV in 2D or 3D [6].

For scanning the mentioned phantom, a modified slice-scanning mode was used to scan a FoV of 65 mm × 29 mm with the frequencies $f_1 = 723.57$ Hz and $f_2 = 16823$ Hz. The scan was performed with an non-isotropic gradient in x and y direction with a maximum strength of 3.05 T/(m·μ_0) and a drive field amplitude of 140 mT/μ_0 (peak-to-peak). The entire acquisition time was 2 sec with 100 averages. For reconstruction a time data based algorithm was used that applies an image-based system matrix approach [7]. A pixel size of 0.5 mm and a reconstruction grid of 57 × 141 was chosen. For calculating the pseudo inverse a truncated singular value deposition algorithm is performed.

II.III. Aachen

The measurements at the RWTH Aachen were performed on a small lifeform demonstrator originally built by Philips Research [8] shown in Fig. 1. The scanner features a gradient of -$G_z = 2 \cdot G_y = 2 \cdot G_x = 5.5$ T/(m·μ_0). Excitation amplitudes of 23/22/8 mT/μ_0 (peak-to-peak) were used in x, y, and z directions, respectively. The data was acquired along a 3D Lissajous trajectory with a repetition time of 21.54 ms. Block averaging over 20 periods lead to an acquisition time of 430.8 ms. The system matrix was measured on a grid of 45 × 33 × 13 voxels covering a FoV of 22 × 16 × 12 mm³ using a 1 × 1 × 1 mm³ delta-sample.

The raw data was reconstructed with the Kaczmarz algorithm with a non-negativity constraint [9]. Only those frequencies with an SNR of at least 2 were used for reconstruction. Reconstruction was performed with 100 iterations. No regularization was applied during reconstruction.

II.IV. Hamburg

The measurements at the UKE in Hamburg were performed with the Bruker preclinical FFP-MPI Scanner (Bruker Biospin MRI GmbH, Ettlingen, Germany) shown in Fig. 1.

A 2D Lissajous sequence was applied in the *xy*-plane (horizontal) of the scanner. For signal detection a custom receive coil developed in [10] was used. The acquisition was performed with a selection field gradient of $-G_z = 2 \cdot G_y = 2 \cdot G_x = 2.5$ T/(m·μ_0) and with an excitation amplitude of 28 mT/μ_0 (peak-to-peak) in the two excitation directions. The acquisition time was 0.6 ms without averaging. The system matrix was measured on a $35 \times 35 \times 1$ grid covering a field of view of $25 \times 25 \times 1$ mm^3 using a $1 \times 1 \times 1$ mm^3 delta-sample.

The same reconstruction method as in Aachen was used with an SNR threshold of 2.3, 10 Kaczmarz iterations and an additional Tikhonov regularization (relative lambda of 10^{-4} [11]).

III. Results

The reconstruction results for each scanner are shown in Fig. 1. For the 3D data measured in Aachen only the central slice through the phantom is shown. As can be seen each scanner is capable of reconstructing the basic shape of the phantom whereas each scanner suffers from different distortions.

IV. Discussion

The results show that different MPI scanners are capable of imaging the essential features of the shown phantom. Each research group manually tuned the acquisition parameters to obtain the best image in terms of spatial resolution while maximizing the temporal resolution by using a minimum number of block averages.

While the basic features of the phantom could be resolved by all scanners one can see various differences in the image quality, the temporal resolution, and the size of the FoV. The image measured in Aachen has the highest spatial resolution due to the highest gradient strength. The Würzburg system has the largest FoV due to its TWMPI concept. The image measured at UKE has a remarkable high spatial resolution for a system with only 1.25 T/(m·μ_0) gradient strength and 0.6 ms acquisition time, but only in 2D. Using a 3D sequence, the phantom could not be resolved at the UKE. The reason for this must be find out and the process is pending.

Besides an initial qualitative comparison of the reconstruction results, it is currently not possible to directly compare the systems themselves, since this would require using the same or equivalent scanning parameter. For a detailed comparison, the spiral phantom would not be suitable. Instead it will be necessary to develop a set of dynamic, resolution and sensitivity phantoms that cover different FoV sizes. Furthermore, reconstruction algorithms would need to be standardized.

V. Conclusions

The comparison of different scanner architectures, imaging sequences, and reconstruction algorithms is a challenging task that has been neglected in most research publications so far. With the current work we made the first step towards comparability of different MPI systems. We plan to develop such a set of phantoms in future work.

REFERENCES

[1] B. Gleich and J. Weizenecker, *Nature*, 435(7046):1217-1217, 2005.
[2] J. Rahmer et al., *BMC Med. Imag.*, 9(1):4. 2009.
[3] T. Knopp et al., *Phys. Med. Biol.*, 62(14):R124. 2017.
[4] L. Wöckel et al. *Proc. on GFW*, 16:120-2, 2017
[5] P. Vogel et al. *IEEE Trans. Med. Imag.*, 33(2):400-407, 2014.
[6] P. Vogel et al. *IJMPI*, 3(2):1706001, 2017.
[7] P. Vogel et al. *IJMPI*, 2(2):1611001, 2016.
[8] J. Weizenecker et al. *Phys. Med. Biol.*, 54(5):L1–L10, 2009.
[9] A. Dax, *SISC*, 14(3):570–584, 1993.
[10] M. Graeser et al., *Sci. Rep.*, 7:6872, 2017.
[11] T. Knopp, et al., *Phys. Med. Biol.*, 55(6):1577-1589, 2010.

Evaluation of Different SPIONs for Their Potential as MPI-Tracers

Stefan Lyer [a,*], Maik Liebl [b], Tobias Bäuerle[c], Michael Uder [c], Arnd Dörfler [d], Frank Wiekhorst [b], Christoph Alexiou [a]

[a] *Universitätsklinikum Erlangen, ENT-Department, Section of Experimental Oncology and Nanomedicine (SEON), Else-Kröner-Fresenius Stiftung-Professorship, Erlangen, Germany*
[b] *Physikalisch-Technische Bundesanstalt, Berlin, Germany*
[c] *Universitätsklinikum Erlangen, Department of Radiology, Erlangen, Germany*
[d] *Universitätsklinikum Erlangen, Department of Neuroradiology, Erlangen, Germany*
[*] *Corresponding author, email: stefan.lyer@uk-erlangen.de*

I. Introduction

The use of SPIONs as contrast agents had limited acceptance in Magnetic resoncance imaging (MRI) due to several reasons. One of the most prevalent ones for sure was the negative (black) contrast based on a signal extinction in T2, T2* and susceptibility sensitive T1 weighted images in MRI. Therefore, radiologists preferred gadolinium based contrast agents with a positive signal enhancement, which is easier to evaluate.

On the other hand, gadolinium based contrast agents have been come under discussion, because it was shown, that multiple administrations could lead to deposition of gadolinium in areas of the brain of humans [1, 2] but also of laboratory animals [3].

Magnetic particle imaging (MPI) facilitates iron oxide nanoparticles as tracers. In this imaging modality, SPIONs lead to a positive contrast [4], which could lead to a better acceptance.

In this work, we therefore aimed on testing and comparing different self-developed nanoparticle systems for their initial MPI-performance by Magnetic Particle Spectroscopy (MPS). MPS can be considered as zero-dimensional MPI with much less technical effort. MPS is capable to provide a sound assessment of the MPI performance. This allows then for further optimization of the tracers for Magnetic Particle Imaging.

II. Material and Methods

II.I. SPION systems used

Three different iron oxid nanoparticle systems were used. The first, SEON[Dex] was prepared by *in situ* precipitation in a dextran solution and subsequent crosslinking of the dextran matrix [5]. For this system, initial testing have been performed for evaluating the MRI-performance, too [6].

The second SPION-system was synthesized by performing wet precipitation and a subsequent coating with the fatty acid lauric acid (SEON[LA]).

The third (SEON[BSA]) was further coated with a serum albumin shell to improve the colloidal stability in salt solutions and especially in blood [7].

II.I. MPS-Measurement

Magnetic particle spectroscopy (MPS) measurements of the SEON systems were performed using a commercial magnetic particle spectrometer (Bruker, Germany) as previously described in detail [8]. MPS detects specifically the non-linear magnetic response of magnetic nanoparticles exposed to an oscillating magnetic field.

For the MPS measurements samples of 10 μL were filled into polymerase chain reaction (PCR) compatible fast reaction tubes (Applied Biosystems, Darmstadt, Germany) and placed into the pick-up coil of the MPS system. The magnetic response of the samples to an AC magnetic field of a frequency f_0 of 25 kHz and an amplitude B_{excit} of 25 mT is recorded for 10 s.

From the time dependent signal, the harmonics spectrum of magnetic moments is obtained by Fourier transformation showing prominent amplitudes at odd multiples of f_0 evoked by the magnetic nanoparticles while the signal at the drive frequency is suppressed by filtering to avoid saturation of the amplifier electronics.

By normalizing the harmonic A_k of the spectrum to the absolute nanoparticle iron content of the sample the specific MPI performance of the tracer is obtained. From the magnetic moment sensitivity of the device (about $5 \cdot 10^{-12}$ Am^2) and the measured A_3 amplitude, we estimated an MNP specific detection limit for the different MNP systems.

III. Results

The MPS-spectrum of SEON^{Dex} shows, that although the MRI-performance is quite well, the signal in MPS is very week. Therefore, we can say that this nanoparticle system is not suitable as tracer for MPI in the present state.

The SEON^{LA}-system seems to be comparable with the performance of Resovist®, with nearly the same values at low harmonic numbers.

The SEON^{BSA}-system, which is basing on the SEON^{LA}-System also showed comparable results like SEON^{LA} and Resovist®.

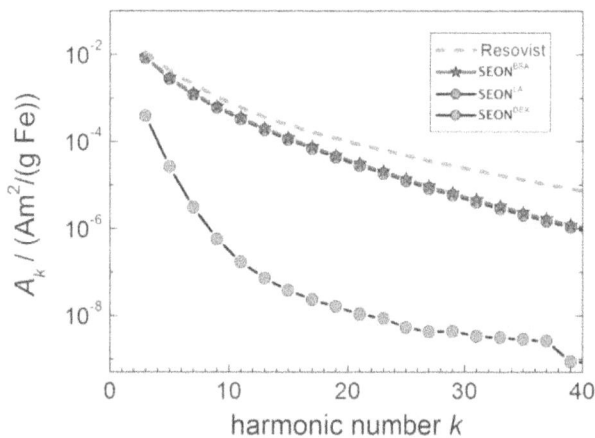

Figure 1: *Normalized MPS spectra at 25 mT of three different nanoparticle systems compared to Resovist®.*

IV. Discussion

In earlier studies, the nanoparticle system showed a tremendously well biocompatibility and a good *in vitro* performance in MRI. Since an excellent *in vivo* biocompatibility is an ultimate prerequisite for SPIONs to be used as contrast agents, we hoped that this system also had a reasonable signal in MPS. Unfortunately, the signal is very low in MPS, therefore it seems to be not suitable under the present MPI hardware preconditions for being used as an MPI tracer.

On the other hand, the spectra of SEON^{LA} and SEON^{BSA} showed signals comparable to Resovist®. Therefore, it is reasonable to have a closer look at these particle systems. Taking into account *in vivo* biocompatibility, the LA-coated nanoparticles did not show very good colloidal stability in blood [7]. But, on the other hand, the further improved system with an additional serum albumin coating showed a very well behavior in blood [7].

V. Conclusions

This work sets the baseline results for the three tested nanoparticle systems regarding their use as MPI-tracers. The results show a week signal of SEON^{DEX} in MPS. Therefore, it cannot be used as MPI-tracer in the present form with the actual MPI-scanners.

The signals of the other two systems based on nanoclusters stabilized with a coating of only lauric acid and serum albumin were comparable with the signal of Resovist®. Taking into account the *in vivo* biocompa-tibility, the

serum albumin coated SEON^{BSA} seem to be the best candidate. Nevertheless, we are interested in how changing different parameters of the synthesis will influence the imaging behavior and biocompatibility. Therefore, we now have started systematically investigating this based on the study presented here.

ACKNOWLEDGEMENTS
For financial support, we would like to thank the DFG (AL552/8-1) and (Wi 4230/1-2).

REFERENCES

[1] M.C.R. Espagnet, B. Bernardi, L. Pasquini, L. Figa-Talamanca, P. Toma, A. Napolitano, Signal intensity at unenhanced T1-weighted magnetic resonance in the globus pallidus and dentate nucleus after serial administrations of a macrocyclic gadolinium-based contrast agent in children, Pediatr. Radiol. 47(10) (2017) 1345-1352.

[2] T. Kanda, Y. Nakai, H. Oba, K. Toyoda, K. Kitajima, S. Furui, Gadolinium deposition in the brain, Magn. Reson. Imaging 34(10) (2016) 1346-1350.

[3] R.J. McDonald, J.S. McDonald, D.Y. Dai, D. Schroeder, M.E. Jentoft, D.L. Murray, R. Kadirvel, L.J. Eckel, D.F. Kallmes, Comparison of Gadolinium Concentrations within Multiple Rat Organs after Intravenous Administration of Linear versus Macrocyclic Gadolinium Chelates, Radiology 285(2) (2017) 536-545.

[4] J. Borgert, J.D. Schmidt, I. Schmale, J. Rahmer, C. Bontus, B. Gleich, B. David, R. Eckart, O. Woywode, J. Weizenecker, J. Schnorr, M. Taupitz, J. Haegele, F.M. Vogt, J. Barkhausen, Fundamentals and applications of magnetic particle imaging, Journal of cardiovascular computed tomography 6(3) (2012) 149-53.

[5] H. Unterweger, R. Tietze, C. Janko, J. Zaloga, S. Lyer, S. Durr, N. Taccardi, O.M. Goudouri, A. Hoppe, D. Eberbeck, D.W. Schubert, A.R. Boccaccini, C. Alexiou, Development and characterization of magnetic iron oxide nanoparticles with a cisplatin-bearing polymer coating for targeted drug delivery, Int J Nanomed 9 (2014) 3659-3676.

[6] H. Unterweger, C. Janko, M. Schwarz, L. Dezsi, R. Urbanics, J. Matuszak, E. Orfi, T. Fulop, T. Bauerle, J. Szebeni, C. Journe, A.R. Boccaccini, C. Alexiou, S. Lyer, I. Cicha, Non-immunogenic dextran-coated superparamagnetic iron oxide nanoparticles: a biocompatible, size-tunable contrast agent for magnetic resonance imaging, Int J Nanomed 12 (2017) 5223-5238.

[7] J. Zaloga, C. Janko, J. Nowak, J. Matuszak, S. Knaup, D. Eberbeck, R. Tietze, H. Unterweger, R.P. Friedrich, S. Duerr, R. Heimke-Brink, E. Baum, I. Cicha, F. Dorje, S. Odenbach, S. Lyer, G. Lee, C. Alexiou, Development of a lauric acid/albumin hybrid iron oxide nanoparticle system with improved biocompatibility, Int J Nanomed 9 (2014) 4847-4866.

[8] W.C. Poller, N. Löwa, F. Wiekhorst, M. Taupitz, S. Wagner, K. Möller, G. Baumann, V. Stangl, L. Trahms, A. Ludwig. Magnetic particle spectroscopy reveals dynamic changes in the magnetic behavior of very small superparamagnetic iron oxide nanoparticles during cellular uptake and enables determination of cell-labeling efficacy. J Biomed Nanotechnol 12 (2016) 337-346.

Session 07 - Posters

Instrumentation II

Excitation and Receive Unit for a Rotating Permanent Magnet Based MPI System

Matthias Weber [a], Justin Ackers [a], Jonas Beuke [a, *], and Thorsten M. Buzug [a]

[a] Institute of Medical Engineering, University of Luebeck, Luebeck, Germany
[*] Corresponding author, email: beuke@imt.uni-luebeck.de

I. Introduction

The simulation, design and construction of customized excitation and receive coils for Magnetic Particle Imaging (MPI) systems is a complex as well as iterative process. This is especially the case if multiple coils and shields have to be considered and optimized. Recently, we presented a second-generation permanent magnet based MPI system (see Fig. 1) that features a field free line (FFL) which drastically reduces the complexity of the utilized excitation and receive coil [1,2]. The key property of this system is the realization of three-dimensional imaging by utilizing only a single excitation and receive channel. Other FFL MPI systems either rely on generating solely projection images [3] or consist out of a complex signal chain [4].

In this paper, we present the development of an optimized shielded excitation and receive unit which is based on the open source simulation framework FEMM (Finite Element Method Magnetics by David Meeker). This approach offers realistic simulation results which hence, simplify the subsequent construction process.

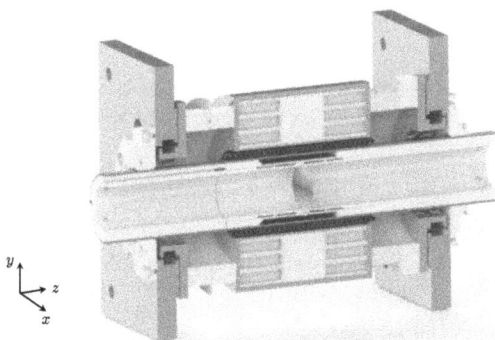

Figure 1: The image above shows a sectional view of our permanent magnet based FFL MPI system.

II. Material and Methods

The gradient field on the x/y-plane featuring the FFL (shown in Fig. 1) solely consists out of magnetic field components pointing in z-direction. It is generated by two Halbach arrays of second order that are circularly aligned around the bore (note that the dipoles are contrary aligned). Hence, it is possible to utilize a solenoid as a drive field coil (DFC) to shift the FFL on the x/y-plane for any angle

of rotation. Accordingly, a cylindrical receive coil (RFC) can be used to acquire the particle signal. Here, the cylindrical design facilitates the straightforward construction of a gradiometric RFC. Since the MPI system features a strong gradient of 5 T/m, it is necessary to include a focus field coil (FFC) which can also be constructed as a solenoid. To minimize external disturbance signals, DFC and RFC are surrounded by a copper shield.

Since all coil geometries as well as the copper shield are rotational symmetric, the simulation of the excitation and receive unit can be reduced to a two-dimensional problem. Here, we use the simulation framework FEMM to analyze and optimize the coil configuration. In FEMM, a sectional view through the coils can be analyzed as it is shown Fig. 2. This view represents the y/z-plane in the MPI system from Fig. 1.

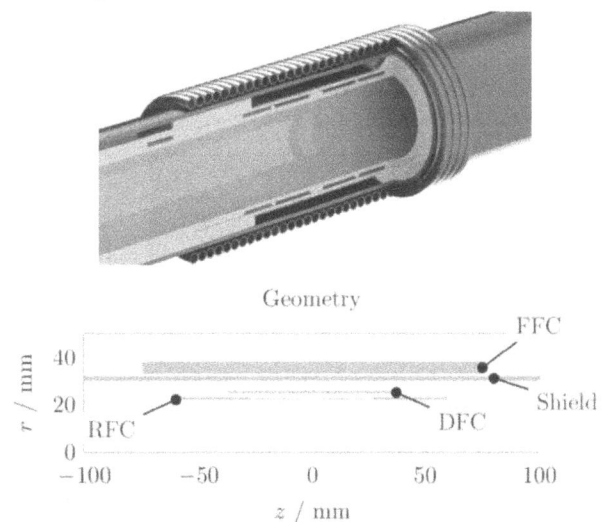

Figure 2: Sectional CAD-view of the excitation and receive unit (top image) and two-dimensional view of the unit as it is represented in FEMM (bottom image).

The RFC is aligned closest to the field of view and consists out of four parts. The left and right part feature two layers of windings and the two inner parts a single layer. Inner and outer part feature opposing winding direction to enable a cancellation of the excitation signal. The DFC surrounds the RFC and is designed for a field amplitude of 20 mT at

60 A peak. The excitation frequency is 25 kHz. Furthermore, the RFC is fitted to the field profile of the DFC in presence of the copper shield since the shield highly influences the field profile (see Fig. 3).

Finally, RFC and DFC are surrounded by the copper shield and the FFC which consists out of hollow copper wire.

III. Results

Fig. 3 shows the simulated fields of the DFC (with and without shielding) and respectively the field of the RFC. As one can see, the copper shielding highly influences the generated magnetic field of the DFC. The flux lines are enclosed inside the copper shield. As a consequence, the field amplitude is dampened and power is dissipated in the shield. However, coupling between DFC and FFC is avoided. Hereafter, only the shielded case is considered.

In our optimized FEMM simulation, a maximum amplitude of 3 V is induced in the RFC by the DFC (B_{pp} = 42 mT, I_{pp} = 120 A, f = 25 kHz, P = 2 kW, L = 48 µH, R = 556 mΩ).

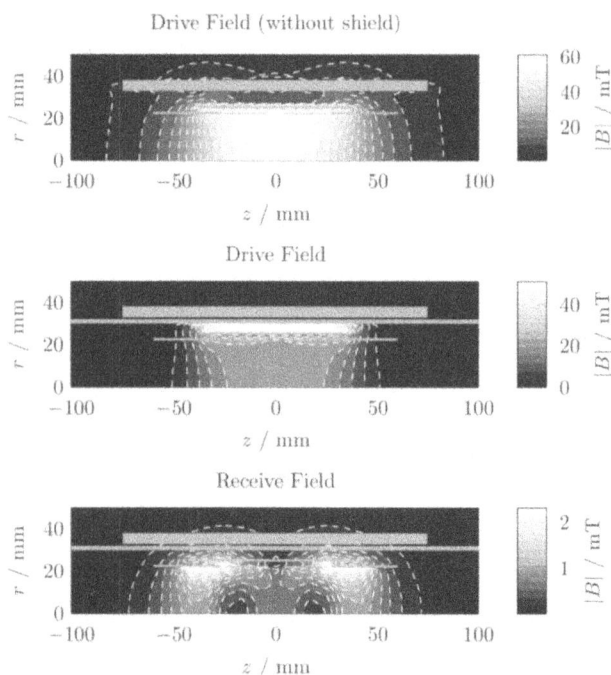

Figure 3: The plots depict the excitation and receive coil unit in a sectional view. The shield highly influences the magnetic field of the DFC at 25 kHz and I_{pp} = 120 A.

Based on the FEMM simulation, a first prototype was constructed with the help of an Ultimaker 3 (PLA material), enameled copper wire (DFC) and Litz wire (RFC).

In a first measurement, we were able to test the gradiometer approach of the RFC. Here, only 14 V were induced by the DFC at I_{pp} = 120 A. Furthermore, the DFC has an inductance of L = 48 µH and a resistance of R = 584 mΩ at 25 kHz.

Fig. 4 shows the constructed RFC with its double layer winding on the left and right and the single layer in the center.

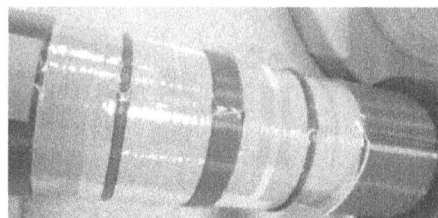

Figure 4: Realized RFC with gradiometer technique.

IV. Discussion

FEMM offers a great framework to analyze rotational symmetric electromagnetic problems. We were able to show that this especially the case for the excitation and receive coil unit in our current permanent magnet based scanner. The DFC and RFC prototype agrees well with the simulation. However, the induced voltage in lab setup is slightly higher than in the FEMM simulation. A further improvement will be possible by constructing the coil holders with CNC technology. Already small geometric inaccuracies as e.g. a shift between DFC and RFC might result in a higher induced voltage. Furthermore, we are currently planning to water-cool the coil and the shield. This will allow for temperature stable instrumentation and the possibility of long time measurements.

V. Conclusions

FEMM is a well-suited and realistic tool to simulate and optimize all important coil parameters for our permanent magnet based FFL MPI scanner. In the future, we will be able to further improve the sensitivity as well as the image quality of our system. As a next step, the development of an FFL MPI head scanner based on FEMM can be carried out.

ACKNOWLEDGEMENTS

We would like to thank Deutsche Forschungsgemeinschaft (DFG, FKZBU 1436/10-1) for their financial support.

REFERENCES

[1] M. Weber, K. Bente, S. Bruns, A. von Gladiss, M. Graeser, and T. M. Buzug. *A 1.4 T/m Field Free Line Magnetic Particle Imaging Device.* 6th International Workshop on Magnetic Particle Imaging (IWMPI), 2016.

[2] M. Weber and T. M. Buzug. *Novel Field Geometry featuring a Field Free Line for Magnetic Particle Imaging.* 7th International Workshop on Magnetic Particle Imaging (IWMPI), 2017.

[3] J. J. Konkle, P. W. Goodwill, O. M. Carrasco-Zevallos, and S. M. Conolly. *Projection Reconstruction Magnetic Particle Imaging.* IEEE Trans. Med. Imaging, 32(2):338-347, Feb. 2013. doi: 10.1109/TMI.2012.2227121.

[4] K. Bente, M. Weber, M. Graeser, T. F. Sattel, M. Erbe, and T. M. Buzug. *Electronic Field Free Line Rotation and Relaxation Deconvolution in Magnetic Particle Imaging.* IEEE Trans. Med. Imaging, 34(2):644-651, Feb. 2015. doi: 10.1109/TMI.2014.2364891

An Acoustic Magnetic Particle Spectrometer

Eric Aderhold [a], Thorsten M. Buzug [a], Thomas Friedrich [a,*]

[a] *Institute of Medical Engineering, Universität zu Lübeck, Lübeck, Germany* [b]
* Corresponding author, email: friedrich@imt.uni-luebeck.de

I. Introduction

In magnetic particle imaging (MPI), the concentration of superparamagnetic iron oxide nanoparticles (SPION) can be resolved spatially. Therefore, a magnetic sinusoidal excitation field of sufficient amplitude causes a periodic change in the particle magnetization. Due to the nonlinear magnetization curve of the SPIONs, the resulting magnetization of the particles shows a spectrum of harmonics. This spectrum is usually measured by means of the voltage it induces in a receive coil. To achieve spatial resolution, gradient fields serve for spatial encoding. Both fields together form a periodically moving field-free point (FFP) within the detection volume. Particles that are sufficiently far away from the FFP are magnetically saturated and do not contribute to the received signal.

A possible alternative to the electromagnetic excitation and detection was proposed by Gleich et al. in 2011 [1]. With a magnetic sample being covered by the trajectory of the FFP, the sample experiences a periodic force due to the periodic change of the magnetic moment. This can lead to sound waves in the surrounding medium. As the force acting on the sample depends on the nonlinear magnetization behavior of the particles, the produced sound will also show a spectrum of harmonics. It is possible to record a system function of the detected sound waves and therefore image reconstruction should be possible. In this paper, it is suggested, to use the described magneto acoustic signal chain to gather various parameters (such as elastic coefficients or temperature) of the biological tissue surrounding a bolus of SPIONs. A change in the recorded spectrum can be expected, when the Brownian relaxation alters due to changes of mechanical properties of the surrounding material, which influences the particle motion and the propagation of the sound wave. In this paper, a basic acoustic magnetic particle spectrometer is described, and experimental data are shown.

II. Material and Methods

The sample cell (see Fig. 1) with field generator, acoustic detector and sample mount are located inside a housing, which serves as an electromagnetic and acoustic shielding, to minimize disturbances from the lab.

In the field generator a pair of coaxially opposing cylindrical NdFeB magnets generate the selection field.

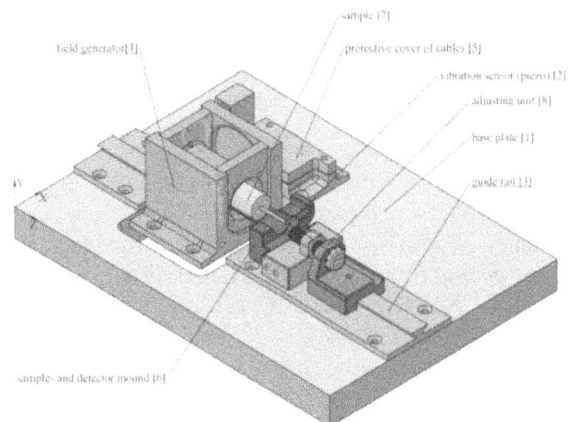

***Figure 1**: Overview of the measuring unit*

The gradient strength in axial direction was measured with a hall probe (LakeShore Gaussmeter 475) to 5.9 T/m. This gradient field is superimposed by the field of a solenoid with 450 turns and an inner diameter of 20 mm. Its impedance was measured to 4.1 Ω at 700 Hz and as this is the optimal range of the used amplifier (AE Techron 2105), it is directly connected without an impedance matching network. The magnetic flux density generated by the empty coil was measured with the hall probe mentioned earlier. Linear regression yields a flux density per current of 9.1 mT/A. The coil was solely excited with 1 A preventing the excessive generation of heat which could lead into thermal problems. The detection is done by the means of a self-made contact microphone, consisting of a commercially available piezoelectric vibration sensor [2]. The voltage signal generated by this vibration sensor is amplified by a low-noise amplifier (SR 560, Stanford Research Systems) and recorded with the sound card of a personal computer.

To guarantee the always same excitation, with the same number of periods and the same phasing, the excitation signal is also generated in the sound card, working in (full) duplex mode. This way excitation- and recording-signal will have the same phase, as well as different recordings among each other, and therefore background correction with previously recorded measurements as well as signal averaging to improve the SNR are possible.

To minimize the recording of the excitation signal, due to direct acoustic interlink between field generator and detector, excitation and detection were spatially separated.

A clearance in the base plate was filled with acoustic absorber foam and the field generator was positioned above, in order to absorb most of the excitation signal. Newly prepared silicone samples, filled with a volume of powdery SPIONs (12.6 mm^3, Fe_3O_4, CAS 1317-61-9), were constructed and placed on the semicircular shell segment of the sample- and detector mount. Thus, the samples are as well acoustically decoupled, which together with the decoupling of the field generator leads to a better resolution of the particle signal.

To enable the measurement of system functions, well defined positions of the sample compared to the FFP are mandatory. Therefore, an adjusting unit, capable of performing a linear feed of 0.05 mm per step is attached to the sample- and detector mount.

III. Results

In order to measure the acoustic response to the magnetic excitation, the sound card generates a sine wave with a frequency of 500 Hz. This voltage signal is amplified by the power amplifier. The gain is set accordingly to apply a current of 1 A in amplitude to the excitation coil. This leads to a resulting flux density of 9.1 mT in amplitude that periodically displaces the FFP by ± 1.72 mm. In a first step, the background signal of the sample without magnetic material and then the magneto acoustic response of the sample filled with SPIONs, is measured. Both voltage signals are subtracted, and the result is averaged 100 times. Fig. 2 shows the resulting signal as well as its spectrum. Repeating these steps for different positions and extracting the amplitudes of the first, second and third harmonic leads to the system function shown in Fig. 3.

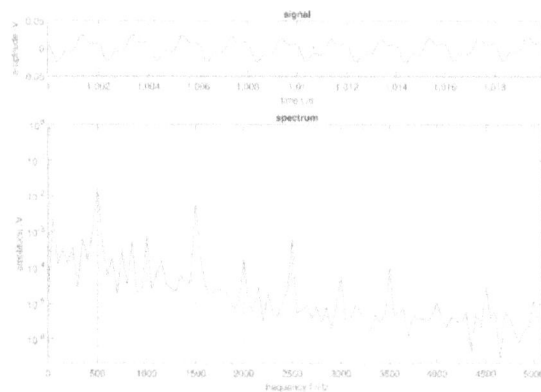

Figure 2: particle signal and spectrum

IV. Discussion

The spectrum shows up to 15 harmonics of the excitation frequency which are clearly distinguishable from the noise floor and from the excitation signal.

The axis of symmetry in the system function of the SPION sample and therefore the FFP without excitation is situated at -0.4 mm. This slight difference to the calculated FFP is due to reading errors on the analog millimeter scale. The recorded system function does not exactly show the expected graph. Nevertheless, in characteristic points

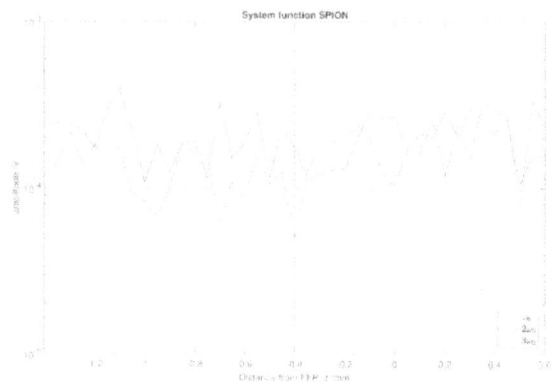

Figure 3: System function of SPION sample

(cf. -0.4 and -0.85 mm) the function shows the same extrema characteristic as predicted by simulations [1].

Additionally, it turned out that the amplitude of the particle signal is also dependent on the excitation frequency and has its maximum between 300 and 500 Hz. As this dependency might be due to the used sample material further tests with different frequencies and different samples should be carried out.

V. Conclusions

Further improvements on the existing spectrometer are conceivable. It seems reasonable to adapt the amplifiers and tailor them exactly to the existing application, or to implement signal filters in the signal chain, both leading to better signal quality.

Fundamentally, it must be analyzed what correlation exists between specific tissue properties and the amplitude spectrum. For this purpose, special samples should be developed that differ in terms of their material properties. By comparing these measurements, conclusions could be drawn.

The presented magneto acoustic spectrometer will be used for further investigations of nanoparticle-matrix interactions, possibly leading to clinical applications and insights for improved diagnostics and therapy.

ACKNOWLEDGEMENTS
This work has been financially supported by the German Federal Ministry of Education and Research (BMBF grant number 13GW0069A aka SAMBA PATI).

REFERENCES
[1] B. Gleich and J. Weizenecker and J. Borgert: *Theory, simulation and experimental results of the acoustic detection of magnetization changes in superparamagnetic iron oxide.* BMC Medical Imaging, 11(1):16, 2011. doi: 10.1186/1471-2342-11-16.
[2] RS-Components. *Datasheet, vibration sensor,* order code 285-784. 2016. http://de.rs-online.com/webdocs/009f/0900766b8009f3f3.pdf

iMPI – inverted Magnetic Particle Imaging

Fabian Piekarek [a,*] **Patrick Vogel** [a,b], **Martin A. Rückert** [a], **Jonathan Markert** [a,c], **Thomas Kampf** [c],
Thorsten A. Bley [b], **Volker C. Behr** [a]

[a] *Department of Experimental Physics 5 (Biophysics), University of Würzburg, 97074 Würzburg, Germany*
[b] *Department of Diagnostic and Interventional Radiology, University Hospital Würzburg, 97080 Würzburg, Germany*
[c] *Department of Diagnostic and Interventional Neuroradiology, University Hospital Würzburg, 97080 Würzburg, Germany*
[*] *Corresponding author, email: Fabian.Piekarek@uni-wuerzburg.de*

I. Introduction

Most Magnetic Particle Imaging (MPI) scanners have a tubular design to analyze three-dimensional objects [1]. For that, a strong gradient represented by a field-free point (FFP) or field-free line (FFL) is generated and steered through the sample to create a non-linear response of magnetic materials [2]. But is that the best and easiest way to study two-dimensional samples?

Since several approaches have been demonstrated for single-sided MPI [3, 4], their aim is to scan objects in 3D. In this abstract, a novel single-sided design for imaging flat two-dimensional samples such as bacteria layers is presented inverting the basic idea of MPI. Instead of a field-free point, a spatially localized field is moved across the sample of encoding.

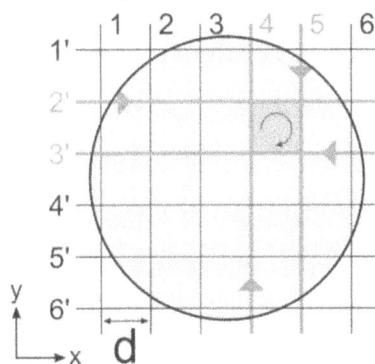

Figure 1: *Scheme of the grid with the circuit pattern for single pixel excitation. At this grid point, the magnetic field is amplified. The current flows through the red wires and the arrows indicate the direction. The grey area represents the global receiving coil (z-direction).*

II. Materials and Methods

The aim is to put a specimen in a constant magnetic (offset) field and amplify certain points with an excitation field modulating the field at specific positions selectively to create higher harmonics. Four wires out of a two dimensional grid [5] consisting of two sets of parallel wires oriented orthogonally with respect to each other form a

loop (see Fig. 1). Due to the offset field (z-direction) and the localized periodical modulation of the magnetic field at this point (marked in red), magnetic material in the vicinity of this 'pixel' generates odd as well as even higher harmonics, which can be measured inductively with a global receive coil (z-direction).

By sequential modulating the field at all points, the image can be rasterized pixel-by-pixel.

II.I. Grid size

The specimen is placed directly on the grid in a Petri dish, giving a distance to the surface (grid) of about 2 mm. In order to achieve maximum field strength at the height h, the wires have to be spaced at a defined wire distance d. In Fig. 2 simulation results of the magnetic field strength for different d at a given height of h=2 mm above the grid is plotted.

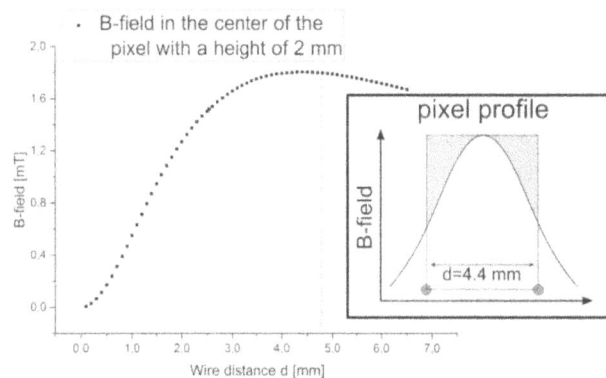

Figure 2: *The graph shows the magnetic field at the center of a 'pixel' in dependence of the wire distance d at a constant height of 2 mm. A maximum occurs at d=4.4 mm. A profile plot of the magnetic field through a pixel with d=4.4 mm is given in the subgraph.*

The graph shows a maximum of the magnetic field at a wire distance of $d_{2\,mm}$=4.4 mm. The subplot indicates the magnetic field profile inside a pixel showing an insufficient covering. To amend the resulting coarse rasterization, the number of wires is doubled reducing the wire distance to

$D=d/2$ (here $D=2.2$ mm) while maintaining the pixel size at $d=4.4$ mm. By using a wire and its second neighbor as a pair (see Fig. 3) the sample can be scanned with sub-pixel resolution.

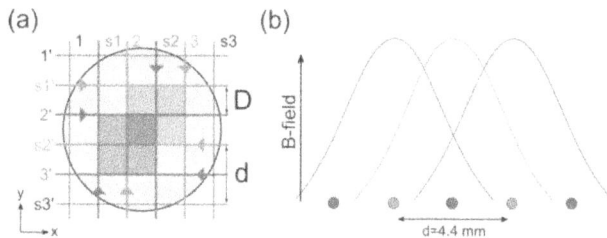

Figure 3: **(a)** *Illustration of a pixel with its subpixels.* **(b)** *Movement of a 'pixel' with sup-pixel resolution by switching the wires #2+#3+#s1'+#s2' to #s1+#s2+#2'+3', etc.*

II.I. Experimental set-up

For the construction of the grid, a wire distance of $D=2.54$ mm is selected (hole spacing of a standard breadboard). To maximize the field strength, the double hole distance of d=5.08 mm is selected for the wiring (see Fig. 3), which fundamentally simplifies the construction of the grid.

III. Results

In an initial experiment the magnetic field profile across a pixel is measured using a robot arm (Dobot Magician, Dobot, China) by moving a tiny receive coil with a diameter of 0.5 mm at a constant height over the board.

Fig. 4 (a) shows the experimental setup consisting of the grid (1) driven by a common audio amplifier (t.amp TA2400, Thomann, Germany), the offset coil (2), the robot arm (3) and the receive coil (4).

The plot in Fig. 4 (b) shows the measured profile of the magnetic field across a pixel with the wire distance of d=5.08 mm.

IV. Discussion

Since magnetic field strength reaches a maximum at a wire distance of 4.4 mm (cf. Fig. 2) there is no point in creating larger pixels. However, by reducing the wire distance an even higher number of sub-pixels should further improve the spatial encoding capability of the system.

V. Conclusion

In this abstract a novel approach for scanning flat 2D samples is presented. Instead of using a FFP or FFL for spatial encoding, localized field modulations are used which resembles a spatially localized version of MPS. This concept offers several new scanning methods such as scanning with sub-pixel resolution (super-resolution) or localized detection of ensemble dispersion.

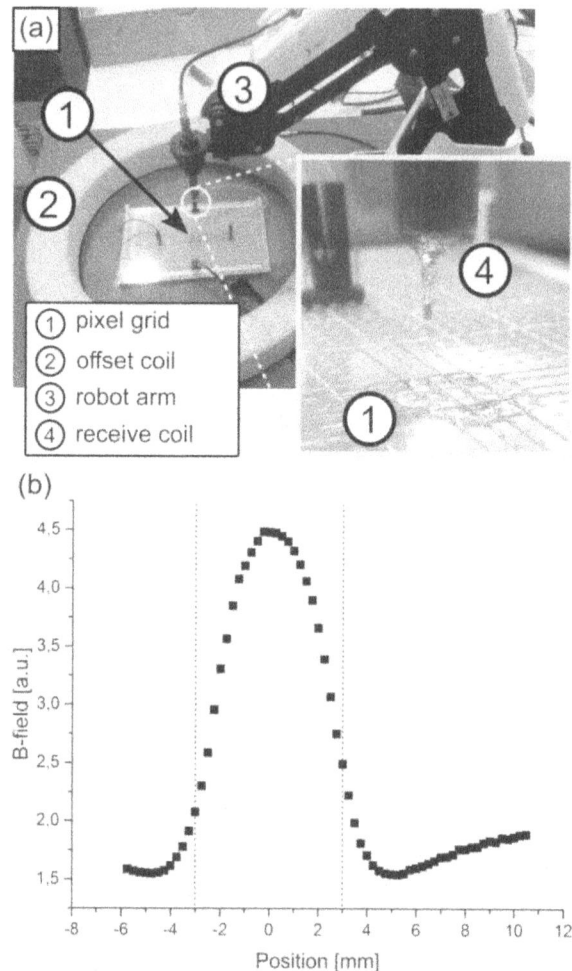

Figure 4: **(a)** *Experimental setup consisting of the breadboard with the grid (1), the offset coil (2), the robot arm (3) moving the tiny receive coil (4) with a diameter of 0.5 mm guided over the grid at a suitable height.* **(b)** *Measurement of the magnetic field profile of a pixel (step size 0.25 mm) with the distance* d=5.08 mm *at a height of 2 mm.*

REFERENCES

[1] T. Knopp, et al., Magnetic Particle Imaging: from proof of principle to preclinical applications, *Phys. Med. Biol.*, vol. 62(14), pp. R124-R178, 2017. DOI: 10.1088/1361-6560/aa6c99

[2] B. Gleich and J. Weizenecker, Tomographic imaging using the nonlinear response of magnetic particles, *Nature*, vol. 435, pp. 1214-7, 2005. Doi:10.1037/nature03808

[3] T. Sattel, et al., Single-sided device for magnetic particle imaging, *Journal of Phys. D: Appl. Phys.*, vol. 42(2):022001, 2008. Doi:10.1088/0022-3727/42/2/022001

[4] A. Tonyushkin, Single-Sided Hybrid Selection Coils for Field-Free Line Magnetic Particle Imaging, *Int. Journal on MPI*, vol. 3(1):1703009, 2017. Doi:10.18416/ijmpi.2017.1703009

[5] C.S. Lee, H. Lee, R.M. Westervelt, Microelectromagnets for the control of magnetic nanoparticles, *Appl. Phys. Lett.*, vol. 79, 3308, 2001. Doi: 10.1063/1.1419049

Hybrid Gradiometer Design for Traveling Wave Magnetic Particle Imaging

Patrick Vogel [a,b,*], Florian Fidler [c], Stefan Herz [b], Fabian Piekarek [a], Jonathan Markert [a,d], Martin A. Rückert [a], Walter H. Kullmann [d], Thorsten A. Bley [b], Volker C. Behr [a]

[a] Department of Experimental Physics 5 (Biophysics), University of Würzburg, 97074 Würzburg, Germany
[b] Department of Diagnostic and Interventional Radiology, University Hospital Würzburg, 97080 Würzburg, Germany
[c] Magnetic Resonance and X-ray Imaging MRB, Fraunhofer Institute for Integrated Circuits IIS, 97074 Würzburg, Germany
[d] Institute of Medical Engineering, University of Applied Sciences Würzburg-Schweinfurt, 97070 Würzburg, Germany
* Corresponding author, email: Patrick.Vogel@physik.uni-wuerzburg.de

I. Introduction

Gradiometer receive coils are an important tool for enhancing the signal quality in experiments measuring varying magnetic fields inductively. Several designs are possible to suppress ambient time varying magnetic fields [1]. The main purpose of a gradiometer is to minimize the influence of environmental disturbances on the acquired signal. The basic gradiometer design uses two solenoids with corresponding signals S_A and S_B assembled in opposite direction to cancel out ambient signal S_{ext} through signal subtraction offering a more sensitive detection of signals S_{sample} from a sample covered by only one of the gradiometer coils (1):

$$S_{sum} = S_A + S_B = S_{ext} - (S_{ext} + S_{sample}) = S_{sample} \quad (1)$$

With such a setup, very sensitive measurements can be performed to obtain small magnetic signals [2].

Since the first publication of Magnetic Particle Imaging [3], several different types of MPI scanners have been presented [4]. The Traveling Wave MPI (TWMPI) approach [5] is a design using a dynamic linear gradient array (dLGA) consisting of several single coil elements [6] for the generation of a strong gradient. For that the elements are driven with a sinusoidal current of a frequency f_z and a phase difference between adjacent coils of $\Delta\phi = 2\pi/N$ with N being the number of elements fitting one period in the dLGA resulting in a sinusoidal magnetic field shape traveling through the FOV. The resulting field free point (FFP) can be steered arbitrarily through the FOV on different trajectories using additional perpendicular saddle coil pairs driven with the frequencies f_x and f_y offering fast 2D and 3D imaging [7] (see Fig. 1 left).

The suppression of the excitation signal is achieved by passive high-pass or band-pass filters [5]. However, in the receiver remaining direct feedthrough can be detected, which compromise the received signal decreasing the signal-to-noise ratio (SNR) and sensitivity especially in experiments using low concentrated tracer material. Graeser et al. [8] showed, that a combination of both passive filtering and gradiometer design can enhance the sensitivity in MPI systems.

II. Material and Methods

To implement a gradiometer setup to a Traveling Wave MPI scanner firstly the magnetic fields of the scanner have to be investigated. In Fig. 1 the central sketch shows the orientation of magnetic fields for dLGA and saddle-coil pairs. While the magnetic field of the dLGA varies along the z-axis, the magnetic field of both saddle coil pairs is constant.

Equation (2) gives the magnetic field components along the symmetry axis (z-axis) depending on time t and position z. The z-component describing the field generated by the dLGA is represented by a perfectly sinusoidal field shape, which is a good approximation [6].

$$\vec{H}(t,z) = \begin{pmatrix} H_x \cdot sin(2\pi f_x t + \varphi_2) \\ H_y \cdot sin(2\pi f_y t + \varphi_3) \\ H_z \cdot sin\left(2\pi f_z t + \frac{2\pi}{l_{dLGA}} \cdot z\right) \end{pmatrix} \quad (2)$$

As mentioned before, the concept of a gradiometer is to cancel out ambient signals. Therefore, the area covered by the receive coil (RC) have to approach zero:

$$\int_{RC} \vec{H}(t,\vec{x}) \, d\vec{x} \to 0 \quad (3)$$

Expression (3) is fulfilled for any given time interval $[T, T+\tau]$.

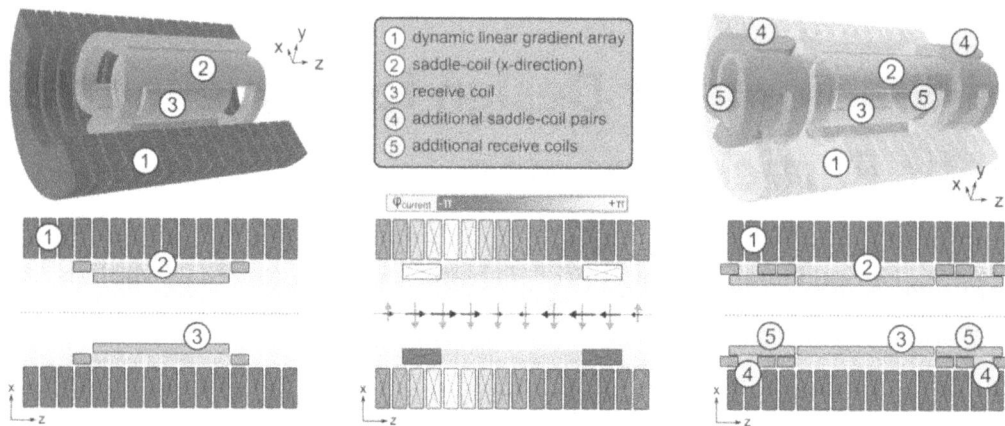

Figure 1: *Left: Sketch of a 2D TWMPI scanner consisting of the dLGA (1), saddle-coil pair (2) and receive coil (3). Center: magnetic field components for a time point along the symmetry axis (z-direction) generated by the dLGA (black) and saddle-coil pair (red). Right: hybrid gradiometer design for TWMPI scanners: additional coils extending the receive coil are used to suppress the dLGA-field (passive gradiometer) and additional saddle-coil pairs compensate the field of the saddle-coils (active gradiometer).*

Passive gradiometer for z-direction

Elongating the receive coil in z-direction until a full period of the sinusoidal magnetic field is covered causes the different induced signals to cancel out each other (see Fig. 1 right (5)) and the condition in (3) can be met (Fig. 1 center).

Active gradiometer for x/y-direction

The elongation of the receive coil does not cancel out residual signals introduced by the saddle-coil pairs because of their constant field across the covered area. The sketch in Fig. 1 right shows an active gradiometer setup, which also compensates the field contributions of the saddle-coils by actively generating an opposite signal.

III. Results

Simulating an entire TWMPI scanner using a home-built simulation environment for MPI [9] allows to validate the concept (see Fig. 2) and determines the parameters, which are required to construct a hybrid gradiometer inset for our TWMPI system.

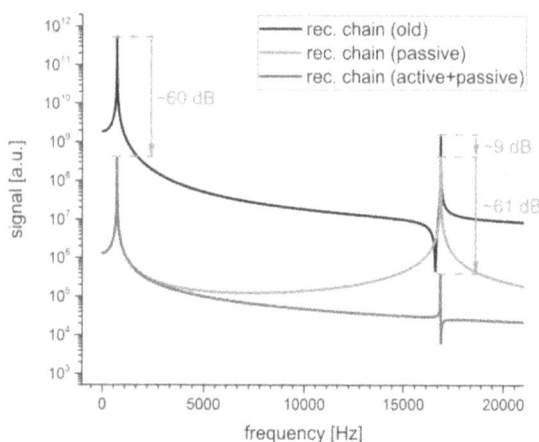

Figure 2: *Comparison of the simulated received signal (f_1=750 Hz, f_2=16800 Hz) without gradiometer (black), passive gradiometer (red) and hybrid gradiometer (blue).*

IV. Discussion

It is possible to extend this approach to 3D without any change by applying an additional set of saddle-coil pairs rotated by 90 degree. Furthermore, this offers the possibility of decoupling the entire system (dLGA, saddle-coil pair 1 and saddle-coil pair 2) by rotating the additional saddle-coil pairs (Fig. 1 right (4)) around the z-axis.

V. Conclusions

A novel concept of hybrid gradiometer design for traveling wave MPI systems (TWMPI) is presented, which allows the suppression of the excitation signals as well as environmental disturbances in the acquired signal by a factor of about 60 dB (Fig. 2).

This approach can provide a cleaner signal (better dynamic range for ADCs) resulting in a better SNR, which is indispensable for *in-vivo* imaging using low concentrated tracer material.

REFERENCES

[1] S. Tumanski, Induction coil sensors – a review, *Meas. Sci. Technol.*, vol. 18:R31, 2007. DOI: 10.1088/0957-0233/18/3/R01

[2] M. Graeser, et al., Towards Picogram Detection of Superparamagnetic Iron-Oxide Particles using a Gradiometric Receive Coil, *Sci. Rep.*, vol. 7:6872, 2017. doi:10.1038/s41598-017-06992-5

[3] B. Gleich and J. Weizenecker, Tomographic Imaging using the nonlinear response of magnetic particles, *Nature*, vol. 435, pp. 1214-7, 2005. Doi: 10.1038/nature03808

[4] T. Knopp, et al., Magnetic Particle Imaging: from proof of principle to preclinical applications, *Phys. Med. Biol.*, vol. 62(14), pp. R124-R178, 2017. DOI: 10.1088/1361-6560/aa6c99

[5] P. Vogel, et al., Traveling Wave Magnetic Particle Imaging, *IEEE TMI*, vol. 33(2), pp. 400-7, 2014. Doi:10.1109/TMI.2013.2285472.

[6] P. Vogel & P. Klauer, et al., Dynamic Linear Gradient Array for Traveling Wave Magnetic Particle Imaging, *IEEE Trans. Magn.*, (in press). Doi: 10.1109/TMAG.2017.2764440

[7] P. Vogel, et al., Real-time 3D Dynamic Rotating Slice-Scanning Mode for Traveling Wave Magnetic Particle Imaging, *Int. Journal on MPI*, vol.3(2):1706001, 2017. Doi:10.18416/ijmpi.2017.1706001.

[8] M. Graeser, et al., Analog receive signal processing for magnetic particle imaging, *Med. Phys.*, vol. 40(4):042303, 2013. DOI: 10.1118/1.4794482

[9] P. Vogel, et al., 3D-GUI Simulation Environment for MPI, *Proc. IWMPI*, p. 95, Lübeck, 2016.

WOTAN – Low Cost Ultra Small Formfactor Console for Magnetic Particle Imaging

Martin A. Rückert [a,*], Patrick Vogel [a,b], Volker C. Behr [a]

[a] Department of Experimental Physics 5 (Biophysics), University of Würzburg, 97074 Würzburg, Germany
[b] Department of Diagnostic and Interventional Radiology, University Hospital Würzburg, 97080 Würzburg, Germany
* Corresponding author, email: Martin.Rueckert@physik.uni-wuerzburg.de

I. Introduction

Since the first publication of Magnetic Particle Imaging (MPI) in 2005 several types of scanners were presented [1, 2]. MPI is based on the nonlinear response of magnetic materials to varying magnetic fields. For imaging, a field free point (FFP) or field free line (FFL) with a strong gradient on the order of 1-7 T/m is moved through the sample covering the volume of interest with a high temporal and spatial resolution. Typical frequencies used for MPI are in the range of 1 kHz and 150 kHz for the excitation fields. The resulting signal frequencies are typically below 1 MHz. This constitutes relatively moderate requirements for the control electronics.

The presented work evaluates the possibility of realizing the complete control unit for a typical 3D MPI scanner on a single microcontroller running 4 transmit and one receive channel. PSoC 5LP is a programmable mixed-signal system on a chip, which extends a microcontroller with programmable logic and a programmable analog system [6]. The latter exceeds the flexibility of any typical microcontroller system. It provides sufficient resources for both the transmit- and receiver chain of a typical 3D MPI scanner on a single chip.

3D imaging results with a Traveling Wave MPI (TWMPI) scanner [3, 4] are demonstrated. The complete source code of the firmware is provided as a github-repository [5].

II. Material and Methods

The control unit for operating a 3D TWMPI scanner was based around the PSoC 5LP chip from Cypress (Cypress Semiconductor Corp, California, USA). The smallest breakout board for the PSoC 5LP delivered by Cypress was used (i.e. the CY8CKIT-059-kit with the CY8C5888LTI-LP097). The setup used for operating the TWMPI scanner is shown in Fig. 1. The four current digital-to-analog converters (IDACs) on the chip were used for driving the four transmit channels of the TWMPI scanner [4], each amplified with audio amplifiers (t.amp TA2400, Thomann, Germany).

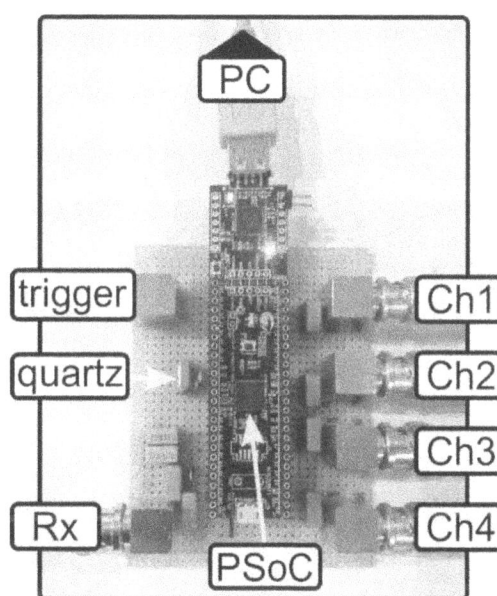

Figure 1: Control module based on the Cypress CY8CKIT-059 breakout board. It provides one receive channel Rx (ADC: 2 MS/s with 12 bit resolution), 4 transmit channels (8 bit resolution, possible sampling rate per channel: 4 MS/s, sampling rate used: 250 kS/s) and one trigger input. The onboard programmer provides a COM-port, which was used for running the TWMPI scanner and retrieving the imaging data via Matlab or Octave.

The IDACs can each operate with up to 4 MS/s and 8 bit resolution. The sampling rate used in this work was 250 kS/s. The two successive approximation register analog-to-digital converters (SAR-ADCs) operate up to 1 MS/s with 12 bit resolution. They were combined to one receive channel with 2 MS/s with 12 bit resolution. The firmware for the control module was written using Creator 4.1 from Cypress. The programmer is included on the breakout board and contains a USB-to-UART interface, which was used for controlling the device via Octave, Matlab (Mathworks Natick, MA, USA) or Python. The duration of one measurement was 15 ms (excluding ramps for starting and ending the sequence smoothly). The resulting 60 kB signal data was transferred in about 5 s using the USB-to-UART on the onboard-programmer with 115200 baud.

Higher transfer rates are possible but typically require extra clock adjustments.

III. Results

A TWMPI described in [3,4] was used for the measurements. The frequencies were set to f_1=723.57 Hz for channel-1 and channel-2, driving the main gradient, and f_2=16823 Hz for channel-3 and channel-4 driving the two perpendicular saddle-coil pairs. The TWMPI system doesn't require any specific frequencies apart from impedance matching, but the image reconstruction methods needs the frequency values with about 5 digit accuracy. The gradient was set to 2 T/m (axial direction).

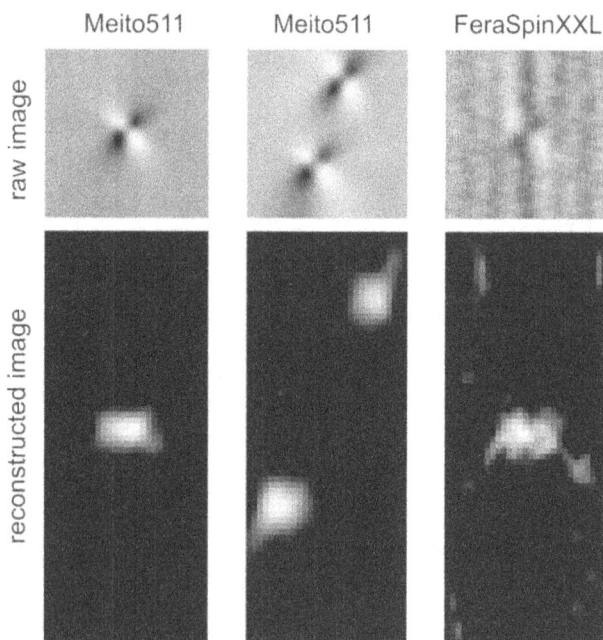

Figure 2: Left: one sample filled with Meito511 (conc. 1 mg (Fe)/ml). Center: two samples filled with Meito511 (same conc.). Right: One sample filled with FeraSpinXXL (conc. 10 µg (Fe)/ml).

For reconstruction, the data were pre-processed (correction of the receive chain distortion) and filtered digitally using a home-built reconstruction environment [7] followed by an image-based reconstruction approach [8].

In Fig. 2 reconstructed images are shown. The first samples filled with Meito511 (Meito Sangyo, Japan) with a concentration of 1 mg (Fe)/ml are well detectable. The signal of the sample filled with FeraSpinXXL (Miltenyi Biotec, Germany) with a concentration of 10 µg (Fe)/ml is in close to the noise level. However, with an averaging of 10 the sample can also be reconstructed.

IV. Discussion

Since the data transfer for only 60 KB is quite slow, for real-time visualization a faster transfer is possible by using the USB 2.0 component on the PSoC instead can be employed. It allows a transfer rate of 12.5 Mbps, which is faster than the transfer rate used here. The slower USB-to-UART provided on the onboard programmer is easier to use while debugging the design because it is on a separate chip.

The tolerance of the oscillators integrated on the chip is in the range of 0.25% and 7%. It is therefore recommendable to add an external quartz, which provides a typical frequency accuracy better than 100 parts per million.

The cost of the entire console is quite low. The breakout board with the PSoC chip is about 15 Euro. The total cost of the shown setup was 57 Euro.

V. Conclusions

A complete control system for the receive- and transmit chain of a 3D TWMPI scanner could be realized based around a single PSoC 5LP chip on a breakout board. The performance matches the requirements of a typical MPI system. It provides a very inexpensive yet powerful plattform for MPI hardware development and could greatly support the hardware development process.

REFERENCES

[1] B. Gleich and J. Weizenecker. Tomographic imaging using the nonlinear response of magnetic particles. *Nature*, 435(7046):1217-1217, 2005. doi: 10.1038/nature03808.

[2] T. Knopp, et al., Magnetic Particle Imaging: from proof of principle to preclinical applications, *Phys. Med. Biol.*, vol. 62(14), pp. R124-R178, 2017. DOI: 10.1088/1361-6560/aa6c99

[3] P. Vogel, et al., Traveling Wave Magnetic Particle Imaging, *IEEE TMI*, vol. 33(2), pp. 400-7, 2014. Doi:10.1109/TMI.2013.2285472.

[4] P. Vogel, et al., Real-time 3D Dynamic Rotational Slice-Scanning Mode for Traveling Wave MPI, *Int. Journal on MPI*, vol.3(2):1706001, 2017. Doi:10.19416/ijmpi.2017.1706001

[5] M.A. Rückert, WOTAN, (2017), GitHub repository, https://github.com/mnruecke/WOTAN

[6] Cypress Semiconductor, PSoC® 5LP: CY8C58LP Family, *Programmable system on a chip.*

[7] P. Vogel, et al., Low Latency Real-time Reconstruction for MPI Systems, *IJMPI*, vol. 3(2):1707002, 2017. Doi: 10.18416/ijmpi.2017.1707002

[8] P.Vogel, et al., Flexible and Dynamic Patch Reconstruction for Traveling Wave MPI, *IJMPI*, vol. 2(2):1611001, 2016. Doi: 10.18416/ijmpi.2016.1611001

Finite Element Analysis of Passive Magnetic Shields for a FFP MPI Scanner

Dilek M. Yalcinkaya [a,*], Alireza Sadeghi-Tarakameh [a,b], Mustafa Utkur [a,b], Emine U. Saritas [a,b,c]

[a] *Department of Electrical and Electronics Engineering, Bilkent University, Ankara, Turkey*
[b] *National Magnetic Resonance Research Center (UMRAM), Bilkent University, Ankara, Turkey*
[c] *Neuroscience Program, Sabuncu Brain Research Center, Bilkent University, Ankara, Turkey*
[*] *Corresponding author, email: mirgun.yalcinkaya@ug.bilkent.edu.tr*

I. Introduction

Imaging scanners that utilize magnetic fields typically require magnetic shielding between various layers of coils. For example, Magnetic Resonance Imaging (MRI) scanners utilize active or passive shields between the gradient coils and the B_0 coil, to avoid inducing long-lasting eddy currents on the cryogen-cooled B_0 coil [1,2]. Likewise, the permanent magnets (PMs) used in Magnetic Particle Imaging (MPI) scanners also need to be shielded from the eddy current inducing effects of the drive coils [3]. If not avoided, these eddy currents can cause a nonlinear magnetization response on the PMs, which can in turn produce harmonics that are picked up by the receive coils, contaminating the nanoparticle signal.

In this work, the finite element (FE) analysis of two different passive copper shield configurations were performed via ANSYS Maxwell. The effectiveness of the two configurations were analyzed and compared.

II. Material and Methods

A passive copper shield placed between the drive coil and the PMs can decrease the number of harmonics produced due to the nonlinear magnetization characteristics of PMs. The same copper shield can also prevent these harmonics from coupling to the receive coil [3]. Here, we analyzed two different passive copper shield configurations, for the case of a field free point (FFP) MPI scanner utilizing disc-shaped PMs. These two configurations are (see Fig. 1):

1) A hollow cylinder copper shield placed around the drive coil.
2) Two separate copper shields wrapped around the surface of each PM.

All simulations were performed in ANSYS Maxwell 14.0 electromagnetic simulation software (Maxwell, ANSYS, Inc., Canonsburg, PA, USA), which simulates low frequency electromagnetic fields using the FE method. Simulations were performed on Intel Core i7-6800K, 3.4 GHz CPU with 128 GB RAM.

First, we created a model for an FFP MPI scanner, having similar sizes and distances as our in-house FFP MPI scanner [4]. The scanner parameters were as follows: two disc-shaped PMs with material type NdFe35, having a 7-cm diameter and 2.5 cm height were placed at a 7.8 cm separation along the x-axis. The drive coil in our FFP scanner has 4-cm inner diameter and 9.7 cm total length, 3 layers with 80 turns in each layer, wound using a 1.2-mm diameter copper wire. This solenoidal coil creates magnetic field along the y-direction. Unfortunately, modelling such a detailed coil structure in Maxwell causes the simulations to significantly slow down. With the goal of speeding up FE analysis while preserving the accuracy of simulations, we have instead modelled the drive coil as three layers of continuous surface currents in clock-wise direction.

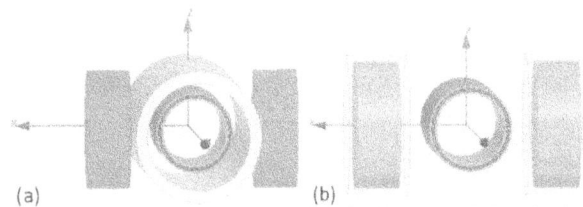

Figure 1: FFP MPI scanner with two different shield configurations. (a) Hollow copper shield placed around the drive coil. (b) Two separate copper shields wrapped around the surface of the PMs.

For the case where the shield is around the drive coil (see Fig. 1a), the length of the copper shield was fixed to 22 cm. For the case where the shield is around PMs (See Fig. 1b), a constant-thickness copper layer covered the surface of both PMs in every direction. For a fair comparison, the thickness of the hollow cylinder and the thickness of the copper layer for the two configurations were set identical at each step. Hence, the free radial distance around the drive coils were identical for both configurations (e.g., for inserting additional coils, such as focus field coils).

To match the operating frequency of our in-house MPI scanner, simulations were carried out at 10 kHz drive field frequency. The permitted simulation error parameters were set to 0.01% for the case where the shield was around the drive coil, and 0.02% for the case where the shield was around the PMs. These two error parameters yielded comparable simulation durations for the two configurations. Ten different shield thicknesses ranging between 0 mm (i.e., no shield case) to 9 mm (the thickness of the shield for our FFP scanner) were simulated for each configuration. Note that the induced eddy currents on the copper shields also counteract the drive field inside the imaging bore. Hence, at each shield thickness, the drive coil currents were adjusted to fix the magnetic field at the isocenter of the scanner to 15 mT. Using the Eddy-Current Solver of Maxwell, the magnetic field on the surface of each PM was measured by averaging the B-field values at 4 sample points at 2-mm radial distances to the surface center of the PM. Next, the B-field values computed for the two PMs were averaged to reach a mean B-field value. These averaging steps were done to increase the reliability of the measurements.

III. Results

Figure 2 shows the B-field attenuation on the surface of the PMs as a function of shield thickness. These values (reported in dB) were normalized to the no-shield case, which yielded 2.1 mT B-field. As expected, B-field attenuation increases with thicker shields for both configurations. While the configuration where the shield is around the drive coil is slightly more effective in attenuating the B-field, the results are largely comparable.

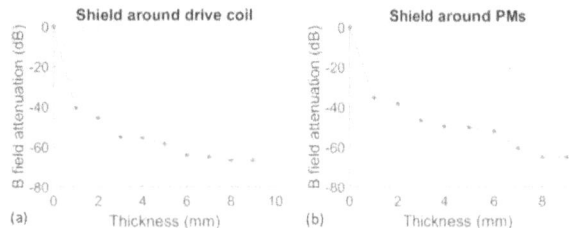

Figure 2: *B-field attenuation on the surface of the PMs as a function of shield thickness for (a) the shield around the drive coil and (b) the shield around PMs.*

As explained in Section II, the drive coil current was adjusted at each shield thickness to fix the drive field amplitude to 15 mT. Figure 3 shows the required drive coil current as a function of shield thickness for the two configurations. Here, the configuration where the shield is around the drive coil requires significantly higher currents as the shield thickness increases, whereas the case where the shield is around the PMs preserves a constant current value.

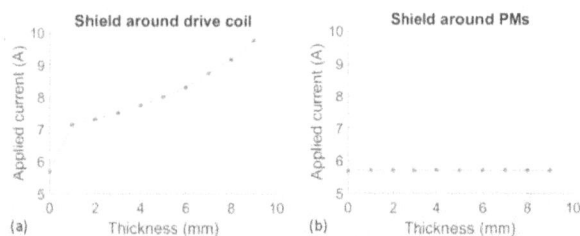

Figure 3: *The required drive coil current to keep the drive field amplitude at 15 mT for (a) the shield around the drive coil and (b) the shield around PMs.*

IV. Discussion

Based on the required currents plotted in Fig. 3, the configuration where the shield is around the PMs is more power-efficient. It provides comparable B-field attenuations at significantly lower drive coil currents, especially for increased shield thicknesses. The skin depth of copper at 10 kHz is approximately equal to 0.65 mm. We see that at around 5 skin depths (~3mm shield thickness), B-field attenuation reaches 50-60 dB for both configurations. To analyze the effects on the time-domain MPI signal, a time-domain transient analysis needs to be performed in Maxwell. This step remains a future work.

The duration of FE analysis is a strong function of the shield thickness, increasing significantly for thicker shields. In addition, simulation durations increase drastically for reduced permitted error values. For example, for the case where the shield was around the drive coil with 3-mm shield thickness, utilizing 0.01% error yielded a simulation time of 4 hours 22 minutes. Reducing the error to 0.005% increased the simulation time to 10 hours 45 minutes. Likewise, for the case when the shield was around the PMs with 4-mm shield thickness, utilizing 0.02% error yielded a simulation time of 1 hour 40 minutes. Using 0.01% error for the same case increased the simulation time to 26 hours 49 minutes. Considering the fact that 10 different shield thicknesses were targeted in this work, 0.01% and 0.02% errors were chosen for the two shield configurations, respectively.

Here, we have analyzed the effects of the passive copper shield in reducing the induced B-field on the PMs. The same shield can also help in reducing the unwanted signal interferences due to other external sources, via shielding the receive coil [5]. This latter effect was not investigated in this work.

IV. Conclusions

In this work, we have analyzed the effectiveness of two different passive copper shield configurations for a FFP MPI scanner. While both configurations are effective in attenuating the B-field induced on the PMs, the case where the shield is around the PMs is more power efficient.

ACKNOWLEDGEMENTS

This work was supported by the European Commission through an FP7 Marie Curie Career Integration Grant (PCIG13-GA-2013-618834), by the Turkish Academy of Sciences through TUBA-GEBIP 2015 program, and by the Science Academy through BAGEP award.

REFERENCES

[1] R. Turner. Gradient coil design: A review of methods. *Magnetic Resonance Imaging*, 11(7):903-920, 1993.
[2] R. Turner and R.M. Bowley. Passive screening of switched magnetic field gradients. *J Phys E: Scientific Instruments*, 19(10):876-879, 1986.
[3] P.W. Goodwill *et al*. An x-space magnetic particle imaging scanner. *Review of Scientific Instruments*, *83*(3), 033708, 2012.
[4] Y. Muslu *et al*. Calibration-Free Relaxation-Based Multi-Color Magnetic Particle Imaging. *arXiv preprint:1705.07624*, 2017.
[5] L. Bauer *et al*. Simulation study of a novel relaxometer shield design. *Proc of International Workshop on Magnetic Particle Imaging (IWMPI)*, 2015.

Session 08 - Talks

Reconstruction II

Exploiting ill-Posedness in Magnetic Particle Imaging - System Matrix Approximation via Randomized SVD

Tobias Kluth[a], Bangti Jin[b]

[a]Center for Industrial Mathematics, University of Bremen, Bremen, Germany
[b]Department of Computer Science, University College London, Gower Street, London WC1E 6BT, UK
* Corresponding author, email: tkluth@math.uni-bremen.de

I. Introduction

In magnetic particle imaging (MPI), measurements are obtained by exploiting particles' nonlinear response to an applied dynamic magnetic field in order to recover the particle concentration. It is frequently modeled by a linear Fredholm integral equation of the first kind. Although highly simplistic, the equilibrium model based on the Langevin function has been used extensively in the literature to predict the signal behavior in MPI [8]. In a 1D field free point (FFP) setup, it was shown that in the limit of large particle diameters, the imaging problem is well-posed [10]. In the multi-dimensional case, the authors analyzed a related problem which is independent of the used FFP trajectory, by assuming multiple scans with nonparallel trajectories at each spatial point, and showed it is severely ill-posed.

Image reconstructions are commonly obtained by variational regularization techniques, and they can benefit enormously from the high temporal resolution which however also requires efficient reconstruction methods [9, 6]. There have been several approaches to accelerate the reconstruction, e.g., sub-sampling the system matrix by excluding frequency bands with small SNR [6] or sparse representations [7], while reducing the influence of the background signal. The problem is then solved preferably by using the algebraic reconstruction technique combined with a nonnegativity constraint. However, the optimal choice of basis functions for sparse recovery is still an open question.

In this presentation, we address the degree of ill-posedness of the inverse problem in MPI in terms of the singular value decay rate from a theoretical perspective. Motivated by these theoretical findings, we propose to use a low-rank approximation of the system matrix, constructed efficiently via randomized singular value decomposition (rSVD), which can be effectively exploited for fast image reconstructions within the context of variational regularization. Numerical results for simulated measurements are presented and compared with the popular algebraic reconstruction technique applied to post-processed system matrices.

II. Methods

II.I Equilibrium model

Let $\Omega \subset \mathbb{R}^d$, $d = 1,2,3$, be an open bounded domain and $T > 0$. The problem is to obtain the concentration c from potentials $\{v_k\}_{k=1,\dots,L}$, $L \in \mathbb{N}$. Using the equilibrium particle model based on the parametrized Langevin function $\mathfrak{L}_\beta : \mathbb{R} \to \mathbb{R}, \mathfrak{L}_\beta(z) = m_0(\coth(\beta z) - 1/(\beta z))$, $\beta, m_0 > 0$, yields the linear forward operator $S : L^2(\Omega) \to L^2(0,T)^L$ mapping the concentration c to the potentials $\{v_k\}_{k=1,\dots,L}$:

$$v_k(t) = -\int_\Omega c(x) s_k(x,t) dx$$
$$s_k = \mu_0 p_k^T \frac{\partial}{\partial t} (\mathfrak{L}_\beta(\|H\|) \frac{H}{\|H\|})$$
$$H(x,t) = g(x) + h(t)$$

for $k = 1, \dots, L$ and with drive field $h : (0,T) \to \mathbb{R}^d$, selection field $g : \Omega \to \mathbb{R}^d$ and coil sensitivity $p_k : \Omega \to \mathbb{R}^d$. The discretized problem is obtained using piecewise constant basis functions in space and time and a Gaussian quadrature rule for approximating the integrals. The system matrix is then generated by computing the discrete Fourier transform of the columns.

II.I Randomized SVD / reconstruction

Given a matrix $S \in \mathbb{C}^{n \times m}$, $n \geq m$, a rank-k approximation of S can be obtained efficiently by randomized SVD [3]. The SVD of S is (U, Σ, V). Let $\Omega \in \mathbb{R}^{m \times (k+p)}$, $k << \min(m, n)$, be a random matrix which entries follow an i.i.d. Gaussian distribution (here $p = 5$). Using the SVD (U, Σ, V) of S yields the random matrix $Y = U\Sigma V^*\Omega$. Let $Q \in \mathbb{R}^{n \times (k+p)}$ be an orthonormal basis for the range of Y which can be computed efficiently by QR factorization. Computing the SVD (W, Σ, V) of $Q^*S \in \mathbb{C}^{(k+p) \times m}$ then yields

$$S_k = U_k \Sigma_k V_k^*$$

with $U_k = [QW]_{:,1:k}$, $\Sigma_k = [\Sigma]_{1:k,1:k}$, $V_k = [V]_{:,1:k}$ ($[X]_{:,1:k}$ denotes taking the first k columns of a matrix $X \in \mathbb{C}^{n \times m}$, $n \geq k$; rows are treated analogously). Due to the size of Q^*S, its SVD can be computed efficiently by standard methods (e.g., Matlab's built-in function).

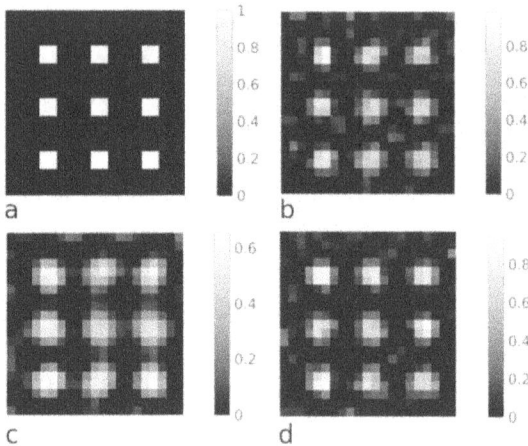

Figure 1: Selected reconstructions with minimal reconstruction error (MSE) for normally distributed noise in time domain $(\mathcal{N}(0,5\|v^\dagger\|/N))$, $v^\dagger \in \mathbb{R}^N$ noisefree signal in time domain): (a) Phantom; (b) randSVD, k = 300; (c) rART 20 %, #iter=2; (d) rART 100 %, #iter=2.

The image reconstruction from the given data $v^\delta \in \mathbb{C}^n$ is obtained by minimizing a standard Tikhonov functional $J_\gamma(c) = \frac{1}{2}\|S_k c - v^\delta\|_2^2 + \frac{\gamma}{2}\|c\|_2^2$, where γ is the regularization parameter. The rank-k SVD and the normal equation together yield a closed-form solution:

$$c_k = \arg\min_{c\in\mathbb{R}_+^m} J_\gamma(c) = P_{\mathbb{R}_+^m} \sum_{i=1}^{k} \frac{\sigma_i}{\sigma_i^2 + \gamma^2} \langle u_i, v^\delta \rangle v_i$$

with inner product $\langle \cdot, \cdot \rangle$ and projection $P_{\mathbb{R}_+^m}$.

III. Results

The estimate for the singular value decay of the corresponding integral operator for $\beta < \infty$ can be derived by using [2, Theorem 3.2]. The regularity of the temporal drive field together with the regularity of the spatial selection field essentially determine the decay rate of the singular values for finite particle diameters $\beta < \infty$ [5, Theorem 4.1 & 4.2]. Smooth functions in typical MPI setups result in an exponential decay of the singular values, indicating a small approximation error when using randomized SVD [3, Theorem 1.2].

We have simulated a 2D FFP scanner setup with excitation frequencies 24.51 kHz and 26.04 kHz in x/y-direction with amplitude 12mT/μ0. Gradient strength is 2 T/m/μ0 and the field of view with a size of 21 mm × 21 mm is discretized in pixels with size 1 mm × 1 mm resulting in a system matrix with 441 columns and 1634 rows. Measurements are simulated with pixel size 0.5 mm × 0.5 mm. Particle parameters can be found in [4].

The computing times (Table 1) and reconstruction results (Figure 1) for the low-rank approximation (randSVD) are compared with a post-processed system matrix (keeping a ratio of frequencies with largest signal energy) reconstruction with the regularized Kaczmarz algorithm (rART) [1, p. 579]. The randSVD results are obtained faster in this test case and show slightly better reconstructions compared with rART 20%.

IV. Discussion

The results indicate that using a low-rank approximation via randomized SVD can be used for image reconstruction with comparable quality while decreasing the computational complexity in the MPI reconstruction, and theoretically this is justified by the severe ill-posed nature of the problem. The randomized SVD is computationally attractive and memory efficient in 3D and also does not require the choice of a particular basis representation. The presented results need to be validated for simulated and real data in 3D. The iterative nature of rART can be disadvantageous in some programming languages and requires further research. Further, a data-driven regularization parameter choice rule is highly desirable for real data experiments in order to achieve good efficiency.

Table 1: Mean computation times over 300 regularization parameters $i = 10^4(1.1)^{-i}$, $i = 0, \ldots, 299$, with Matlab on an Intel(R) Core(TM) i5-6200U CPU@ 2.30GHz with 8GB DDR4-RAM.

randSVD (k)	100	200	300	400
Time [ms]	0.45	0.83	1.45	1.90

rART (#iter)	1	2	3	4
20% / time [ms]	5.83	10.58	14.63	19.41
100% / time [ms]	25.37	49.42	72.02	93.66

ACKNOWLEDGEMENTS

T. Kluth is supported by the Deutsche Forschungsgemeinschaft (DFG) within the framework of GRK 2224/1.

REFERENCES

[1] A. Dax. On row relaxation methods for large constrained least squares problems. *SIAM J. Sci. Comp*, 14(3):570–584, 1993.

[2] M. Griebel and G. Li. On the decay rate of the singular values of bivariate functions. INS preprint No. 1702, University of Bonn, 2017.

[3] N. Halko, P.-G. Martinsson, and J. A. Tropp. Finding structure with randomness: Probabilistic algorithms for constructing approximate matrix decompositions. *SIAM Rev.* 53(2):217–288, 2011.

[4] T. Kluth and P. Maass. Model uncertainty in magnetic particle imaging: Nonlinear problem formulation and model-based sparse reconstruction. *Int. J. Magnet. Particle Imag.*, 3(2), 2017.

[5] T. Kluth, B. Jin, G. Li. On the degree of ill-posedness of multi-dimensional magnetic particle imaging. Preprint, arXiv:1712.05720v1, 2017.

[6] T. Knopp and M. Hofmann. Online reconstruction of 3D magnetic particle imaging data. *Phys Med Biol*, 61(11): N257–67, 2016.

[7] T. Knopp and A. Weber. Local system matrix compression for efficient reconstruction in magnetic particle imaging. *Adv. Math. Phys.*, 2015:Article ID 472818, 7 pages, 2015.

[8] T. Knopp, N. Gdaniec, and M. Möddel. Magnetic particle imaging: from proof of principle to preclinical applications. *Phys. Med. Biol.* 62(14):R124, 2017.

[9] J. Lampe, C. Bassoy, J. Rahmer, J. Weizenecker, H. Voss, B. Gleich, and J. Borgert. Fast reconstruction in magnetic particle imaging. *Phys Med Biol*, 57(4):1113–1134, 2012.

[10] T. März and A. Weinmann. Model-based reconstruction for magnetic particle imaging in 2D and 3D. *Inv. Probl. Imag.* 10(4):1087–1110, 2016.

MPI Reconstruction Using Structural Prior Information and Sparsity

Christine Bathke [a,*], Tobias Kluth [a], Peter Maaß [a]

[a] *Center for Industrial Mathematics, University of Bremen, Bibliothekstr. 1, 28359 Bremen*
[*] *Corresponding author, email: cbathke@uni-bremen.de*

I. Introduction

Magnetic Particle Imaging is a new imaging modality that promises a lot of interesting features like a high temporal resolution and no harmful radiation. Apart from technical advances, image reconstruction methods tailored to MPI are crucial. Tikhonov regularization using the Kaczmarz method is the most commonly used method for image reconstruction in MPI - and for good reasons: it is computationally cheap, easy to implement and fast. However, more sophisticated techniques exist, that use additional assumptions on the tracer concentration to be reconstructed. Those assumptions can come from another modality, e.g. MRI, or specify the desired look of the image, e.g. smooth or sharp. In the past few years some efforts have been made to include one type of these assumptions at a time [10],[1],[8].

In this talk, we aim at combining them both, structural information from a second modality and sparsity of the MPI tracer concentration, to further improve reconstruction quality. If edges are present in the prior information, we can assume that they are likely to show up in the MPI reconstruction as well. Therefore, we encourage our algorithm to favour those edges over edges not present in the prior information with a modified TV penalty. This edge information is what we call structural information. Since MPI is often combined with MR images to conclude on the actual location of the reconstructed tracer in the patient [9], this structural information is usually available. Also, there are efforts to combine both modalities, MPI and MRI, into one scanner [6]. Our second assumption is that the tracer reconstruction is sparse, i.e. has only few nonzero entries. This is reasonable because the iron oxide nanoparticles are confined to the injected tracer fluid which in turn is restricted to the blood vessels. Therefore, the whole background should be zero.

II. Material and Methods

The Kaczmarz method minimizes the functional

$$\arg\min_{c\in\mathbb{R}_+^N} \frac{1}{2} \| Sc - u \|_2^2 + \alpha \| c \|_2^2. \qquad (1)$$

where $S \in \mathbb{C}^{K\times N}$ is the system matrix in frequency space, $u \in \mathbb{C}^K$ are the Fourier coefficients of the measurements and $c \in \mathbb{R}_+^N$ is the tracer concentration to be reconstructed. The first term links the tracer concentration to the model,

while the second one ensures smooth minimizers. The regularization parameter $\alpha > 0$ is used to balance these two.

The $\|\cdot\|_2$-norm in equation (1) promotes overall smooth images, i.e. it not only smoothes out noise but also edges. To retain sharp edges we propose to use a total variation like term as well a l_1-norm to promote sparsity [7] in the image resulting in the following functional

$$\arg\min_{c\in\mathbb{R}_+^N} \frac{1}{2} \| Sc - u \|_2^2 + \alpha \mathrm{dTV}(c) + \beta \| c \|_1. \qquad (2)$$

The directional TV-term

$$\mathrm{dTV}(c) = \sum_n \left\| \left(I - \frac{\nabla v_n \nabla v_n^T}{\|\nabla v_n\|_2^2+\varepsilon} \right) \nabla c_n \right\|_2 \qquad (3)$$

allows to include additional information $v \in \mathbb{R}^N$ from a second modality [5]. For magnetic particle imaging this could be MRI.

To solve the above minimization problem, we used ADMM (Alternating Direction Method of Multipliers) [3] to split the problem in two subproblems and use iterative soft thresholding [4] and a gradient projection method [2] to solve the resulting subproblems.

III. Results

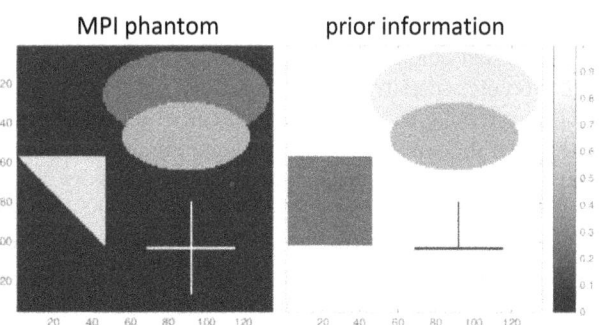

Figure 1: Phantom used for MPI simulation and corresponding prior information. For the prior information the contrast has been inverted and some edges have been added/removed.

III.I Simulation

To test our reconstruction method, we simulated MPI measurements in a 2D FFP scanner using the Langevin model and the phantom depicted in Fig. 1. This phantom contains homogenous areas as well as straight and round edges and fine lines. We used the excitation frequencies

24.51kHz and 26.04kHz in x/y-direction with amplitude $12\text{mT}/\mu_0$ and a gradient strength of $2\text{T/m}/\mu_0$. The field of view, having a size of $27\text{mm} \times 27\text{mm}$, is discretized in pixels with size $0.5\text{mm} \times 0.5\text{mm}$ resulting in a system matrix with 2916 columns and 2388 rows. Measurements are simulated with a pixel size of $0.2\text{mm} \times 0.2\text{mm}$.

For the particle simulation, we used the diameter $d = 30\text{nm}$, the saturation magnetization $M_S = 0.6\text{T}/\mu_0$ and the temperature $T = 293\text{K}$.

We added 5%of Gaussian noise on the time signal.

III.II Reconstruction

Our results using the Kaczmarz algorithm and our proposed method, both with nonnegativity projection, are shown in Fig. 2. As regularization parameters we used $\alpha = 1.5$ for the Kaczmarz method and $\alpha = 1 \cdot 10^{-1}, \beta = 4 \cdot 10^{-4}$ for the other functional. The prior information we used in the TV term (3), as shown in Fig. 1 on the right, differs slightly from the true MPI solution shown on the left. Hence, we can observe how our algorithm behaves when edges that should be present in the reconstruction of the phantom do not exist in the prior information and vice versa.

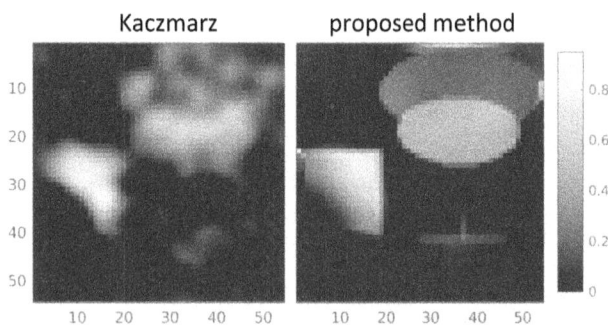

Figure 2: *Reconstruction results for data with 5% Gaussian noise generated using the phantom in Fig. 1: Reconstruction parameters were $\alpha = 1.5$ (left) and $\alpha = 1 \cdot 10^{-1}, \beta = 4 \cdot 10^{-4}$ (right).*

As we can see in Fig. 2, the proposed method shows clearly superior results compared to the Kaczmarz method. The TV term that contains prior information and the l_1-norm, that promotes sparsity, are able to reconstruct sharp images while supressing noise. Our method can also produce fine lines as of the cross in the bottom right corner. The edges that are present in the prior information appear very sharp in the reconstruction (on the right of Fig. 2), the bottom edge that is not present in the prior information is not reconstructed. Edges that are not available in the additional information remain blurred, i.e. the long side of the triangle. This feature is reconstructed better with the Kaczmarz method on the left of Fig. 2, which does not produce a perfectly straight but less blurry line.

IV. Conclusion

We showed in a simulation of a 2D FFP scanner that choosing sophisticated penalty terms can significantly improve reconstruction. The directional TV term recovers sharp edges if they are available in given additional information, as has been shown in [1]. In addition, the sparsity penalty reduces background artefacts and makes the image look clearer. The proposed method can be easily extended to 3D; also other penalty terms could be added or swapped.

The potential of this method to reconstruct delicate structures like human vessels has to be validated on real data. Furthermore, a parameter choice rule depending on the given data is desirable, since two regularization parameters need to be balanced.

ACKNOWLEDGEMENTS

C. Bathke is supported by the Deutsche Forschungsgemeinschaft (DFG, project MA 1657/24-1) and the Chinesisch-Deutsche Zentrum fuer Wissenschaftsfoerderung (project GZ 1025). T. Kluth acknowledges funding from the Deutsche Forschungsgemeinschaft (DFG) within the framework of GRK 2224/1.

REFERENCES

[1] C. Bathke, T. Kluth, C. Brandt, and P. Maaß. Improved image reconstruction in magnetic particle imaging using structural a priori information. *International Journal on Magnetic Particle Imaging*, 3(1):1–10, 2017.
[2] A. Beck and M. Teboulle. Fast Gradient-Based Algorithms for Constrained Total Variation Image Denoising and Deblurring Problems. *IEEE Transactions on Image Processing*, 18(11):2419–2434, 2009.
[3] S. Boyd. Distributed Optimization and Statistical Learn- ing via the Alternating Direction Method of Multipliers. *Foundations and Trends® in Machine Learning*, 3(1):1–122, 2011.
[4] I. Daubechies, M. Defrise, and C. De Mol. An iterative thresholding algorithm for linear inverse problems with a sparsity constraint. *Communications on Pure and Applied Mathematics*, 57(11):1413–1457, 2004.
[5] M. J. Ehrhardt and M. M. Betcke. Multi-Contrast MRI Reconstruction with Structure-Guided Total Variation. *SIAM Journal on Imaging Sciences*. 9(3):1084–1106, 2016.
[6] J. Franke, U. Heinen, H. Lehr, A. Weber, F. Jaspard, W. Ruhm, M. Heidenreich, and V. Schulz. System Characterization of a Highly Integrated Preclinical Hybrid MPI-MRI Scanner. *IEEE Transactions on Medical Imaging*, 35(9):1993–2004, 2016.
[7] B. Jin and P. Maaß. Sparsity regularization for parameter identification problems. *Inverse Problems* 28(12), 2012.
[8] T. Kluth and P. Maaß. Model uncertainty in magnetic particle imaging: Nonlinear problem formulation and model-based sparse reconstruction. *International Journal on Magnetic Particle Imaging*, 3(2):1–10, 2017.
[9] J. Salamon, M. Hofmann, C. Jung, M. G. Kaul, and F. Werner. Magnetic Particle/Magnetic Resonance Imaging: In-Vitro MPI-Guided Real Time Catheter Tracking and 4D Angioplasty Using a Road Map and Blood Pool Tracer Approach. *PLOS ONE*, 11(6), 2016.
[10] M. Storath, C. Brandt, M. Hofmann, T. Knopp, J. Salamon, A. Weber, and A. Weinmann. Edge preserving and noise reducing reconstruction for magnetic particle imaging. *IEEE Transactions on Medical Imaging*, 36(1):74–85, 2016.

Direct Reconstruction of Lissajous MPI Data using Chebyshev Compressed System Matrices

Martin Möddel [a,b]*, **Leonard Schmiester** [c,d], **Wolfgang Erb** [e], **Tom Hauswald** [b], **Tobias Knopp** [a,b]

[a] *Section for Biomedical Imaging, University Medical Center Hamburg-Eppendorf, Hamburg, Germany*
[b] *Institute for Biomedical Imaging, Hamburg University of Technology, Hamburg, Germany*
[c] *Institute of Computational Biology, Helmholtz Zentrum München, Neuherberg, Germany*
[d] *Chair of Mathematical Modeling of Biological Systems, Technical University Munich, Garching, Germany*
[e] *Department of Mathematics, University of Hawai'i at Mānoa, Honolulu, USA*
* *Corresponding author, email: m.hofmann@uke.de*

I. Introduction

Lissajous type magnetic particle imaging (MPI) sequences offer high acquisition rates of up to 40 frames/s for field of views in the order of $30{\times}30{\times}15$ mm³. Compared to Cartesian sequences, where a number of highly efficient reconstruction algorithms exist [1,2,3,4], real time Lissajous type data reconstruction is much more challenging. In [1] the authors used the structure of the MPI imaging operator, which includes a weighted Chebyshev transformation and an additional convolution, to derive a direct reconstruction formula for 1D MPI data.

Unfortunately, an equivalent formulation has not been found for Lissajous type imaging equations so far. Nevertheless, the 2D system function shows high similarity to tensor products of weighted Chebyshev polynomials [1]. Reconstruction of Lissajous type MPI data therefore relies on a calibration-based method where the system function is measured at discrete positions and the acquired system matrix is used for image reconstruction [5]. Due to the size of the dense system matrix image reconstruction is usually much slower than the data acquisition. Therefore, it was a key finding that the system matrix can be approximated by a sparse coefficient matrix and a unitary transformation matrix allowing for fast image reconstruction [6].

In our recent work [7], we investigated the Chebyshev transformation for matrix compression and showed that it can provide better reconstruction results for very high compression rates compared to the commonly applied Cosine transformation if the domain of the Chebyshev polynomials is matched to the area of the field free point (FFP) trajectory. Moreover we derived a direct reconstruction method for the limiting case where a single coefficient per matrix row was used to represent the MPI system matrix in Chebyshev space.

The restriction of the domain of the Chebyshev polynomials to the FFP trajectory leads to artifacts from signal sources outside the domain. In this work, we propose to reduce such artifacts and further improve compression rates by introducing a heuristically chosen convolution kernel.

II. Materials and Methods

In MPI various static and oscillating magnetic fields encode the spatial distribution of magnetic nanoparticles (MNPs) into voltage signals measured with multiple receive coils. The static fields define the scanner topology amongst which there are field free point and field free line scanners having static fields with a single zero field point or line respectively. In this work we consider FFP scanners, which for simplicity are assumed to have a single receive channel only.

Lissajous type sequences excite the magnetic nanoparticles by moving the FFP along a Lissajous trajectory as sketched in Fig. 1a. The bounding box of this trajectory is the so-called drive-field field of view (DF-FOV). It is the region, where the signal response of MNPs is strongest. However, signal is not exclusively generated within the DF-FOV. Therefore, the region in which the signal is still distinguishable from the noise floor is bounded by the system function field of view (SF-FOV) and we denote the region outside the DF-FOV but still inside the SF-FOV as the overscan region.

The relation between the distribution of the MNPs c and the Fourier transformed voltage signal induced in the receive coil u is given by

$$u = Sc, \qquad (1)$$

where S is the so called system matrix [5]. The reconstruction of an unknown particle distribution involves the solution of a least squares problem with Equation (1) as the data term. Due to the size of the dense system matrix reconstruction is usually slow. Using a suitable basis transformation matrix B one can factorize the system matrix into $\hat{S} = SB$ with a sparse coefficient matrix $\hat{S}$ which can be compressed by removing all but the largest coefficients per matrix row [6]. For Lissajous type system matrices most of the signal is located inside the DF-FOV [1] as shown in Figure 1b for a single frequency component. In [7] we used a basis transform based on Chebyshev polynomials of the second kind with the spatial domain restricted to the DF-FOV.

The restriction of the domain of the Chebyshev polynomials causes an increasing approximation error towards the edges of the DF-FOV and in the overscan region as can be seen in Figure 1b and 1c. To improve the overall compression and lower the approximation error we introduce a convolution with a Gauss kernel into the Chebyshev model as shown in Figure 1d. The width of the kernel is optimized with respect to the overall compression rate.

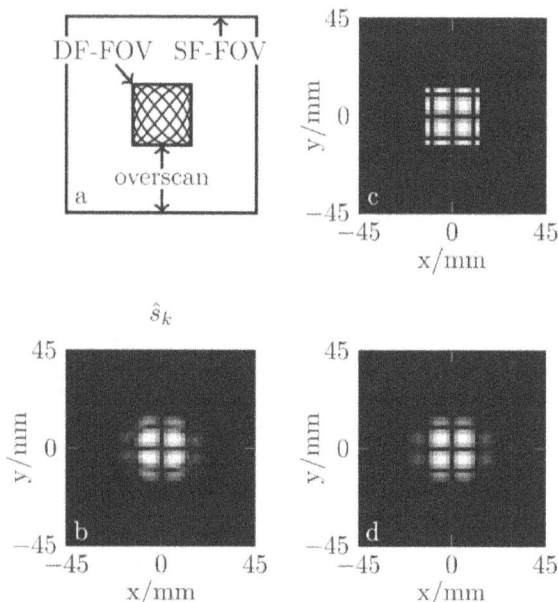

Figure 1: Graphical illustration of the drive-field field of view (DF-FOV), the system function field of view (SF-FOV) and the overscan region (a).The idea of matrix compression is to represent the frequency components of the system function $\hat{s}_k$ (b) in a suitable basis. Restriction of the Chebyshev basis to the DF-FOV (c) yield a better compression for high compression rates, but introduce errors at the DF-FOV edges. These can be reduced by convolving the elements of the Chebyshev basis with a Gauss kernel (d).

Using the compressed coefficient matrix $\hat{S}^\Gamma$ the system of equations (1) can be approximated by $u = \hat{S}^\Gamma B^{-1} c$ which can be solved efficiently. From $\hat{S}^1$ a direct reconstruction method can be derived. To this end, we remove all zero columns from $\hat{S}^1$ and replace all linear dependent rows by a single prevalent one. This results in a diagonal matrix P. For simplicity we chose the row with the largest absolute coefficient. We obtain the direct reconstruction formula $c = BZP^{-1}Z^T u$, where Z is the sparse matrix describing the row and column reduction of $\hat{S}^1$.

III. Discussion

Our results show that the restriction of the Chebyshev polynomials to the DF-FOV yields a good approximation of the system function for high compression rates [7]. In a

direct comparison with the restricted compression based on the discrete cosine transformation (DCT) as introduced in [6] the Chebyshev based compression outperforms the DCT based compression for high compression rates of one and two coefficients per matrix row. For lower compression rates the DCT performs better than the Chebyshev based compression.

Reconstructions of phantom measurements with 2D Lissajous excitation using both the Chebyshev and the DCT compressed matrices compare very well to a reconstruction with the dense system matrix as long as the phantom is located in the center of the DF-FOV. Introducing a heuristically chosen convolution operator into the matrix compression the approximation at the drive field edges and the overscan region can be improved significantly. Due to the better overall approximation reconstruction artifacts at the edges of the DF-FOV are reduced significantly. Using the limiting case of only one coefficient per row in the coefficient matrix, we could derive a direct reconstruction method that shows comparable image quality compared to a reconstruction that uses the dense system matrix.

Reconstruction of 2D Lissajous data with P and $\hat{S}^1$ offered a 66 fold speed-up compared to a dense reconstruction, i.e. a reconstruction speed about twice as long as the acquisition rate. Since the speed-up scales with dimension real-time capable reconstruction should be feasible for 3D Lissajous trajectories.

ACKNOWLEDGEMENTS

The authors thankfully acknowledge the financial support by the German Research Foundation (DFG, grant number KN 1108/2-1).

REFERENCES

[1] J. Rahmer, J. Weizenecker, B. Gleich and J. Borgert. Signal encoding in magnetic particle imaging. *BMC Medical imaging*, 9, 4, 2009. doi: 10.1186/1471-2342-9-4.

[2] P. W. Goodwill and S. M. Conolly. The X-space formulation of the magnetic particle imaging process: 1-D signal, resolution, bandwidth, SNR, SAR, and magnetostimulation. *IEEE Trans Med Imaging*, 29(11), 1851-9. 2010. doi: 10.1109/TMI.2010.2052284.

[3] P. W. Goodwill and S. M. Conolly. Multidimensional x-space magnetic particle imaging. *IEEE Trans Med Imaging*, 30(9), 1581-90. 2011. doi: 10.1109/TMI.2011.2125982.

[4] J. J. Konkle, P. W. Goodwill, D. W. Hensley, R. D. Orendorff, M. Lustig, S. M. Conolly. A Convex Formulation for Magnetic Particle Imaging X-Space Reconstruction. *PLoS One*, 10(10), e0140137. 2011. doi: 10.1371/journal.pone.0140137.

[5] B. Gleich and J. Weizenecker. Tomographic imaging using the nonlinear response of magnetic particles. *Nature*, 435(7046), 1214-7. 2005. doi: 10.1038/nature03808.

[6] J. Lampe, C. Bassoy, J. Rahmer, J. Weizenecker, B. Gleich and J. Borgert. Fast reconstruction in magnetic particle imaging. *Phys Med Biol*, 57(4), 1113-34, 2012. doi: 10.1088/0031-9155/57/4/1113.

[7] L. Schmiester, M. Möddel, W. Erb and T. Knopp. Direct Image Reconstruction of Lissajous-Type Magnetic Particle Imaging Data Using Chebyshev-Based Matrix Compression. *IEEE Trans Comp Imaging*, 3(4), 671-681, 2017. doi: 10.1109/TCI.2017.2706058.

A Generalized Reconstruction Technique for Non-Cartesian X-Space MPI

Ali Alper Ozaslan [a,b,c*], **Ahmet Alacaoglu [d]**, **Omer Burak Demirel [a,b,c]**, **Tolga Çukur [a,b,c]**, **Emine Ulku Saritas [a,b,c]**

[a] *Department of Electrical and Electronics Engineering, Bilkent University, Ankara, Turkey*
[b] *National Magnetic Resonance Research Center (UMRAM), Bilkent University, Ankara, Turkey*
[c] *Neuroscience Program, Sabuncu Brain Research Center, Bilkent University, Ankara, Turkey*
[d] *Laboratory for Information and Inference Systems (LIONS), EPFL, Lausanne, Switzerland*

* Corresponding author, email: ozaslan@ee.bilkent.edu.tr

I. Introduction

In Magnetic Particle Imaging (MPI), signal acquisition is achieved via sweeping the Field Free Point (FFP) on a specified trajectory [1]. With x-space reconstruction technique, typically a Cartesian trajectory is used [2-4], where the drive field is applied in 1D while the focus field covers the target field-of-view (FOV). In contrast, non-Cartesian trajectories are widely utilized together with system function reconstruction approach [5,6]. Recently, we have demonstrated a partitioning approach for x-space reconstruction of Lissajous trajectories, where the trajectory was separated into two parts of nearly orthogonal scan directions [7]. However, this approach only works for trajectories that can be partitioned into different directions.

In Magnetic Resonance Imaging (MRI), reconstruction from non-Cartesian k-space data is performed using optimized gridding reconstructions [8,9]. Accordingly, data points lying on a non-Cartesian trajectory in k-space are convolved with an optimized gridding kernel, and the outcomes of the convolution operation are sampled and accumulated on the Cartesian grid. In this work, we adapt MRI gridding algorithms to x-space MPI. The proposed algorithm is a generalized reconstruction technique for non-Cartesian x-space MPI and is trajectory independent. Here, we demonstrate this algorithm for a Lissajous trajectory.

II. Material and Methods

II.I. Theory

The proposed gridding algorithm, adapted to x-space MPI, can be stated as follows:

$$\hat{m}(x,y) = \frac{\left[\left(m(x,y)s(x,y)\right) * c(x,y)\right] \cdot \mathrm{III}\left(\frac{x}{\Delta x}, \frac{y}{\Delta y}\right)}{\left[s(x,y) * c(x,y)\right] \cdot \mathrm{III}\left(\frac{x}{\Delta x}, \frac{y}{\Delta y}\right)} \quad (1)$$

where,

$$s(x,y) = \sum_i \delta(x - x_i, y - y_i) \quad (2)$$

Here, $m(x,y)$ is the ideal MPI image, $s(x,y)$ is the 2D non-Cartesian sampling function sampled at positions (x_i, y_i) on the FFP trajectory, $c(x,y)$ is the gridding kernel, and $\mathrm{III}(x/\Delta x, y/\Delta y)$ is a 2D comb function.

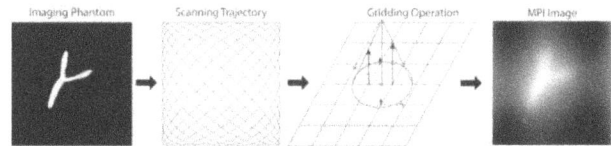

Figure 1: *Schematic of the proposed reconstruction technique, demonstrated for a Lissajous trajectory.*

Fig. 1 visually summarizes the proposed reconstruction technique for the example of a Lissajous trajectory. First, MPI signal is obtained by scanning the FOV with the Lissajous trajectory. Performing a speed compensation on the MPI signal yields the sampled data, $m(x,y)s(x,y)$. Then, each data point on the non-Cartesian trajectory is convolved with the gridding kernel. This step is repeated for all data points, accumulating the data onto the Cartesian grid. In the denominator of Eq. 1, the same steps are repeated for the case when $m(x,y) = 1$, i.e., gridding ones. This second step provides density compensation for the scanning trajectory. The resulting image, $\hat{m}(x,y)$, is the final x-space MPI image.

As opposed to MRI gridding algorithms, the reconstruction is performed directly in image domain for x-space MPI. Hence, while MRI gridding algorithms can leave certain k-space pixels unfilled, the gridding in MPI must spread the data to all pixels on the Cartesian grid. Furthermore, the resolution of the MRI images is directly dictated by the extent of the acquired k-space, which in turn determines the grid size. In contrast, there is no strict information that determines the grid size in x-space MPI. Hence, image size and kernel width are critical parameters for achieving high-quality x-space MPI images via the proposed technique. Here, these two parameters (i.e., $(\Delta x, \Delta y)$ and $c(x,y)$) are computed automatically from the FFP trajectory, without any external intervention (details not included).

II.II. Simulations

To evaluate the performance of the proposed technique, MATLAB simulations were performed using a custom MPI toolbox. An FFP scanner with selection field gradients of (3, 3, -6) T/m/μ_0 in the (x, y, z) directions, drive field amplitude of 30 mT and 25-nm diameter nanoparticles were assumed. A Lissajous trajectory with a frequency ratio of 17/16 was generated using a base frequency of 2.5 MHz [10]. An imaging phantom of 2×2 cm^2 (shown in Fig. 1, left) was utilized. Based on the trajectory, the proposed algorithm automatically chose an image size of 197×197 and a kernel width of 20×20. The fundamental frequency was filtered out before image reconstruction steps.

For comparison purposes, two different techniques were implemented:

1) All data points together with the trajectory were fed to a scattered interpolation algorithm, for directly interpolating the data onto a Cartesian grid.
2) The Lissajous trajectory was partitioned into two segments with nearly orthogonal directions. An image for each partition was generated using scattered interpolation, and the resulting images were averaged. Details of this second technique can be found in [7].

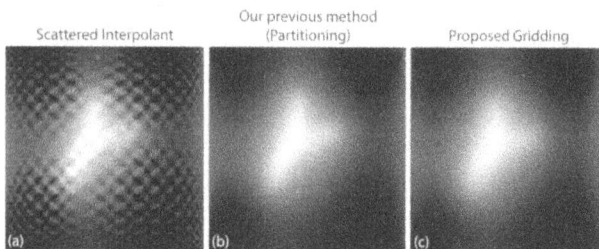

Figure 2: *Simulation results. (a) Scattered interpolation results suffer from severe artifacts. (b) Results of partitioning the trajectory into two directions, followed by scattered interpolation. (c) Results of the proposed generalized reconstruction technique for non-Cartesian x-space MPI.*

III. Results

Fig. 2 shows the resulting MPI images for the proposed technique and the comparison methods. Directly performing a scattered interpolation causes severe artifacts in the image. Since the x-space images from different scan directions are blurred via different point spread functions (PSFs) [2], the data from nearby points on a trajectory can be inconsistent. This inconsistency results in the artifacts seen in Fig. 2a. As shown in Fig. 2b, partitioning of the trajectory solves this problem, as each partition contains data from similar scan directions. However, slight vertical/horizontal stripe artifacts remain, potentially due to inconsistencies between the partitioned images. Fig. 2c shows the result of the proposed technique, which does not suffer from any artifacts. As a trade-off of the proposed algorithm, the image in Fig. 2c is slightly blurred when compared to Fig. 2b.

IV. Discussion

The proposed technique and the partitioning based technique provide visually similar results for the Lissajous trajectory. An important advantage of the proposed technique is that it can be applied to any scanning trajectory (e.g., spiral or radial trajectories), whereas the partitioning based technique can only be applied to trajectories that can be separated into a few directions (e.g., Lissajous trajectory). To overcome blurring caused by the PSF of the imaging system and/or the convolution kernel, a subsequent equalization filter [11] or Wiener deconvolution can be applied on the resulting images.

V. Conclusion

In this work, we presented a reconstruction scheme for non-Cartesian x-space MPI, and demonstrated our results for the example of a Lissajous trajectory. This technique can also be applied to other scanning trajectories such as bi-directional Cartesian, spiral, or radial Lissajous trajectories. The algorithm automatically determines the image size and kernel width for gridding operations, making it a generalized algorithm for non-Cartesian x-space MPI.

ACKNOWLEDGEMENTS
This work was supported by the European Commission through an FP7 Marie Curie Career Integration Grant (PCIG13-GA-2013-618834), by the Turkish Academy of Sciences through TUBA-GEBIP 2015 program, and by the Science Academy through BAGEP award.

REFERENCES
[1] B. Gleich and J. Weizenecker. Tomographic Imaging using the Nonlinear Response of Magnetic Particles. *Nature*, 435(7046): 1214-127, 2005. doi: 10.1038/nature03808.
[2] P. Goodwill and S. Conolly. Multidimensional X-Space Magnetic Particle Imaging. *IEEE Transactions on Medical Imaging*, 30 (9): 1581-1590, 2011. doi: 10.1109/TMI.2011.2125982.
[3] E.U. Saritas *et al.*, Magnetic Particle Imaging (MPI) for NMR and MRI Researchers. *J Magn Reson*, 229:116-126, 2013. doi:10.1016/j.jmr.2012.11.029.
[4] P. Goodwill *et al.*, X-Space MPI: Magnetic Nanoparticles for Safe Medical Imaging. *Advanced Materials*, 24 (28): 3870-3877, 2012. doi: 10.1002/adma.201200221.
[5] T. Knopp *et al.*, Trajectory Analysis for Magnetic Particle Imaging. *Phys Med Biol.*, 54:385-397, 2009. doi: 10.1088/0031-9155/54/2/014.
[6] J. Rahmer *et al.*, Signal encoding in magnetic particle imaging: properties of the system function. *BMC Med Imaging*, 9 (4). 2009. doi: 10.1186/1471-2342-9-4.
[7] A. Alacaoglu *et al.*, Nonlinear Scanning in X-Space MPI. *Proc of International Workshop on Magnetic Particle Imaging(IWMPI)2016*, 74.
[8] P. Beatty, D. Nishimura and J. Pauly, Rapid gridding reconstruction with a minimal overlapping ratio. *IEEE Transactions on Medical Imaging*, 24 (6): 799 – 808, 2005. doi: 10.1109/TMI.2005.848376.
[9] J. Jackson *et al.*, Selection of a Convolution Function for Fourier Inversion using Gridding (Computerised Tomography Application). *IEEE Transactions on Medical Imaging*, 10 (3): 473-478, 1991. doi: 10.1109/42.97598.
[10] F. Werner *et al.*, First experimental comparison between the Cartesian and the Lissajous trajectory for magnetic particle imaging. *Phys Med Biol.*, 2017 May 7;62(9):3407-3421. doi: 10.1088/1361-6560/aa6177.
[11] K. Lu *et al.*, Reshaping the 2D MPI PSF to be isotropic and sharp using vector acquisition and equalization. *2015 5th International Workshop on Magnetic Particle Imaging (IWMPI)*, Istanbul, 2015, pp. 1-1. doi: 10.1109/IWMPI.2015.7106994.

Influence Of A Changing Tracer Distribution On Joint Image And Background Reconstruction

Marcel Straub [a,*], Volkmar Schulz [a,b]

[a] *Department of Physics of Molecular Imaging Systems, Institute of Experimental Molecular Imaging, RWTH Aachen University, 52074 Aachen, Germany*
[b] *Philips Research Europe*
[*] *Corresponding author, email: marcel.straub@pmi.rwth-aachen.de*

I. Introduction

Magnetic Particle Imaging (MPI) as well as other imaging modalities suffer from a background signal. Usually, the background signal is measured before/after the sample measurement. However, the background of some MPI scanners [1] changes over time and cannot be easily modelled. Thus, during prolonged measurements, i.e. more than 20 s, the linear interpolation between two background measurements becomes improper in several cases. This renders prolonged measurements unfeasible because it necessitates a periodical removal of the sample from the field of view (FOV) to remeasure the background signal. Furthermore, for imaging immobilized SPIONs in cells, the background substraction technique [1] reduces the sensitivity and the image quality [2].

To cope with the changing background, we developed an algorithm [3] that uses a well defined shift of the scanner FOV between two consecutively recorded volumes (see Fig. 1 left) to jointly estimate background and tracer distribution. We assume that background and tracer distribution do not change during this FOV shift. Hence, any signal change is a result of the well-known FOV shift. This assumption seems justified due to the fast MPI acquisition time of about 20 ms per volume.

We formulate the reconstruction of the measurement signals $u_i \in \mathbb{C}^{N_{\text{freq}}}$, which only differ by a well-known shift r_i of the FOV and measurement noise, as a regularized least squares problem. With the system matrix $S \in \mathbb{C}^{N_{\text{pos}} \times N_{\text{freq}}}$, the estimated SPION concentration distribution $c \in \mathbb{R}^{N_{\text{pos}}}$ with $N_{\text{pos}} = N_x \times N_y$ voxels, the estimated

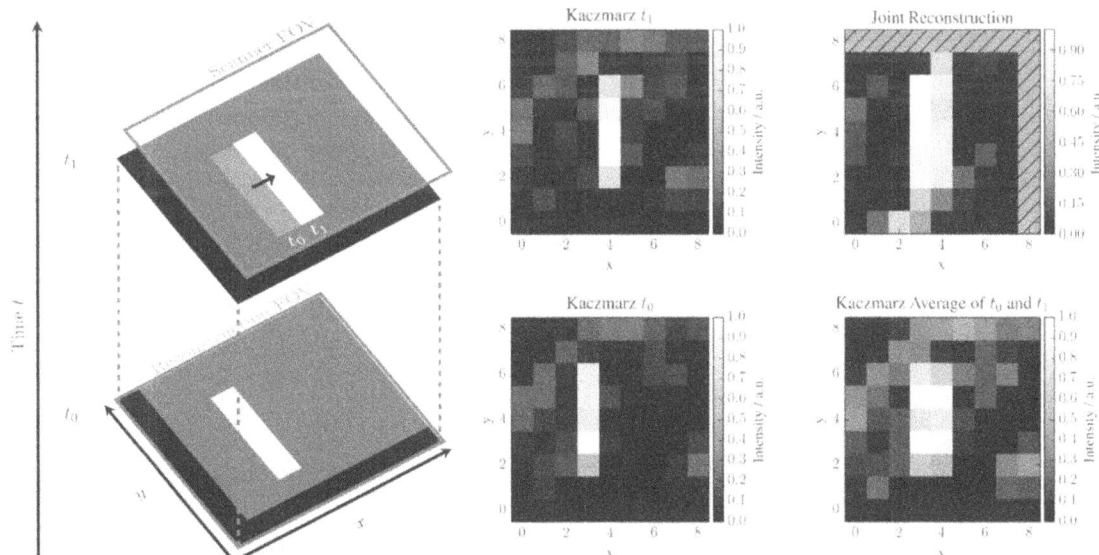

Figure 1: *(left) Illustration of the joint reconstruction method. From time t_0 to t_1, the scanner FOV is shifted by one voxel in x and y direction. The reconstruction FOV is the common subset of voxels. During the shift of the scanner FOV, the sample is also moved by one voxel in x direction. (center column) The reconstruction result for the Kaczmarz reconstruction with non-negativity constraint for time points t_0 and t_1. Besides background subtraction, a background is still visible in the reconstructed image. (right, bottom) Reconstruction of the average of the t_0 and t_1 measurement. (right, top) Joint reconstruction of t_0 and t_1 to a single image. In contrast to the averaged Kaczmarz reconstruction, the background in the image is reduced. However, a smearing resulting from the shift of the Scanner FOV in x and y direction is visible. The smearing in y direction solely results from the FOV*

background $b \in \mathbb{C}^{N_{\text{freq}}}$ and the L_2 regularization factor $\alpha \in \mathbb{R}^{\geq 0}$ this reads:

$$\sum_{i=0}^{1} \|(Sc(r_i) - u_i + b)\|_2^2$$
$$+ \alpha \|c\|_2^2 + \beta \|b - b_{\text{init}}\|_2^2 \rightarrow \min \quad (1)$$

The term $\beta \| b - b_{\text{init}} \|_2^2$ with the parameter $\beta \in \mathbb{R}^{\geq 0}$ describes the background structure as a prior and is based on a previously measured background signal b_{init}.

In this paper, we present a simulation study of the influence of sample movement on this reconstruction method.

II. Material and Methods

We determine the influence of sample movement on our algorithm by simulation. Thereto, we simulate the MPI signal generated by the sample for a movement by one and two pixels in x-direction between two consecutive volumes. During the simulation of a single frame the tracer distribution is kept static. The MPI signal is simulated by forward projecting a spatial phantom concentration distribution c_{true} with a measured system matrix S into the MPI signal domain u_{true}: $u_{\text{true}} = S \cdot c_{\text{true}}$. The MPI signal u, which is used for reconstruction, is gained by superimposing simulated gaussian noise $n \in \mathbb{C}^{N_{\text{freq}}}$ and a background signal b to u_{true}. The background signal b is gained from an actual background measurement series. The reconstruction is seeded with a background signal b_{init} that is linearly interpolated between the first and the last measurement of the background measurement series. The simulation data is also reconstructed with the Kaczmarz algorithm with non-negativity constraint [4]. Thereto, the simulated signal u is background corrected by subtracting b_{init}.

The image quality of the joint recontruction method is evaluated by using the Mean Absolute Error (MAE) between c and c_{true}. The MAE of the moved concentration distribution is normalized by the MAE of the static concentration distribution.

III. Results

Fig. 1 (center column) shows the resulting images of the reconstruction with the Kaczmarz algorithm for both scanner FOVs, i.e. timepoints t_0 and t_1, respectively. Fig. 1 (right, bottom) shows the Kaczmarz reconstruction of the average of the single images (center column). All mentioned images feature a clearly visible image domain background. Fig. 1 (right, top) shows the image resulting from the joint reconstruction of simulated signals. In contrast to Fig. 1 (right, bottom), the resulting image features a smearing of the tracer distribution in y direction. Fig. 2 shows the MAE of the moved tracer distributions relative to the MAE of the static tracer distributions. An increase of the MAE for an increased movement is clearly visible. This effect is higher for a higher signal SNR.

IV. Discussion

In general, the image quality is improved by our reconstruction technique. In the case of a changing tracer

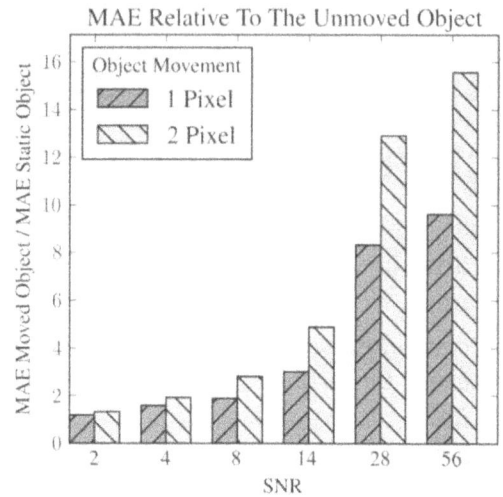

Figure 2: *Relative Mean Absolute Error (MAE) for a simulated one and two voxel movement of the sample in x direction for different SNR values. The MAE is normalized to the MAE of the static sample simulation.*

distribution between consecutive frames, smearing artifacts in the direction of the applied FOV shift are introduced. This is reflected by an increased relative MAE. With increasing tracer dynamic the MAE and the visibility of reconstruction artifacts increase, too. For small changes of the tracer distribution, the introduced artifacts are small and the suppression of the background artifacts is still evident.

To avoid the smearing artifacts, it seems reasonable to apply our algorithm only for frames with minimal changes of the tracer distribution. The so estimated background signal can be used for conventional background subtraction in combination with Kaczmarz reconstruction during highly dynamic episodes.

V. Conclusions

We examined the influence of a changing tracer distribution on our reconstruction method. We showed that a change of the tracer distribution leads to smearing artifacts in the direction of the applied FOV shift. For small changes of the tracer distribution, the background is still reduced and the smearing artifacts are comparable to those of averaging over consecutive volumes.

ACKNOWLEDGEMENTS

This research project is supported by the START-Program of the Faculty of Medicine, RWTH Aachen.

REFERENCES

[1] K. Them, M. G. Kaul, C. Jung, M. Hofmann, T. Mummert, F. Werner, and T. Knopp, "Sensitivity Enhancement in Magnetic Particle Imaging by Background Subtraction," IEEE Transactions on Medical Imaging, vol. 35, no. 3, pp. 893–900, 2016.

[2] K. Them, J. Salamon, P. Szwargulski, S. Sequeira, M. Kaul, C. Lange, H. Ittrich and T. Knopp, "Increasing the sensitivity for stem cell monitoring in system-function based magnetic particle imaging," Phys. Med. Biol., vol. 61, no. 9, pp. 3279-3290, 2016.

[3] M. Straub and V. Schulz, "Joint Reconstruction of Tracer Distribution and Background in Magnetic Particle Imaging," Accepted for publication in IEEE Transactions on Medical Imaging, 2017.

[4] A. Dax, "On Row Relaxation Methods for Large Constrained Least Squares Problems," SIAM Journal on Scientific Computing, vol. 14, no. 3, pp. 570–584, 1993.

Reconstruction of an Object Moved Continuously Through the Field of View in MPI

Patryk Szwargulski [a,b,*], Nadine Gdaniec [a,b], Martin Möddel [a,b], Matthias Graeser [a,b], Tobias Knopp [a,b]

[a] Section for Biomedical Imaging, University Medical Center Hamburg-Eppendorf, Hamburg, Germany
[b] Institute for Biomedical Imaging, Hamburg University of Technology, Hamburg, Germany
* Corresponding author, email: p.szwargulski@uke.de

I. Introduction

Magnetic Particle Imaging (MPI) is a highly sensitive [1, 2, 3] and fast imaging technique [1, 4]. The field of view (FoV) in MPI is defined as the ratio of the drive-field (DF) amplitude to the selection-field strength. Due to the risk of peripheral nerve stimulation, the DF amplitude is limited to about 3 mT for human applications [5, 6] leading to a limited FoV size of few cubic centimeters. To overcome this limitation, focus fields [7] and/or object movements can be used [8]. While electromagnetic FoV movements are in general favorable, focus field shifts come at the cost of an increased electrical power loss of the system. Moreover, they lead to distortions of the scanning trajectory, which need to be accounted for in the reconstruction process. We will therefore investigate object movements as an alternative in this work.

The object can be moved stepwise [9] or continuously through the FoV as shown in Fig. 1 (a). To enlarge the FoV based on continuously acquired data, an adaptation of the system matrix is required. To this end we will apply an approach that has been proposed for continuous focus field movement in [10] and can be equally applied for object movements. We evaluate the approach on phantom data.

II. Material and Methods

II.I. Correction of the movement

Under the assumption of a 3D field-free point (FFP) MPI scanner with sinusoidal excitations with frequencies $f_x = 2.5/102$ MHz, $f_y = 2.5/96$ MHz, and $f_z = 2.5/99$ MHz the FFP follows a Lissajous trajectory during one cycle with the period length T as shown in Fig. 1 (b).

The MPI signal equation is given by

$$u(t) = \int_\Omega c(r) \underbrace{(-\mu_0)\frac{\mathrm{d}}{\mathrm{d}t}m(r,t) \cdot p(r)}_{s(r,t)} \ \mathrm{d}^3 r \qquad (1)$$

whereby $u(t)$ is the induced voltage signal, $c(r)$ is the particle distribution inside the scanner bore Ω, and $s(r,t)$ is the system function including the vacuum permeability μ_0,

$p(r)$ is the coil sensitivity, and $m(r,t)$ is the magnetic moment.

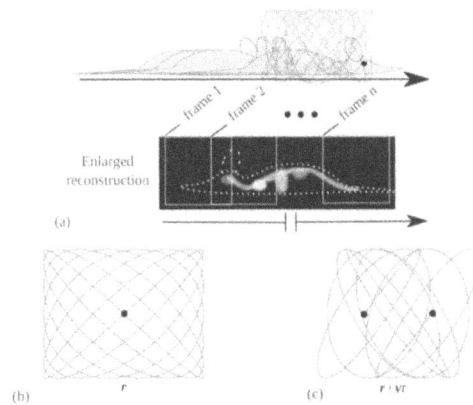

Figure 1: Schematic visualization of the approach and required correction. The imaged object is moved through a static FoV (a). An exemplary static FFP trajectory is shown in (b). The moving object results in a distortion of the FFP trajectory (c) that needs to be corrected.

A moving object induces inconsistencies in the acquired data. These can be described by spatial shifts $\tilde{r} = r + vt$, where $t \in [0,T]$ and v is the velocity of the object. Alternatively, the moving object can be interpreted as an elongation of the FFP-trajectory as presented in Fig. 1 (c). If the movement is included into the signal equation (1) it changes to

$$u(t) = \int_\Omega c(\tilde{r}) \underbrace{(-\mu_0)\frac{\mathrm{d}}{\mathrm{d}t}m(\tilde{r}-vt, t) \cdot p(\tilde{r}-vt)}_{s(\tilde{r}-vt,t)} \ \mathrm{d}^3\tilde{r},$$

where $s(\tilde{r}-vt,t)$ is the shifted system function.

II.II. Experimental Setup

For the experiments a preclinical 3D FFP MPI scanner (Bruker Biospin MRI GmbH, Ettlingen, Germany) with a gradiometric receive coil [2] was used. All scans were performed with a gradient strength of $G_z = 2 \cdot G_y = 2 \cdot G_x = 2$ T/(m·μ_0) and with a 3D sinusoidal excitation with an amplitude of 12 mT/μ_0 in all directions. In the experiment, we compare the effects on the reconstructed images of continuously moving versus stepwise shifting the phantom. A 5.5 cm long spiral mounted on a 3D printed robot holder was used as a phantom and is shown in Fig. 2. The spiral was made of a tube filled with diluted Resovist (62.5 mmol(Fe)/L). The stepwise motion in increments of 2 mm took about 30 s including 50 frames at each position, whereas the continuous motion was performed at 54 mm/s (1.16 mm/frame) with a total scan time of 1.01 s.

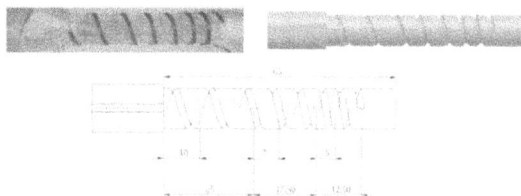

Figure 2: Shown is the final spiral phantom (top) the CAD model (center) and the schematic representation (bottom).

The data has been reconstructed using the implicit joint multi-patch approach proposed in [11]. Here, a static measured system matrix has been used and adapted for the correction of the movement. To validate the effect of the correction the quotient of the maximal signal and the standard derivation of the noise (signal to noise ratio) for the reconstructed images has been calculated.

III. Results

In the upper part of Fig. 3 the reconstruction results of the phantom experiments as maximum intensity projection of the xz plane are shown. The reconstruction result of the step-wise moved phantom (a) is given as a ground-truth. The result of the continuously moved object without (b) and with an additional system matrix correction (c) is also shown. An axial profile at the marked positions through the reconstructed image of the spiral for each case is shown in the lower part of Fig. 3.

The correction of the system matrix improves the image quality of the reconstruction results for a continuously moved object leading to similar image quality as for the stepwise moved object. This is underlined by the calculated signal to noise ratios for each image. Those are 46 for the stepwise moved image, 34 for the continuously moved without and 41 with an additional system matrix adaption.

IV. Discussion

The reconstruction results of the phantom experiments demonstrate that a continuous movement during acquisition is possible without high distortions. The proposed correction reduces the motion artifacts resulting in a better signal to noise ratio of the image. With a look to faster shifts and/or for combined move and focus field measurements, the correction will be very important.

V. Conclusions

In this work we proposed to enlarge the FoV in MPI by a continuous external movement of the object. Due to the continuous movement the reconstruction includes motion artifacts. Those are corrected by modifying the system matrix such that the movement is compensated. It could be shown, that the proposed method is a valid alternative to enlarge the FoV also for 3D scanners with and without focus fields.

ACKNOWLEDGEMENTS

The authors thankfully acknowledge the financial support by the German Research Foundation (DFG, grant number KN 1108/2-1) and the Federal Ministry of Education and Research (BMBF, grant number 05M16GKA). Further the authors want thank Dr. Jürgen Rahmer for fruitful discussions.

REFERENCES

[1] B. Gleich and J. Weizenecker. Tomographic imaging using the nonlinear response of magnetic particles. *Nature*, 435(7046):1217-1217, 2005.

[2] M. Graeser et al. Towards Picogram Detection of Superparamagnetic Iron-Oxide Particles Using a Gradiometric Receive Coil. *Sci. Rep.* 7:6872, 2017.

[3] H. Arami et al. Tomographic magnetic particle imaging of cancer targeted nanoparticles. *Nanoscale*, pp. –, 2017.

[4] J. Weizenecker et al. Three-dimensional real-time in vivo magnetic particle imaging. *Phys. Med. Biol.* 54(5):L1 – L10, 2009.

[5] E. U. Saritas et al. Magnetostimulation limits in magnetic particle imaging. *IEEE TMI*, 32(9):1600–1610, 2013.

[6] I. Schmale et al. Human PNS and SAR study in the frequency range from 24 to 162 kHz. *3th IWMPI*. 1-1, 2013.

[7] B. Gleich et al. Fast MPI demonstrator with enlarged field of view. *In Proc. ISMRM*, 18:218, 2010.

[8] P. W. Goodwill and S. M. Conolly. Multi-dimensional x-space magnetic particle imaging. *IEEE TMI* 30(9):1581 – 1590, 2011.

[9] P. Szwargulski et al. Enlarging the field of view in MPI using a moving table approach. *In Proc. SPIE*, 10578-51. 2017.

[10] J. Rahmer et al. Automated Derivation of Sub-Volume System Functions for 3D MPI with Fast Continuous Focus Field Variation. *4th IWMPI*, 97, 2014.

[11] P. Szwargulski et al. Fast Implicit Reconstruction of Focus Field Data in MPI. *6th IWMPI*, 176, 2017.

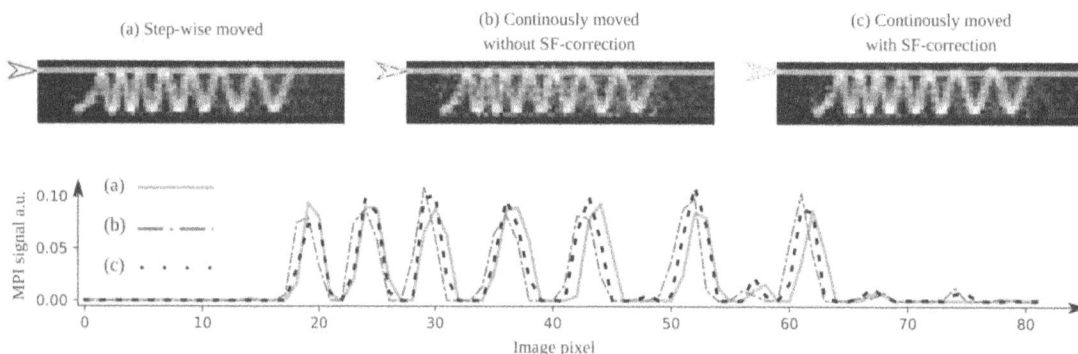

Figure 3: Results of the phantom experiments. Maximum intensity projection of the step-wise moved (a), the continuously moved without SF correction (b) and with SF correction (c) is shown in the upper part. In the lower part, profiles for all cases are shown.

Session 09 - Talks

Applications II

Temperature Dependence of MPI Spectra

James Wells[*], Norbert Löwa, Hendrik Paysen, Olaf Kosch, Lutz Trahms, Frank Wiekhorst

Physikalisch - Technische Bundesanstalt, Abbestraße 2, 10587 Berlin, Germany
[*] Corresponding author, email: james.wells@ptb.de

I. Introduction

Magnetic nanoparticles (MNPs) in liquid suspension exhibit a wide variety of dynamic behaviours when exposed to alternating magnetic fields. These responses depend on many contributing factors; these include the type of MNPs, the suspension medium used, and the amplitude and frequency of the applied field [1].

Recently studies have demonstrated detectable temperature dependences in the spectra obtained by magnetic particle spectrometry (MPS) [2], and magnetic particle imaging (MPI) [3]. These works primarily concentrated on the development and implementation of new technologies such as remote thermometry via monitoring the relaxation behaviours of particles under AC fields [4], or the development of thermally resolved MPI to aid in magnetic hyperthermia cancer therapy [5]. While these concepts have been demonstrated in limited cases, using specific MNP types, a wider study of the variations in temperature dependent behaviours between different MNP systems has yet to be undertaken.

MPS and MPI measurements are usually conducted on liquid suspensions of MNP. Here, the particles may be subject to both Néel and Brownian relaxation. The respective contributions depend on the MNP composition, local environment and applied fields. The two relaxation types have distinct temperature dependences [6]. Differing contributions from the relaxation types in each MNP system result in unique spectral temperature dependences.

We present an experimental study of temperature dependences in spectra obtained using temperature-controlled MPS for two MNP systems. We also present initial temperature-dependence results obtained from MPI scanner measurements using a specially built temperature-controlled sample holder.

II. Material and Methods

II.I. Magnetic particle spectrometry

A commercial MPS spectrometer (MPS-3, Bruker) with built-in control of the sample temperature was used. The MPS provides a single-axis excitation (25 kHz, 12 mT). Sample temperatures can be varied between 296 K and 318 K (magnetic hyperthermia therapy typically utilizes temperatures between 315 K and 318 K) as higher temperatures may damage the calibration of the MPS pick-up coil. Separate background measurements at each temperature were used to compensate for any thermal drift within the system.

II.II. MPI scanner

MPI scanner measurements were conducted using a Bruker MPI 25/20 FF system installed at the Charité Berlin. Temperature dependent results using a single-axis excitation and no selection field were previously published [6]. To test the behaviours of the MNP under real MPI imaging conditions, a 3-axis field excitation was employed with frequencies of 2.5 MHz divided between 102/96/99 in the x/y/z axes and amplitude of 12 mT. A selection field gradient of 2.5/1.25/1.25 T/m in x/y/z axes was used. All data was recorded using the x-axis receive coil. Raw measurements without transfer function removal were used.

Temperature dependent MPI measurement acquisition was achieved by implementing a purpose-built temperature-controlled sample holder. The holder uses a water pump with built-in heater (situated outside MPI scanner's shielded room) which circulates a continuous stream of water to maintain the sample at a constant temperature. Using the heater unit currently available, temperatures from room temperature up to 323 K can be achieved.

II.III Particle Systems studied

We report the temperature dependence of MPS and MPI spectra produced by two commercial iron-oxide MNP systems, each of which is marketed as a potential MPI tracer. Results and analysis from additional MNP systems will be presented at the conference.

Ferucarbotran (FCT) (Meito Sangyo, Japan) - A colloidal solution of multicore MNPs; comprising superparamagnetic iron oxide cores coated in carboxydextran. FCT is characterized by a broad distribution of hydrodynamics sizes in the range 5 – 80 nm.

Synomag (SYN) (Micromod Partikel Technologie GmbH, Germany) - Iron oxide nanoparticles in aqueous buffer suspension with COOH surface functionalization. The average hydrodynamic diameter is approximately 30 nm.

MNP samples consisted of 30 μL of suspension inside a non-magnetic container. The same MNP sample and container used in the MPS studies were used for the MPI scanner measurements.

II.IV Spectra Changes

The ratio between the fifth and third harmonics (A_5/A_3) of the MNP spectra obtained using MPS and MPI was used to probe the changes in the MNP dynamics with increasing temperature. For MPI measurements (3-axis excitation), the harmonics were measured at multiples of the x-axis excitation frequency, as the data was collected in this axis. The A_5/A_3 does not give complete information about a particle system's spectra, but a simple indication of the rate at which the spectra decays in the higher harmonics. The temperature dependence of other key spectral parameters will be presented and discussed at the IWMPI conference.

III. Results

The temperature dependence of the A_5/A_3 obtained via MPS for each MNP system is presented in Fig 1. Significant differences are observed in both the magnitude and polarity of the changes for the two MNP systems. The A_5/A_3 of FCT rises with increasing temperature, indicating that the MPI imaging quality of this tracer may improve at higher temperatures. Conversely, the A_5/A_3 of SYN is observed to decrease with increasing temperature, this indicates that less signal is detected in the higher frequency components at higher temperatures, and so imaging quality may be reduced. The underlying cause for this fundamental difference is currently unclear, however similar differences were previously reported in similar measurements of other particle systems [7]. Detailed analysis of these results, and additional measurements from other MNP systems will be presented at the IWMPI conference.

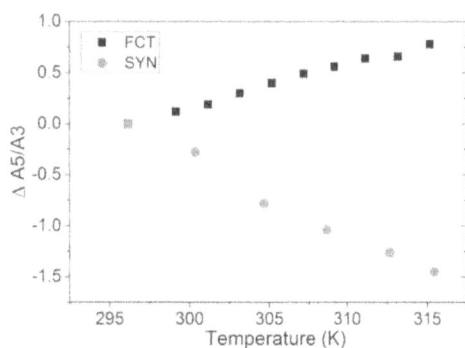

Figure 1: *MPS results showing the changes in A_5/A_3 ratio with increasing temperature for FCT and SYN particles.*

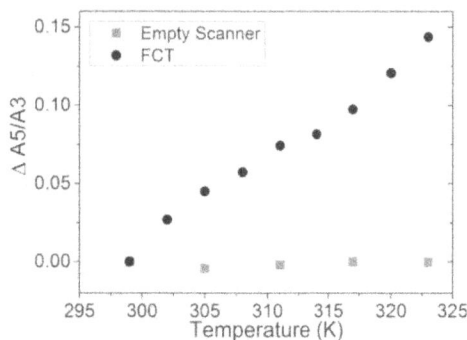

Figure 2: *Initial MPI temperature dependences obtained using FCT, compared with empty scanner measurement. Measurements for the remaining particle systems will be completed before IWMPI 2018 and presented along with a full discussion and analysis.*

Results so-far obtained using the temperature controlled platform for the MPI scanner are presented in figure 2. The changes in A_5/A_3 with increasing temperature are plotted for both a measurement of a pure water sample ("Empty scanner"), and for a sample of FCT. The empty scanner measurement shows negligible variation with increasing temperature, this indicates that the heat escaping from the temperature-controlled sample holder is not causing any drift within the MPI scanner electronics. The FCT measurement shows a clear increase in A_5/A_3 with increasing temperature, which agrees with the MPS result. The amplitude of the observed change in the MPI measurement is significantly smaller than in the MPS (around one tenth). The likely cause for this difference is related to the use of multi-axis excitation and additional selection field gradient in the MPI scanner as compared with the single-axis excitation of the MPS. The multi-axis excitation results in a broader distribution of signal between the frequency components, and thus lower amplitudes in the individual harmonics.

V. Conclusions

We have demonstrated non-negligible and MNP-specific thermal dependences in the spectra produced by two iron-oxide MNP systems with potential for use as MPI tracers. Temperature dependences were observed in both MPS (single-axis excitation) and MPI scanner (3-axis excitation). The differing effects in the particle systems studied highlight our need for advanced understanding of the properties which govern the complexities of the spectral response of a given MNP system to a given field excitation. Improvements in our understanding of these processed will aid the development of higher quality, and more reliable MPI results, as well as aiding in the development of novel and high-impact technologies including temperature-resolved MPI. With further analysis of the existing results, and additional measurements, we will develop a deeper understanding of the causes for the observed behaviours.

ACKNOWLEDGEMENTS

The financial support of the DFG research grants "quantMPI: Establishment of quantitative Magnetic Particle Imaging" (TR 408/9-1) and "AMPI: Magnetic particle imaging: Development and evaluation of novel methodology for the assessment of the aorta in vivo in a small animal model of aortic aneurysms" (SHA 1506/2-1) is gratefully acknowledged.

REFERENCES

[1] L. M. Bauer et al. Magnetic particle imaging tracers: state-of-the-art and future directions. J. Phys. Chem. Lett., 2015, 6 (13), pp 2509-2517

[2] E. Garaio et al. Harmonic phases of the nanoparticle magnetization: An intrinsic temperature probe. *Appl. Phys. Lett.* 107 , 123103 (2015)

[3] C. Stehning et al. Simultaneous magnetic particle imaging (MPI) and temperature mapping using multi-colour MPI. *IJMPI*, 2, 2 (2016)

[4] D. B. Reeves and J. B. Weaver. Magnetic nanoparticle sensing: decoupling the magnetization from the excitation field. J Phys D Appl Phys. 2014; 47(4): 045002

[5] D. Hensley et al. Combining magnetic particle imaging and magnetic fluid hyperthermia in a theranostic platform. *Phys. Med Biol.* 62, 9 (2017)

[6] J. Dieckhoff et al. Magnetic-field dependence of Brownian and Neel relaxation times. *J. Appl. Phys.* 119, 043903 (2016)

[7] J. Wells et al. "Temperature dependence in magnetic particle imaging" AIP Advances 8, 056703 (2018)

Spatial and Temperature Resolutions of Magnetic Nanoparticle Temperature Imaging with a Scanning Magnetic Particle Spectrometer

Jing Zhong [a,*], Meinhard Schilling[a], and Frank Ludwig[a]

[a] Institut für Elektrische Messtechnik und Grundlagen der Elektrotechnik, TU Braunschweig, Braunschweig, Germany
* Corresponding author, email: j.zhong@tu-braunschweig.de

I. Introduction

Non-invasive and *in-vivo* temperature imaging is crucial to biomedical applications [1]. Recently, magnetic nanoparticle (MNP) thermometry has been reported for non-invasive temperature measurement, but only for the integral, average temperature of a MNP sample [2-5]. In 2005, magnetic particle imaging (MPI) was firstly introduced to directly measure the spatial distribution of MNP concentration [6]. Then, MPI was used to estimate the spatial distribution of MNP temperatures with temperature dependent MPI image intensity and an approach of color MPI [7-9]. Additionally, a scanning magnetic particle spectrometer (SMPS) was designed to simultaneously measure the spatial distributions of MNP concentration and temperature [10].

This paper investigates the temperature and spatial resolutions of MNP temperature imaging with a SMPS. A multi-line phantom is used to perform experiments to image the spatial distributions of MNP concentration and temperature. The spatial and temperature resolutions of the MNP temperature imaging are discussed.

II. Material and Methods

A SMPS, consisting of a mechanical scanner and a magnetic particle spectrometer (MPS), was designed to locally measure MNP harmonics [10]. The MPS consists of a Helmholtz coil and a gradiometric pickup coil with a diameter of about 2.5 mm and a length of about 3 mm. The measured i^{th} harmonic $u_i(x, y)$ is a convolution of the coil sensitivity $s(x, y)$ and the ith harmonic $M_i(x, y, \varphi, T)$ generated by local MNPs

$$u_i(x,y) = i\omega \cdot s(x,y) * M_i(x,y,\varphi,T), \quad (1)$$

where $M_i(x, y, \varphi, T)$ depends on MNP concentration φ and temperature T, and $s(x, y)$ depends only on the geometry of the gradiometric pickup coil, which is defined as the point spread function (PSF). A deconvolution based on the PSF enables the images of MNP harmonics generated by local MNPs, which can be used for MNP concentration and

temperature imaging. In this paper, the 1st and 3rd harmonics are measured to realize MNP concentration and temperature imaging. The simultaneous algebraic reconstruction technique (SART) is used to perform the deconvolution, where a parameter K_{max} is set to stop the iteration. The measured 1st and 3rd harmonics are independently deconvolved by the SART. Then, the harmonic ratios, independent of MNP concentration, are used to calculate MNP temperature images.

III. Results

The MNP phantoms are filled with SHP-30, purchased from Ocean NanoTech. Ltd. Corp. (San Diego, USA). A water tube with cycling water by a pump was used to change the temperature profile of the phantom (see Fig. 1a). The water temperature was controlled in a water bath at about 346K (about 73 °C). An ac magnetic field with amplitude of 10 mT and frequency of 2004 Hz is applied. A multi-line phantom (see Fig. 1a) was scanned with the SMPS. Each line in the phantom has a length of 8 mm and a width of 1 mm. The distances between adjacent two lines are 0.5 mm, 1.0 mm, 1.5 mm, 2.0 mm, 3.0 mm and 4.0 mm. The scanning field of view (FOV) is 10 mm × 22 mm in x- and y-directions with a scanning step of 0.2 mm. The scanning time amounts to about 15 min.

Figures 1b and 1c show the measured 1st and 3rd harmonics whereas Fig. 1d and 1e depict the deconvolved 1st and 3rd harmonics. It indicates that the deconvolution improves the spatial resolution. To investigate the spatial and temperature resolutions, different K_{max} values are applied in the deconvolution. The deconvolved 1st and 3rd harmonics at the middle of the images shown in Fig. 1 are used to calculate the concentration φ and temperature T, shown in Fig. 2. Fig. 2a displays the curve of normalized concentration φ versus y (φ-y curve) whereas Fig. 2b displays the curve of temperature T versus y (T-y curve). Herein, the temperature was calculated with the harmonic ratio of the 3rd to 1st harmonic amplitude $R_{3rd/1st}$ and a calibration curve of temperature versus $R_{3rd/1st}$. Note that $K_{max} = 0$ means that the harmonics are the measured ones without deconvolution. A threshold is applied in the calculation of harmonic ratio. If the MNP concentration is lower than the threshold, the calculated temperature is set to be room temperature (about 295 K).

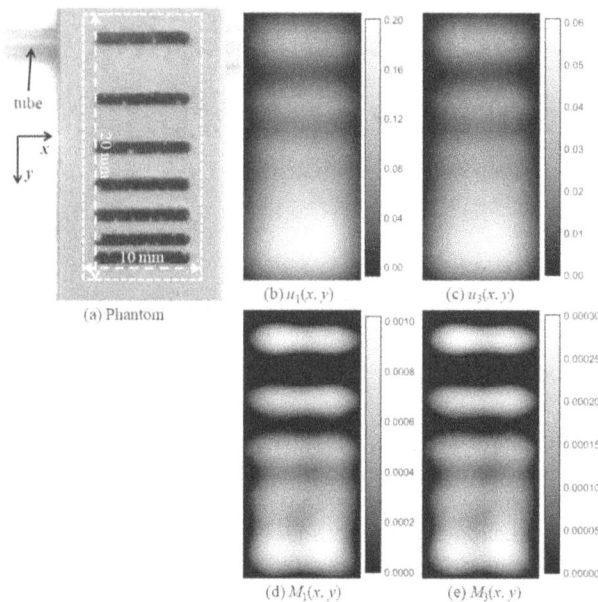

(a) Phantom   (b) $u_1(x, y)$ (c) $u_3(x, y)$

(d) $M_1(x, y)$ (e) $M_3(x, y)$

Figure 1: (a) A photo of the multi-line phantom. (b) and (c) show the measured 1st and 3rd harmonics. (d) and (e) show the deconvolved 1st and 3rd harmonics. K_{max}=100 is applied in the deconvolution. The scanning FOV is 10 mm × 22 mm with a scanning step of 0.2 mm.

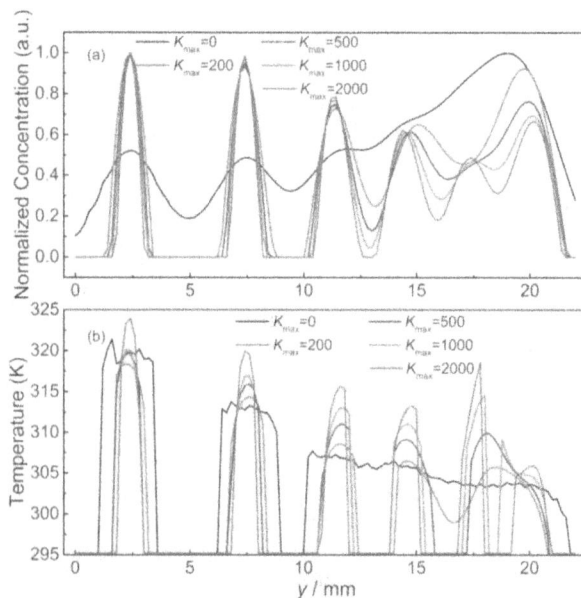

Figure 2: (a) Normalized concentration φ versus y curves with different K_{max} values. (b) Temperature versus y curves with different K_{max} values. Symbols represent experimental results whereas solid lines are guides to the eye.

IV. Discussion

The φ-y curves shown in Fig. 2a indicate that the spatial resolution increases with increasing K_{max}. For $K_{max} = 0$, the φ-y curve shows about 3 or 4 peaks, resulting in a spatial resolution of between 2 and 3 mm. For $K_{max} = 200$, the φ-y curve shows about 5 peaks, meaning that the spatial

resolution is about 2 mm. For $K_{max} = 1000$ or 2000, the deconvolved image shows 6 peaks, resulting in a spatial resolution of about 1 mm. However, the deconvolved image with a higher K_{max} cannot distinguish the two lines with a distance of 0.5 mm. Thus, the highest spatial resolution achievable with the given setup is about 1 mm.

The T-y curves displayed in Fig. 2b show that temperature expectedly decreases with increasing the distance between the hot-water tube and the MNP sample. For $K_{max} = 0$, the fluctuation in the temperature mainly comes from the measurement noise, as shown by the black solid line in Fig. 2b. With increasing K_{max}, the oscillation in temperature worsens, meaning that the measured temperature will have a high oscillation and consequently a worse resolution. Therefore, a higher K_{max} allows a higher spatial resolution, but a low temperature resolution.

V. Conclusions

This paper investigates the spatial and temperature resolutions of MNP temperature imaging with a scanning magnetic particle spectrometer. Experimental results show that the deconvolution increases the spatial resolution, but worsens the temperature resolution. The highest achievable spatial resolution is about 1 mm.

ACKNOWLEDGEMENTS

Financial support from the Alexander von Humboldt Foundation is acknowledged.

REFERENCES

[1] B. Thiesen and A. Jordan, Clinical applications of magnetic nanoparticles for hyperthermia, *Int. J. Hyperthermia*, 24 (6): 467-474, 2008. doi: 10.1080/02656730802104757.

[2] J. B. Weaver, A. M. Rauwerdink and E. W. Hansen, Magnetic nanoparticle temperature estimation, Med. Phys. 36 (5): 1822-1829, 2009. doi: 10.1118/1.3106342.

[3] M. Zhou, J. Zhong, W. Liu, Z. Du, Z. Huang, M. Yang, and P. C. Morais, Study of magnetic nanoparticle spectrum for magnetic nanothermometry, *IEEE Trans. Magn.*, 51 (9): 6101006, 2015. doi: 10.1109/TMAG.2015.2434322.

[4] J. Zhong, J. Dieckhoff, M. Schilling, and F. Ludwig, Influence of static magnetic field strength on the temperature resolution of a magnetic nanoparticle thermometer, *J.Appl. Phys.*, 120 (14): 143902, 2016. doi: 10.1063/1.4964696.

[5] J. Zhong M. Schilling, and F. Ludwig, Magnetic nanoparticle thermometry independent of Brownian relaxation, *J. Phys. D: Appl. Phys.*, in press. doi: 10.1088/1361-6463/aa993d.

[6] B. Gleich and J. Weizenecker. Tomographic imaging using the nonlinear response of magnetic particles. *Nature*, 435(7046): 1217-1217, 2005. doi: 10.1038/nature03808.

[7] K.Murase, M. Aoki, N. Banura, K. Nishimoto, A.Mimura, T. Kuboyabu, and I. Yabata. Usefulness of magnetic particle imaging for predicting the therapeutic effect of magnetic hyperthermia. *Open J.Med. Imag.*, 5(2):85–99, 2015. doi:10.4236/ojmi.2015.52013.

[8] J. Rahmer, A. Halkola, B. Gleich, I. Schmale and J. Borgert. First experimental evidence of the feasibility of multi-color magnetic particle imaging. *Phys. Med. Biol.*, 60 (5): 1775–1791, 2015. doi:10.1088/0031-9155/60/5/1775.

[9] C. Stehning, B. Gleich, and J. Rahmer. Simultaneous magnetic particle imaging (MPI) and temperature mapping using multi-color MPI. *Int. J.Magnetic Particle Imaging*, 2(2): 1612001, 2016. doi: 10.18416/ijmpi.2016.1612001.

[10] J. Zhong, M. Schilling, and F. Ludwig. Magnetic nanoparticle temperature imaging with a scanning magnetic particle spectrometer. *Small, Submitted.*

Influence of Magnetic Nanoparticle Mobility on the Harmonic Response Studied by Magnetic Particle Spectroscopy

S. Draack [a,*], T. Viereck [a], F. Ludwig [a], and M. Schilling [a]

[a] Institut für Elektrische Messtechnik und Grundlagen der Elektrotechnik, Technische Universität Braunschweig, Braunschweig, Germany
* Corresponding author, email: s.draack@tu-bs.de

I. Introduction

Magnetic Particle Spectroscopy (MPS) is a spectral characterization method determining both the linear and the non-linear magnetization properties of magnetic nanoparticles (MNP). MPS provides a powerful tool to characterize MNP and thus to examine their suitability as tracer for Magnetic Particle Imaging (MPI) [1]. Especially with regard to mobility [2] or multi-color MPI [3], MPS allows one to investigate the influence of environmental parameters, such as dynamic viscosity and temperature, on the harmonic spectrum. To investigate the influence of dynamic viscosity and binding state on spectral changes of measurement data, MPS measurements were performed using a model-like particle system dispersed in various water-glycerol mixtures. The experimental results are compared to numerical simulations.

II. Material and Methods

For typical field strengths in MPS, a sinusoidal magnetic excitation field forces the magnetization of the particles periodically into saturation. Due to the particles' non-linear magnetization curve, the magnetization response includes higher harmonics which provide sensitive information not only on the particles' magnetic moments but also about their dynamics and binding state. The institute's custom-built MPS setups provide drive-field peak amplitudes up to 30 mT. The frequency can be adjusted in a range from 100 Hz to 25 kHz in our low-frequency setup, which additionally allows temperature-dependent measurements between -14 °C and 114 °C [4], while the high-frequency setup supports excitation frequencies from 10 kHz to 100 kHz.

To systematically study impacts of MNP properties on MPS and MPI signal generation, a model-like particle system with well-known particle properties is required. An important requirement for the investigation of particle mobility is that MNP are thermally blocked, i.e., that the Brownian mechanism dominates the dynamics. Its mean core diameter of 25 nm with narrow distribution and comparatively small hydrodynamic mean diameter

suggests Ocean NanoTech SHP-25 as a model system to investigate particle-matrix interactions and to clarify MPS and MPI signal generation including particle dynamics. Mathematical models are examined for their suitability for describing the measurement data and compared to each other.

For low excitation frequencies, the dynamics of thermally blocked MNP in Newtonian liquids are dominated by the Brownian relaxation process. Therefore, the spectra in MPS measurements significantly modulate with varying matrix properties. The following MPS measurements were performed using a drive field peak amplitude of 25 mT and an excitation frequency of 1 kHz.

III. Results

Fig. 1 shows the spectral magnitude of the odd higher harmonics for six different glycerol-water mixtures of Ocean NanoTech SHP-25 samples, each with the same iron concentration.

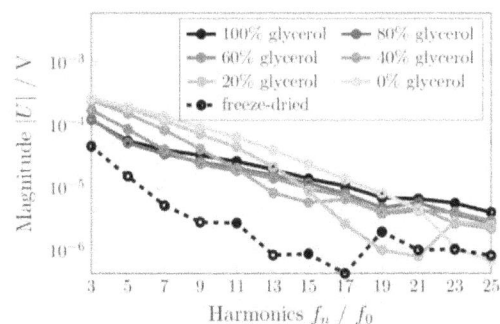

Figure 1: Spectral magnitude of odd higher harmonics of Ocean NanoTech SHP-25 for different glycerol-water mixtures and a freeze-dried (mannitol) reference sample, acquired in a MPS measurement at peak field amplitude $\mu_0 H = 25$ mT and frequency $f_0 = 1$ kHz.

Additionally, the harmonics of a freeze-dried (D-Mannitol) reference sample is shown, which also contains the same iron concentration. The measurement points of the higher harmonics are linked via linear interpolations to better distinguish different samples. The harmonic spectra display a very complex behavior with crossings despite the monotonous change in viscosity.

A different illustration of the low-order odd harmonics ($3 f_0$ to $11 f_0$) as a function of the dynamic viscosity of the matrix [5] is shown in the first row of Fig. 2. The representation of the real and imaginary part of the magnetic susceptibility which is proportional to the induced voltage in our gradiometric pick-up coil is well-known from AC susceptibility (ACS) measurements.

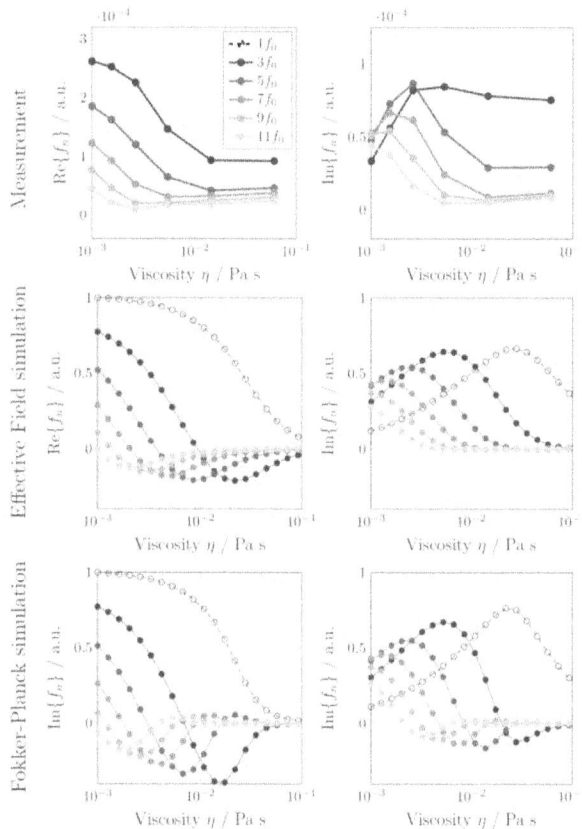

Figure 2: *Measured (first row) real and imaginary parts of the odd higher harmonics depending on the dynamic viscosity of the suspension matrix as well as simulation data using the Effective Field method (second row) and the Fokker-Planck equation (third row) for Brownian relaxation only.*

To explain the measured observations, simulations of mathematical models were performed. The center row and the bottom row of Fig. 2 show the Effective Field method [6] and the Fokker-Planck equation [7] simulation results for the given particle properties.

IV. Discussion

As can be seen from Fig. 1 the lower harmonics decrease with higher viscosity of the matrix, whereas the higher harmonics increase by trend. The lower the viscosity of the water-glycerol mixture, the larger is the contribution of particles relaxing via Brownian rotation. Therefore, the lower harmonics in the MPS magnitude spectra which are dominated by the particle contribution relaxing via Brownian rotation exhibit an emphasized signal amplitude.

A more familiar and perhaps easier-to-understand representation of the measured data which is similar to ACS measurements of the fundamental only can be achieved by plotting real and imaginary parts of each higher harmonic over the dynamic viscosity. The effect of dynamic viscosity on the magnetic behavior of thermally blocked MNP can approximately be explained by using well-known simulation models like the Effective Field model (see second row in Fig. 2), including the field-dependent Brownian relaxation time, or the Brownian Fokker-Planck equation (see third row in Fig. 2) which intrinsically includes the magnetic field dependency. As can be seen from Fig. 2, both the Effective Field model and the Fokker-Planck equation explain the measured data very well. Nevertheless, some deviations are discernable which are caused by the additional Néel contribution. Both models consider only Brownian relaxation. However, the investigated sample SHP-25 also includes particles relaxing via the Néel relaxation mechanism leading to measurable signals even at very high viscosities. In addition, the fraction of MNP relaxing via the Néel mechanism is expected to change with viscosity.

V. Conclusions

Since the Brownian rotation is directly related to matrix properties, multiparametric MPS measurements on model-like MNP/matrix systems allow one to investigate the influence of environmental parameters, such as viscosity and temperature, on the harmonic generation. Currently available non-linear models describe measurement data only incomplete, as one of the possible relaxation modes is always neglected. Further developments of coupled models are necessary to enable a model-based reconstruction and the establishment of MPI as a quantitative imaging modality.

ACKNOWLEDGEMENTS
Financial support by the German Research Foundation, DFG Priority Program 1681 (SCHI383/2-1, VI892/1-1) and from "Niedersächsisches Vorab" through the "Quantum- and Nano-Metrology (QUANOMET)" initiative within project NP-2 are acknowledged.

REFERENCES
[1] B. Gleich and J. Weizenecker. *Tomographic imaging using the nonlinear response of magnetic particles.* Nature 435:30, 2005. doi: 10.1038/nature03808.

[2] T. Viereck, C. Kuhlmann, S. Draack, M. Schilling, and F. Ludwig. *Dual-frequency magnetic particle imaging of the Brownian contribution.* J. Magn. Magn. Mater. 427:156-161, 2017. doi: 10.1016/j.jmmm.2016.11.003

[3] J. Rahmer, A. Halkola, B. Gleich, I. Schmale, J. Borgert. *First experimental evidence of the feasibility of multi-color magnetic particle imaging.* Phys. Med. Biol. 60:5, 2015. doi: 10.1088/0031-9155/60/5/1775

[4] S. Draack, T. Viereck, C. Kuhlmann, M. Schilling, and F. Ludwig. *Temperature-dependent MPS measurements.* Int. J. Magn. Part. Imag. 3, No. 1, 2017. doi: 10.18416/ijmpi.2017.1703018

[5] T. Wawrzik, T. Yoshida, M. Schilling, and F. Ludwig. *Debye-Based Frequency-Domain Magnetization Model for Magnetic Nanoparticles in Magnetic Particle Spectroscopy.* IEEE Trans. Magn. 51, 2015. doi: 10.1109/tmag.2014.2332371

[6] D. B. Reeves and J. Weaver. *Approaches for modeling magnetic nanoparticle dynamics.* Crit. Rev. Biomed. Eng. 42(1):85-93, 2014. doi: 10.1615/CritRevBiomedEng.2014010845

[7] R. J. Deissler, Y. Wu, and M. A. Martens. *Dependence of Brownian and Néel relaxation times on magnetic field strength.* Med. Phys. 41 (1), 2014. doi: 10.1118/1.4837216

Relaxation-Based Calibration-Free Multi-Color MPI for FFL Scanners: A Simulation Study

Yavuz Muslu [a, b*], Emine Ulku Saritas [a, b, c]

[a] *Department of Electrical and Electronics Engineering, Bilkent University, Ankara, Turkey*
[b] *National Magnetic Resonance Research Center (UMRAM), Bilkent University, Ankara, Turkey*
[c] *Neuroscience Program, Sabuncu Brain Research Center, Bilkent University, Ankara, Turkey*
[*] *Corresponding author, email: ymuslu@ee.bilkent.edu.tr*

I. Introduction

In X-space magnetic particle imaging (MPI), the ideal signal is defined as the Langevin response of the nanoparticles to an oscillating drive field [1], [2]. While in theory an instantaneous response is expected from the nanoparticles, in practice a delay process called relaxation takes place [3]. This process causes a lagging and widening in the time-domain MPI signal. In image domain, the effect of relaxation is seen as a blurring along the scan direction. The differences in both the underlying Langevin response and relaxation times of different nanoparticles have recently been exploited for multi-color MPI, with the purpose of identifying nanoparticle types or environmental conditions such as temperature and viscosity [4]-[9].

In a previous study, we proposed a calibration-free method for generating multi-color images from relaxation time constants estimated directly from the time-domain MPI signal [10] and provided an experimental demonstration on our in-house field free point (FFP) MPI scanner [11]. Here, we show that this calibration-free relaxation-based multi-color MPI technique can be extended to field free line (FFL) scanners, by leveraging a modified projection reconstruction (PR) algorithm.

II. Material and Methods

The proposed relaxation time constant estimation method in [11] utilizes a periodic FFP trajectory, where the resulting time-domain MPI signal shows symmetry between the positive and negative cycles. This symmetry property also applies to FFL scanners that use a periodic trajectory. Here, we briefly show what the estimated time constants correspond to for projection imaging, and how the underlying 2D relaxation map can be recovered.

II.I. PR in X-space MPI

To express the projection x-space MPI data, we start with a change of coordinates:

$$x(s) = l \cdot \cos\theta - s \cdot \sin\theta \qquad (1)$$

$$y(s) = l \cdot \sin\theta + s \cdot \cos\theta \qquad (2)$$

Here, l and s denote the rotating spatial coordinates, which can be used to express the projection data in terms of the particle distribution, i.e.,

$$g(l, \theta) = \int_{-\infty}^{\infty} c(x(s), y(s)) ds \qquad (3)$$

Here, $c(x, y)$ denotes the particle distribution in Cartesian coordinates, and $g(l, \theta)$ denotes its projection at projection angle θ. It was previously shown that the 1D projection x-space MPI image at angle θ can then be expressed as [12]:

$$IMG_p(x_s(t), \theta) = g(l, \theta) * \dot{\mathcal{L}}[kGl]|_{l=x_s(t)} \qquad (4)$$

In this equation, $\dot{\mathcal{L}}[\cdot]$ denotes the derivative of the Langevin function, i.e., the 1D point spread function in x-space MPI [12]. The final x-space MPI image, $IMG(x, y)$, can then be reconstructed via filtered backprojection [13], i.e.,

$$IMG(x, y) = FBP\left(IMG_p(x_s(t), \theta)\right) \qquad (5)$$

Here, FBP denotes the filtered backprojection operation.

II.II. Proposed Modified PR for Relaxation Map

To reconstruct the 2D relaxation map, first we need to model the 1D relaxation maps obtained from the projections. By the nature of our relaxation time constant estimation method, the 1D relaxation maps of the projections can be expressed as the average of $\tau(x, y)$ values along the FFL, weighted by the corresponding pixel intensities:

$$\tau_p(l, \theta) = \frac{\int_{-\infty}^{\infty} \tau(x(s), y(s)) \cdot IMG(x(s), y(s)) ds}{\int_{-\infty}^{\infty} IMG(x(s), y(s)) ds} \qquad (6)$$

Here, $\tau_p(l, \theta)$ is the measured relaxation sinogram, and $\tau(x, y)$ is the desired 2D relaxation map.

In the standard utilization of the filtered backprojection algorithm, the measured projections should correspond to the line integrals of the underlying 2D function. Since this is not the case in Eq. 6, a direct filtered backprojection would lead to an erroneous 2D relaxation map. To overcome this problem, we propose the following modified projection reconstruction algorithm. First, we multiply the sinogram $IMG_p(x_s(t), \theta)$ by the relaxation sinogram $\tau_p(l, \theta)$, and apply filtered backprojection. We then divide the result of this step by the final x-space MPI image, i.e.,

$$\tau(x, y) = \frac{FBP\left(IMG_p(x_s(t), \theta) \cdot \tau_p(l, \theta)\right)}{IMG(x, y)} \quad (7)$$

This process yields the estimated 2D relaxation map, $\tau(x, y)$.

II.III. Simulations

MATLAB simulations were performed to demonstrate the FFL implementation of multi-color MPI. The following parameters were utilized: (6, 0, -6) T/m selection field gradients in (x, y, z) directions, 15 mT drive field at 10 kHz, 25 nm nanoparticle diameter. The fundamental harmonic of the MPI signal was filtered out, and white Gaussian noise was added with signal-to-noise ratio of 100. Projections were taken with 3° angular steps. Two different nanoparticle distributions were assumed, with τ=1.1 μs and τ=2.9 μs. To demonstrate that the proposed method can handle different nanoparticle concentrations, a concentration ratio of 2:1 was selected between the 1.1-μs and 2.9-μs particles.

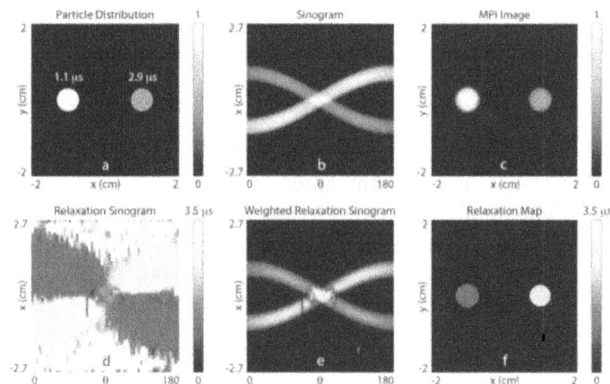

Figure 1: (a) Phantom used in the simulations. The nanoparticle distributions on the left and right have τ =1.1 μs and τ =2.9 μs, respectively. (b) Sinogram, $IMG_p(x_s(t), \theta)$, obtained from FFL scanning. (c) 2D x-space MPI image reconstructed via filtered backprojection. (d) Measured relaxation sinogram, $\tau_p(l, \theta)$. (e) Weighted relaxation sinogram obtained via multiplying (b) and (d). (f) 2D relaxation map reconstructed via the proposed algorithm.

III. Results

Figure 1 shows the results of the proposed technique. The top row demonstrates the PR results for the x-space MPI image, and the bottom row shows the results of the modified PR algorithm. When generating the 2D relaxation map shown in Fig. 1f, a final thresholding was applied based on the MPI image to remove the background regions. A numerical inspection of the resulting 2D relaxation map shows that the relaxation time constants are estimated with less than 6% error.

IV. Discussion

Here, we have used two distinct nanoparticles with different relaxation times to demonstrate the proposed

technique. The results showed reliable estimation of the underlying time constants. However, inhomogeneous mixtures of different nanoparticle distributions (e.g., a gradual transition region from one nanoparticle type to the other) may result in unreliable estimations [11]. In the case of FFL scanners, the projection operation may further increase the probability of encountering this problem, as the signal contributions from different regions along the FFL can also create the same effect. Therefore, a recovery algorithm may be needed to correctly identify the time constants for those regions. Handling of these special cases and experimental demonstration of the proposed technique remains as future work.

V. Conclusions

In this work, we demonstrated that relaxation-based calibration-free multi-color MPI can be extended to FFL scanners. To enable this extension, we proposed a modified projection reconstruction algorithm, that incorporates both the projection data from x-space imaging, and the estimated time constants for the projections.

ACKNOWLEDGEMENTS

This work was supported by the Scientific and Technological Research Council of Turkey through a TUBITAK 3501 Grant (114E167), by the European Commission through an FP7 Marie Curie Career Integration Grant (PCIG13-GA-2013-618834), by the Turkish Academy of Sciences through TUBA-GEBIP 2015 program, and by the BAGEP Award of the Science Academy.

REFERENCES

[1] B. Gleich and J. Weizenecker. Tomographic imaging using the nonlinear response of magnetic particles. *Nature*, 435(7046):1217-1217, 2005. doi: 10.1038/nature03808.

[2] P. Goodwill and S. M. Conolly. The x-space formulation of the magnetic particle imaging process: 1-D signal, resolution, bandwidth, SNR, SAR, and magnetostimulation. *IEEE Trans Med Imaging*, vol. 29, no. 11, pp. 1851–1859, 2010.

[3] L. R. Croft et al. Relaxation in x-space magnetic particle imaging. *IEEE Trans Med Imaging*, vol. 31, no. 12, pp. 2335-2342, 2012.

[4] J. Rahmer et al. First experimental evidence of the feasibility of multi-color magnetic particle imaging. *Phys Med Biol*, vol. 60, no. 5, p. 1775-1791, 2015.

[5] D. Hensley et al. Preliminary experimental x-space color MPI. *5th international workshop on magnetic particle imaging*. Istanbul, 2015, p. 10

[6] A. M. Rauwerdink and J. B. Weaver. Viscous effects on nanoparticle magnetization harmonics. *J Magn Magn Mater*, vol. 322, no. 6, p. 609-613, 2009.

[7] M. Utkur et al. Relaxation-based viscosity mapping for magnetic particle imaging. *Phys Med Biol*, vol. 62, no. 9, p. 3422, 2017.

[8] J. B. Weaver et al. Magnetic nanoparticle temperature estimation. *Med Phys*, vol. 36, no. 5, p. 1822-1829, 2009.

[9] T. Wawrzik et al. Effect of brownian relaxation in frequency-dependent magnetic particle spectroscopy measurements. *3rd international workshop on magnetic particle imaging*. Berkeley, 2013, p.1

[10] Y. Muslu et al. Calibration-free color mpi. *6th international workshop on magnetic particle imaging*. Lubeck, 2016, p. 10.

[11] Y. Muslu et al. Relaxation-Based Calibration-Free Multi-Color MPI. arXiv:1705.07624 [physics.med-ph], 2017.

[12] P. Goodwill et al. Projection x-space magnetic particle imaging. *IEEE Trans Med Imaging*, vol. 31, no. 5, p. 1076-1085, 2012.

[13] J. J. Konkle et al. Projection reconstruction magnetic particle imaging. *IEEE Trans Med Imaging*, vol. 32, no. 2, p. 338-347, 2013.

Characterization of Single-Core Magnetic Nanoparticles as Tracer for Mobility MPI

Frank Ludwig [a,*], Hilke Remmer [a], Sebastian Draack [a], and Thilo Viereck [a]

[a] Institut für Elektrische Messtechnik und Grundlagen der Elektrotechnik, TU Braunschweig, Braunschweig, Germany
* Corresponding author, email: f.ludwig@tu-bs.de

I. Introduction

Recently, several approaches to extend the capability of Magnetic Particle Imaging (MPI) towards a simultaneous imaging of the spatial distribution of the magnetic nanoparticle (MNP) mobility (e.g., viscosity of the medium or MNP binding state) or temperature were proposed [1,2]. The simultaneous imaging of the spatial distribution of MNP concentration and MNP mobility proposes that the dynamics of a significant portion of MNPs is dominated by the Brownian mechanism, i.e., the physical rotation of the whole MNP in a time-varying magnetic field. Although MNP suspensions from several manufacturers were identified to provide a better harmonic signal than the "gold standard" Resovist, not much attention was paid on their suitability as tracer for mobility MPI.

In this contribution, we characterize the commercially available single-core MNP system PrecisionMRX® from Imagion Biosystems applying different dynamic magnetic techniques, such as ac susceptometry and multiparameter magnetic particle spectroscopy (MPS). To verify that the dynamics of a significant portion of MNPs is dominated by the Brownian mechanism, MNPs suspended in pure DI water and in DI water/glycerol mixtures are compared.

II. Material and Methods

The MNPs have nominal core diameters of 24.4 nm (from SAXS measurements) and either carboxyclic acid or mPEG shells. The nominal hydrodynamic diameter (intensity-weighted Z-average estimated by DLS) amounts to 83.8 nm for the mPEG-coated and 42.8 nm for the carboxylic-acid-functionalized MNP (note that the number-weighted DLS median diameter should be lower than the intensity-weighted one). The iron content of the as-received samples amounts to 5 mg(Fe)/mL. The measured saturation magnetization of $4.38 \cdot 10^5$ A/m is about 92% of the bulk value of magnetite [3] being a very high value for single-core iron-oxide nanoparticles of this size. For the viscosity series, 15 µL of MNP suspension were mixed with 135 µL of different ratios of DI water/glycerol.

III. Results

Figure 1 depicts the imaginary part of the ac susceptibility (ACS) spectrum measured on a 150 µL sample of the as-received suspension with mPEG-coated MNPs. Obviously, the imaginary part exhibits two maxima: one at around 1 kHz and one at about 100 kHz. The spectra resemble those measured on single-core MNPs from the University of Washington and LodeSpin Labs [4]. To model the measured spectra, the generalized Debye model, including lognormal distributions of core and hydrodynamic diameter, is applied [5]. The core diameter d_c is related to the Néel relaxation time, while the hydrodynamic size d_h determines the Brownian one. Fixing the median core diameter to 24.4 nm, the measured spectra can be modelled very well, but the obtained median number-weighted hydrodynamic diameter of 91 nm is significantly larger than the intensity-weighted value from DLS measurements. To solve this problem, a bivariate lognormal distribution function $f(d_c, d_h)$ is introduced, correlating core and hydrodynamic diameters. For a correlation coefficient $\rho = 0.7$ a median hydrodynamic diameter of 70 nm is found, in fair agreement with the DLS result. Both, distributions of core and hydrodynamic diameter are with a standard deviation of about 0.15 very narrow.

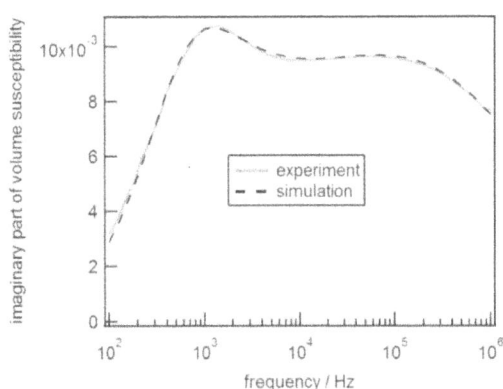

Figure 1: Spectrum of imaginary part of AC susceptibility measured on PrecisionMRX MNPs with mPEG coating along with modelled spectrum.

To verify that the double peak structure results from the coexistence of Brownian rotation (maximum at 1 kHz) and Néel relaxation (maximum around 100 kHz), measurements on suspensions with different viscosities were performed. The low-frequency maximum clearly shifts with increasing viscosity to lower frequencies – as expected from the scaling of the Brownian relaxation time with viscosity – while the position of the high-frequency maximum remains unchanged.

As expected due to the smaller hydrodynamic diameter, the carboxylic-acid-coated PrecisionMRX MNPs show a Brownian maximum in the ACS imaginary part at around 10 kHz. As for the mPEG-coated ones, the low-frequency maximum shifts to smaller frequencies when increasing the viscosity while the maximum around 100 kHz remains unchanged.

MPS spectra measured at different frequencies of the excitation field show that the rate of decrease in harmonic amplitude becomes steeper as the drive frequency was increased, caused by MNP dynamics. MPS measurements between 1 kHz and 25 kHz and with 25 mT drive field amplitude on mPEG-coated Precision MRX samples with viscosities ranging from 1 mPa·s for DI water to 4.9 mPa·s for 48 w% glycerol show only marginal differences between the harmonic spectra. For comparison, – due to their smaller Brownian relaxation time – an effect of viscosity on MPS spectra is discernable for the carboxylic-acid-coated MNPs which becomes more pronounced with decreasing drive field frequency (Fig. 2).

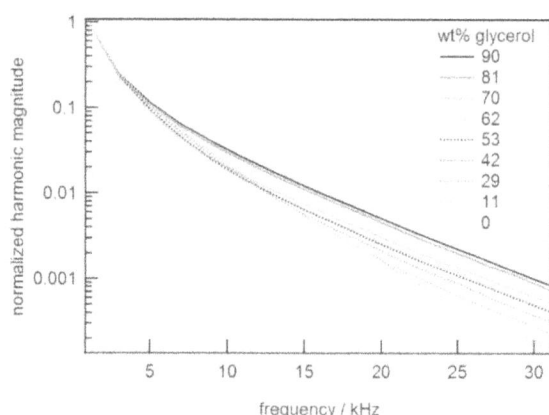

Figure 2: MPS spectra measured at 1 kHz on diluted PrecisionMRX MNPs with carboxylic-acid shell suspended in water-glycerol mixtures of different viscosities.

IV. Discussion

The refined ACS model shows that the double peak structure in the imaginary part of the PrecisionMRX MNP suspension does not conflict with the nominal single-core nature. While the low-frequency maximum is caused by the Brownian rotation of thermally blocked single-core MNPs, the high-frequency maximum can be attributed to the internal Néel relaxation of MNPs. The significant Néel contribution despite the relatively large core diameters of 24.4 nm is caused by the comparably small anisotropy constant $K = 3.7$ kJ/m^3.

The fact that a significant Brownian contribution is seen in ACS spectra but not in MPS can be attributed to the different ac field amplitudes. While the ACS measurements were performed at a field amplitude of 95 µT, the MPS spectra were recorded at 25 mT amplitude. While both Brownian and Néel relaxation times decrease with increasing ac field strength, the latter one decreases much stronger [6]. As the analysis of ACS spectra has shown, the low-field relaxation time of the nanoparticles is close to the crossover between Brownian and Néel time constants. Thus, it can be expected that the dynamics at 25 mT field amplitude is dominated by the internal Néel relaxation so that differences in the matrix viscosity are not seen which is in agreement with [7]. Due to the smaller hydrodynamic diameter of the carboxylic-acid-coated MNPs, some viscosity effect on the MPS spectra is observed for low excitation frequencies.

V. Conclusions

The studied MNP system PrecisionMRX from Imagion Biosystems – either coated with mPEG or with carboxylic acid – is well suited as tracer material for MPI. The relatively high core diameters, combined with a high saturation magnetization, provide large magnetic moments of about $3.3 \cdot 10^{-18}$ A·m^2, causing a steep magnetization curve and a narrow point-spread function (PSF). The comparably small anisotropy constant of 3.7 kJ/m^3 causes that the majority of MNP can follow the drive field in MPI for frequencies up to at least 25 kHz. While the ACS spectra, recorded in the small-field limit, provide a significant contribution of Brownian-dominated particles to the spectrum, at field amplitudes, relevant for MPI and MPS, the majority of mPEG-coated PrecisionMRX MNPs follow the drive field via the Néel mechanism. Due to the lower hydrodynamic diameter and thus smaller Brownian relaxation time, the effect of viscosity is slightly higher for carboxylic-acid-coated PrecisionMRX MNPs.

ACKNOWLEDGEMENTS

Financial support by the German Research Foundation, DFG Priority Program 1681 (LU800/4-2, SCHI383/2-1) and from "Niedersächsisches Vorab" through the "Quantum- and Nano-Metrology (QUANOMET)" initiative within project NP-2 are acknowledged.

REFERENCES

[1] J. Rahmer, A. Halkola, I. Schmale, B. Gleich, and J. Borgert, Phys. Med. Biol. 60, 1775 (2015).
[2] T. Viereck, C. Kuhlmann, S. Draack, M. Schilling, and F. Ludwig, J. Magn. Magn. Mater. 427, 156 (2017).
[3] Z. W. Tai, D. W. Hensley, E. C. Vreeland, B. Zheng, and S. M. Connolly, Biomed. Phys. Eng. Express 3, 035003 (2017).
[4] F. Ludwig, C. Kuhlmann, T. Wawrzik, J. Dieckhoff, A. Lak, A. P. Kandhar, R. M. Ferguson, S. J. Kemp, and K. M. Krishnan, IEEE Trans Magn. 50, 5101804 (2014).
[5] F. Ludwig, C. Balceris, C. Jonasson, and C. Johansson, IEEE Trans Magn. 53, 6100904 (2017).
[6] J. Dieckhoff, D. Eberbeck, M. Schilling, and F. Ludwig, J. Appl. Phys. 119, 043903 (2016).
[7] M. Utkur, Y. Muslu, and E. U. Saritas, Phys. Med. Biol. 62, 3422 (2017)

Viscosity Mapping through Relaxation Effects for Functional Magnetic Particle Imaging

Mustafa Utkur [a,b,*], Yavuz Muslu [a,b], Emine Ulku Saritas [a,b,c]

[a] *Department of Electrical and Electronics Engineering, Bilkent University, Ankara, Turkey*
[b] *National Magnetic Resonance Research Center (UMRAM), Bilkent University, Ankara, Turkey*
[c] *Neuroscience Program, Sabuncu Brain Research Center, Bilkent University, Ankara, Turkey*
[*] *Corresponding author, email: mustafa.utkur@bilkent.edu.tr*

I. Introduction

Magnetic particle imaging (MPI) is a promising imaging modality for in vivo functional imaging, including viscosity mapping. Previously, measuring viscosity through the harmonic ratio of nanoparticle's magnetization curve was suggested [1]. Another study looked into using relaxation-induced nanoparticle delays to estimate their mobility [2]. Recent color MPI approaches have shown that different nanoparticles can be differentiated via their MPI responses, which further suggests that MPI could be used to map different environmental conditions [3-5]. In fact, studies on MPI cell tracking applications have shown that the nanoparticles have altered response when they are in cells vs. water [6, 7]. While the exact reasons for these changes in nanoparticle response are not well understood, one potential explanation is the increased viscosity within the cell environment when compared to water.

Recently, we have proposed a relaxation-based viscosity mapping technique for MPI, where we directly estimate a relaxation time constant from the time-domain nanoparticle signal [8]. In this work, we extend our technique to multi-color imaging experiments using our in-house field free point (FFP) MPI Scanner. We compare the performance of the proposed technique in distinguishing different viscosity environments at drive field frequencies of 1.1 kHz and 10 kHz.

II. Material and Methods

II.I. Theory

For a repetitive scanning trajectory that scans a field-of-view (FOV) back and forth, the ideal MPI signal can be separated into positive and negative half cycles that possess mirror symmetry [5, 8]. However, this symmetry breaks down due to relaxation delays. Previously, a phenomenological model for the relaxation-delayed signal was presented as follows [10]:

$$s_{received}(t) = s_{ideal}(t) * \frac{1}{\tau} e^{-\frac{t}{\tau}} u(t) \qquad (1)$$

Here, τ is the relaxation time constant, $s_{ideal}(t)$ is the nanoparticle signal without relaxation, and $u(t)$ is the Heaviside step function. This model was shown to provide a very good fit to the experimental data from a magnetic particle spectrometer (MPS) for various drive field frequencies and amplitudes, and it was also validated via imaging experiments on an MPI scanner at 25 kHz [10].

Based on the model given above, we have previously proposed a technique to directly estimate τ from the nanoparticle signal, through the recovery of the underlying mirror symmetry [8]:

$$\tau = \frac{S_{pos}^*(f) + S_{neg}(f)}{i2\pi f \left(S_{pos}^*(f) - S_{neg}(f) \right)} \qquad (2)$$

Here, $S_{pos}(f)$ and $S_{neg}(f)$ are the Fourier transforms of the positive and negative half-cycles of the received signal, and the superscript star sign denotes conjugation operation. Importantly, estimating the relaxation time constant through this technique does not require any prior information about the nanoparticle response.

Our previous work on a magnetic particle spectrometer (MPS) setup has shown that the drive field amplitude and frequency strongly affect the viscosity mapping capabilities of this relaxation-based technique [8]. The results suggested that frequencies around 1 kHz may be more suitable for one-to-one mapping. In this work, we perform multi-color imaging experiments on a FFP scanner to compare how well the proposed method can distinguish nanoparticles in different viscosity environments at 1.1 kHz and 10 kHz drive fields.

II.II. Experimental Setup

Our in-house FFP MPI scanner is shown in Figure 1. The selection field gradients are (-4.8, 2.4, 2.4) T/m in (x, y, z) directions. In this scanner, the drive coil is in z-direction. This water-cooled coil is wound using a capillary copper tube of 3/2 mm outer/inner diameters with 3 layers and 40 turns at each layer. The receive coil, which directly fits inside the drive coil, has a single layer of Litz wire wound into a three section gradiometer geometry. This receive coil has 34 turns in the middle section and 17 turns on the side sections. Overall, the MPI scanner has an imaging FOV of $1 \times 1 \times 10$ cm^3.

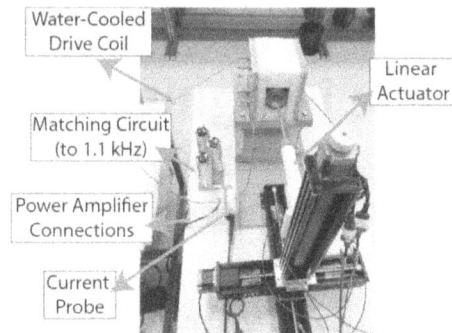

Figure 1: *Our in-house FFP MPI scanner. The arrows indicate different components of the scanner. The water-cooled drive coil is matched to the power amplifier (AE Techron 7224) through two different capacitive circuitries, for 1.1 kHz and 10 kHz.*

II.III. Sample Preparation

Three different glycerol/water mixtures were prepared with a total volume of 20 µL. Deionized water was utilized in the preparation of all samples. To avoid concentration bias in the results, the prepared samples had identical nanoparticle concentrations: each mixture contained 5 µL of undiluted Perimag nanoparticles (Micromod GmbH, Germany) at 151.8 mmol Fe/L. The resulting glycerol percentages were 0% (i.e., water only), 25%, and 45% by volume. The corresponding viscosity levels, measured using a rheometer, were 0.94 mPa•s, 2.23 mPa•s, and 5.2 mPa•s, respectively. Note that these viscosity levels are within the biologically relevant range, as cell cytoplasm was previously reported to have 1-2 mPa•s viscosity [11], and the viscosity of blood was reported to vary between 1.3-7.8 mPa•s [12]. For imaging experiments, these three samples were placed in a phantom at 2 cm separations (see Fig. 2a).

III. Results

The imaging results showing the relaxation maps at two different drive field frequencies, 1.1 kHz and 10 kHz, are presented in Fig. 2. The estimated relaxation time constants were mapped at 15 mT-peak drive field amplitude for both frequencies. The relaxation map at 10 kHz shows nearly uniform relaxation values for the samples at different viscosity levels, showing insensitivity to viscosity at this relatively high frequency. At a lower frequency of 1.1 kHz, the relaxation time constants decrease with increasing viscosity (from left to right), which is consistent with our previous results [8].

IV. Discussion

Currently, the most common drive field frequency in MPI is 25 kHz. In theory, high drive field frequencies provide higher signal-to-noise ratio, since the signal is received inductively. However, lower drive field frequencies may be more sensitive to relaxation-based functional imaging capabilities of MPI. The results in Fig. 2 suggests that lower frequencies around 1 kHz are more suitable than higher frequencies for viscosity mapping with MPI.

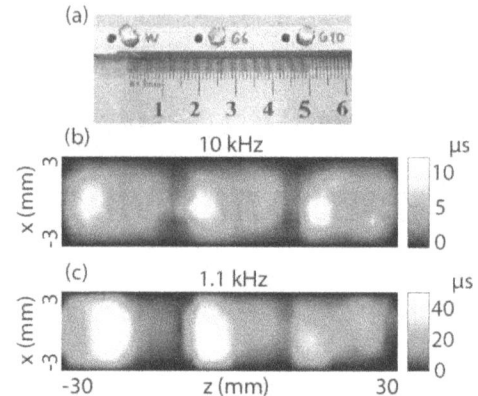

Figure 2: *Imaging experiment results at 15 mT-peak drive field. (a)The prepared samples at three different viscosity levels. From left to right: 0%, 25%, and 45% glycerol by volume. (b) Relaxation map at 10 kHz, and (c) relaxation map at 1.1 kHz. The proposed technique shows better viscosity mapping capabilities at 1.1 kHz when compared to 10 kHz.*

V. Conclusions

In this work, we have shown the viscosity mapping potential of MPI through a relaxation-based multi-color imaging technique. Our experimental results suggest that lower drive field frequencies around 1 kHz are more suitable for distinguishing nanoparticles in different viscosity environments.

ACKNOWLEDGEMENTS

This work was supported by the Scientific and Technological Research Council of Turkey (TUBITAK 114E167), by the European Commission through FP7 Marie Curie Career Integration Grant (PCIG13-GA-2013-618834), by the Turkish Academy of Sciences through TUBA-GEBIP 2015 program, and by the BAGEP Award of the Science Academy.

REFERENCES

[1] A. M. Rauwerdink and J. B. Weaver. Viscous effects on nanoparticle magnetization harmonics. J. Magn. Magn. Mater. 322(6):609-613,2010, http://dx.doi.org/10.1016/j.jmmm.2009.10.024

[2] T. Wawrzik et. al., Estimating particle mobility in MPI. 3rd Int. Workshop on Magnetic Particle Imaging (IWMPI) (Berkeley), 2016, http://dx.doi.org/10.1109/IWMPI.2013.6528372

[3] J. Rahmer et. al., First experimental evidence of the feasibility of multi-color magnetic particle imaging. Phys. Med. Biol.,60(5):1775-91, 2015. doi: 10.1088/0031-9155/60/5/1775.

[4] D. Hensley et. al., Preliminary experimental X-space color MPI. 5th Int. Work. Magn. Part. Imaging (IWMPI), 2015.

[5] Y. Muslu et. al., Calibration-Free Color MPI. Proc. of the 6th Int. Workshop on Magnetic Particle Imaging (IWMPI), 2016.

[6] B. Zheng et. al., Magnetic Particle Imaging tracks the long-term fate of in vivo neural cell implants with high image contrast. Sci. Rep.,5(14055), 2015. http://dx.doi.org/10.1038/srep14055

[7] K. Them et. al., Increasing the sensitivity for stem cell monitoring in system-function based magnetic particle imaging Phys. Med. Biol., 61(9):3279, 2016. http://dx.doi.org/10.1088/0031-9155/61/9/3279

[8] M. Utkur et. al., Relaxation-based viscosity mapping for magnetic particle imaging. Phys. Med. Biol., 62(9):3422, 2016, https://doi.org/10.1088/1361-6560/62/9/3422

[9] M. Utkur et. al., Relaxation-Based Viscosity Mapping in Different Viscous Environments. Proc. of the 7th Int. Workshop on Magnetic Particle Imaging (IWMPI), 2017.

[10] L. R. Croft et. al., Relaxation in X-space magnetic particle imaging. IEEE Trans. Med. Imaging, 31(12):2335-2342, 2012, http://dx.doi.org/10.1109/TMI.2012.2217979

[11] M. K. Kuimova et. al., Imaging intracellular viscosity of a single cell during photoinduced cell death. At. Chem.,1:69-73, 2009. http://dx.doi.org/10.1038/nchem.120

[12] B. Pirofsky. The determination of blood viscosity in man by a method based on Poiseuille's law. J. Clin. Invest., 32(4):292–298, 1953. http://dx.doi.org/10.1172/JCI102738

Discriminating Nanoparticle Size Using Multi-Spectral MPI

Martin Möddel [a,b,*], Carolyn Shasha [c], Patryk Szwargulski [a,b], Eric Teeman [c],
Kannan M. Krishnan [c], Tobias Knopp [a,b,*]

[a] Section for Biomedical Imaging, University Medical Center Hamburg-Eppendorf, Hamburg, Germany
[b] Institute for Biomedical Imaging, Hamburg University of Technology, Hamburg, Germany
[c] Department of Materials Sciences & Engineering, Roberts Hall, University of Washington, Seattle, USA
[*] Corresponding author, email: m.hofmann@uke.de

I. Introduction

The possibility for multicolor image reconstruction by separating the MPI signal from particles of different types has recently been demonstrated [1]. Possible applications of multicolor MPI include e.g. distinguishing between particles coated on a catheter and particles flowing in the blood [2]. Here, we discuss differentiation of particles based purely on their size using multiple types of tailored single-core particles with distinct narrow core-size distributions. The signal from particles of differing sizes can be separated into different channels and then assigned to different colors, resulting in a multicolor image.

The optimal size range for MPI nanoparticle tracers is 20-28 nm in core diameter [3,4]. Below ~20 nm, particles require a higher applied field strength to saturate, resulting in lower recorded signal. Above ~28 nm, the phase lag between the drive field and particle response becomes large and the particle can no longer follow the field, also resulting in lowered signal. Due to this size restriction, a size-based differentiation approach requires highly monodisperse particles with carefully controlled size, as well as a highly sensitive signal separation technique.

For particles in this size range under an applied ac field, a combination of Néel rotation (flipping of the magnetic moment within the particle) and Brownian rotation (rotation of the entire particle to align with the field) will occur. Typically, the particle dynamics and resulting signal are described in terms of equilibrium timescales associated with each relaxation process; however, this description has limited applicability for the field conditions required for MPI (amplitudes ~10 mT, frequencies ~25 kHz), in which non-equilibrium behavior will dominate. For particles ~25 nm in diameter, a nontrivial combination of Brownian rotation and Néel rotation occurs [5]. Consequently, stochastic simulations of Langevin equations are employed in order to predict size-dependent nanoparticle behavior [6].

The harmonic spectrum of the recorded MPI signal is highly sensitive to numerous particle characteristics, including size. Previous simulations have predicted the possibility of size-based particle differentiation in 1D by examining the spectral response [6]. In this work, we take advantage of the sensitivity of the spectral response in order to demonstrate particle size discrimination in 2D.

II. Material and Methods

Magnetite nanoparticles were synthesized according to a thermal decomposition process using an iron oleate precursor, as described in detail in [7]. Three particle samples were fabricated, with core diameters (distribution parameters) of 23.8 nm (0.05), 25.2 nm (0.09), and 27.6 nm (0.1). Particle sizes were assumed to follow a log-normal distribution, and were determined from TEM images. The nanoparticle cores were coated with a poly(ethylene glycol) PEG-based amphiphilic polymer, resulting in respective hydrodynamic sizes (distribution parameters) of 53.0 nm (0.1), 53.6 nm (0.1), and 69.0 nm (0.1). Particles were then dispersed in distilled water at a concentration of 0.9 mgFe/mL.

From each particle sample a cubic 1 mm³ delta sample was prepared and used for MPI measurements. These were obtained on the preclinical MPI system (Bruker) at the University Medical Center Hamburg-Eppendorf. All measurements were performed using a gradient field of 2 $T\mu_0^{-1}m^{-1}$ in z-direction and 1 $T\mu_0^{-1}m^{-1}$ in x- and y-directions. For excitation a 2D sinusoidal drive field with field strengths of 12 $mT\mu_0^{-1}$ in x- and y-directions and frequencies of 2.5/102 MHz and 2.5/96 MHz respectively were used. The resulting drive-field field of view had a size of 24×24 mm². The period length of a single drive field cycle was 653 μs.

For each sample a system matrix was acquired on a 30×30 mm² Cartesian grid with a pixel size of 1×1 mm² and 4000 averaged measurements per grid position. For a series of measurements, a triangular sample holder was used which allowed positioning of the samples in the xy-plane with a mutual distance of 9.3 mm. The samples were measured pairwise, altogether amounting to a total of four measurements. For each measurement a total of 5000 frames were captured.

Multi-channel reconstruction was performed using the system matrix based approach presented in [1]. Prior to reconstruction each measurement was reduced by block averaging chunks of 200 frames. Moreover, a frequency selection was applied to the Fourier domain data. For each measurement three channels c_i were obtained by 100 iterations of the Kaczmarz algorithm solving the Thikonov regularized least squares problem

$$\operatorname*{argmin}_{c_1,c_2,c_3}\| \sum_{i=1}^{3} \mathbf{S}_i \mathbf{c}_i\|_2^2 + \lambda \sum_{i=1}^{3} \|\mathbf{c}_i\|_2^2. \quad (1)$$

Here $\mathbf{S}_i$ are the three system matrices and λ is the manually optimized regularization parameter.

III. Results

In total, three channels were obtained per reconstruction, each corresponding to a system matrix of a specific particle core-size as can be seen in Figure 1. In all reconstructed images the strongest signal contribution could be found in the channel matching the sample. However, we also observed leakage of signal into the channels corresponding to non-matching system matrices and therefore a non-perfect signal separation. This leakage may be attributable to the nonzero size distributions of the nanoparticle samples, which predicts some overlap in particle size among samples. The strength of the signal leakage depended on the size of the particles. Smaller particles leaked more signal into the channels of larger particles than the other way around. Moreover, the overall signal strength in each channel was reduced compared to data obtained with a mono-spectral reconstruction.

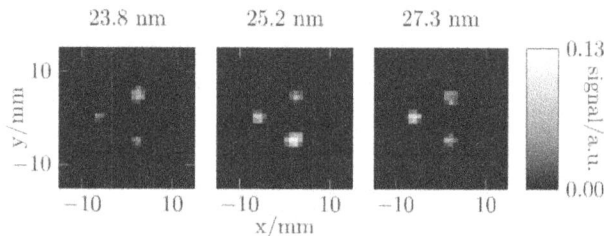

Figure 1: The signal distribution within the three reconstruction channels is shown for the joint measurement of all samples. All three 23.8nm (bottom right), 25.2 nm (top right), and 27.3 nm (center left) contribute signal to each channels. The strongest signal can be observed, where sample and channel match.

The qualitative signal separation, i.e. the contrast of the signals from the different sources, correlated with the chunk size of the block averaging prior to the reconstruction and therefore with the SNR of the measurement. A source discrimination was achieved by summing up the signal in the region around a signal source for each channel and mapping these onto the three types of particles.

IV. Discussion

Our results show that it is possible to reliably discriminate three samples containing nanoparticles with different sizes all with the same iron concentration. Due to the fact that the 27.6 nm particles had a much larger hydrodynamic size, the signal discrimination cannot solely be accounted to the core-size for all particles. However, the first two core-sizes had very similar hydrodynamic size and could be separated quite well, which provides strong evidence for a core-size based signal separation.

A separation with samples of known and fixed particle concentration does not necessarily require the multi-spectral approach, as spectral changes usually lead to an increase or decrease of the mono-spectral MPI signal. Nevertheless, it is an important step towards the separation of samples with varying concentrations and a quantification of the mixing ratio of mixtures of different size particles.

V. Conclusions

In this work, by synthesizing single-core nanoparticles with a high degree of size control, we were able to differentiate between particles with only 1-2 nm variations in core-size diameter based on multicolor MPI.

ACKNOWLEDGEMENTS
C. Shasha was supported by NSF Grant No. DGE-1256082 and a Sigma Xi Grant-in-aid of Research. T. Knopp thankfully acknowledge the financial support by the German Research Foundation (DFG, grant number KN 1108/2-1) and the Federal Ministry of Education and Research (BMBF, grant number 05M16GKA). K. M. Krishnan acknowledges the Alexander von Humboldt Forschungspreis 2016.

REFERENCES
[1] J. Rahmer, A. Halkola, B. Gleich, I. Schmale, and J. Borgert. First experimental evidence of the feasibility of multi-color magnetic particle imaging. *Physics in Medicine and Biology*, 60(5), 1775, 2016.
[2] J. Haegele, S. Vaalma, N. Panagiotopoulos, J. Barkhausen, F. M. Vogt, J. Borgert, and J. Rahmer J. Multi-color magnetic particle imaging for cardiovascular interventions. *Physics in Medicine and Biology*, 61(16), N415, 2016.
[3] R. M Ferguson, A. P. Khandhar, H. Arami, L. Hua, O. Hovorka, and K. M. Krishnan. Tailoring the magnetic and pharmacokinetic properties of iron oxide magnetic particle imaging tracers. *Biomedizinische Technik/Biomedical Engineering*, 58(6), 493-507, 2013.
[4] R. M. Ferguson, A. P. Khandhar, S. J. Kemp, H. Arami, E. U. Saritas, L. R. Croft, J. Konkle, P. W. Goodwill, A. Halkola, J. Rahmer, J. Borgert, S. M. Conolly. and K. M. Krishnan. Magnetic particle imaging with tailored iron oxide nanoparticle tracers. *IEEE Transactions on Medical Imaging*, 34(5), 1077-1084, 2015.
[5] S. A. Shah, D. B. Reeves, R. M. Ferguson, J. B. Weaver, and K. M. Krishnan. Mixed Brownian alignment and Néel rotations in superparamagnetic iron oxide nanoparticle suspensions driven by an ac field. *Physical Review B*, 92(9), 094438, 2015.
[6] C. Shasha, E. Teeman, and K. M. Krishnan. Harmonic Simulation Study of Simultaneous Nanoparticle Size and Viscosity Differentiation. *IEEE Magnetics Letters*, 8, 1-5, 2017.
[7] S. J. Kemp, R. M. Ferguson, A. P. Khandhar, and K. M. Krishnan. Monodisperse magnetite nanoparticles with nearly ideal saturation magnetization. *RSC Advances*, 6(81), 77452-77464, 2016.

Session 10 - Posters

Instrumentation III

Preliminary Design of Hybrid of Magnetic Particle imaging and Optical Multimodality Imaging System for Small Animals

Hui Hui [a, b], Kun Wang [a, b], Wenting Shang [a, b], Xin Yang [a, b], Jie Tian [a, b*]

[a] *Key Laboratory of Molecular Imaging, Institute of Automation, Chinese Academy of Sciences, Beijing, 100190, China*
[b] *Beijing Key Laboratory of Molecular Imaging, Institute of Automation, Beijing, 100190, China*
* Corresponding author, email: jie.tian@ia.ac.cn; tian@ieee.org

I. Introduction

Multimodality imaging is a growing research field because it can provide comprehensive medical imaging [1]. PET/CT is a typical multimodality imaging technology that combines structural imaging and functional imaging together. This technique has been widely used in clinical applications. Molecular imaging is a powerful technique that can monitor biomedical and chemical events of specific molecular process in vivo [2]. It is widely applied for biomedical applications. However, each molecular imaging modality has its drawbacks. Therefore, hybrid of different molecular imaging modalities are developed for earlier detection and characterization of disease applications [3].

In the last decade, a new imaging modality called Magnetic particle imaging (MPI) has been growing fast because of the ability to detection of nanomolar concentrations of super-paramagnetic iron oxide (SPIO) nanoparticles [4-5]. Recently, multimodality molecular imaging with two modalities are prevalent [6-7], even tri-modal imaging has been investigated [8]. In this work, we present our design of a hybrid of MPI and optical multimodality imaging system.

II. Hardware Structure Design

The hardware structure is key part of our multimodality system. We have integrated the devices of five modalities into one system. Fig. 1 shows the schematic of our system. The animal holder has interface anesthetic gases input and output pipes to keep the mouse under anesthesia during the imaging process.

All the optical molecular imaging devices are mounted on the gantry. The gantry is connected with a servo motor. So that, all the imaging devices can be rotated during multimodal image acquisition. The position of the animal holder is controlled by three motorized stages.

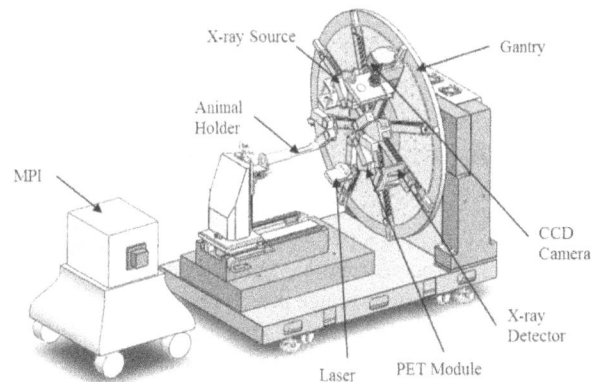

Figure 1: *Schematic of hybrid MPI and optical multimodality imaging system. MPI system is perpendicular to the gantry of optical multimodality imaging system. Animal holder can move forward and backward to take small animal into the FOV of optical multimodality imaging system and MPI respectively.*

The X-ray source and X-ray flat panel detector are used for computed tomography (CT) imaging. The charge-coupled Device (CCD) camera is used for collecting signals of Cerenkov luminescence imaging (CLI), bioluminescence imaging (BLI) and fluorescence molecular imaging (FMI). Eight PET flat panel detectors are formed as a ring to detect gamma photons. Each image device is mounted on a translation stage so that the field of view (FOV) can be adjusted for different samples.

III. Multimodality Imaging Data Acquisition

In this section, we introduce the data acquisition flow of our system. At the beginning of the experiment, optical multimodality imaging probes are injected into the mouse via tail intravenous injection. Then, the anaesthetized mouse isu put on the holder. The translation stages move the animal holder into the field of view of the optical imaging devices. Then the system is started to acquire PET data, After that, the optical molecular imaging data and CT data are acquired sequentially.

During the PET data acquisition, the X-ray source, X-ray detector, CCD camera and laser are located to the periphery while the PET detectors are moved to the center to form a ring. While the mouse is centered at this ring. Thus, those detectors can detect gamma rays emitted from the mouse.

After PET data acquisition, we perform optical molecular imaging and CT data collection. We perform optical molecular imaging first, which includes CLT, BLT and FMT. The data acquisition of BLT is similar with CLT. While for the FMT, the laser source is used to excite the fluorecent proteins targeted to lesion. The CCD camera will detect the emission light of the markers. After molecular image data collection, we collect CT projection data. We acquire 360 projection views at 1 degree interval. When all the optical molecular imaging data have been acquired, MPI imaging is performed with i.v. injection of SPIO nanoparticles. Finally, three-dimentional reconstruction is performed for the optical multimodalities as well as MPI by our development of reconstruction software.

III. Multimodality Images Processing Software

We have designed all-in-one software for three-dimensional reconstruction, multimodality image registration, and further image processing. This software is based on our previous work for multimodal medical imaging [9]. This framework provides a unified software framework for image reconstruction. It contains CT and optical molecular image reconstruction. Medical Imaging ToolKit (MITK) and three-dimensional Medical Image Processing and Analyzing system (3DMed) are two tools developed by our group [10]. MITK is a C++ library for integrated medical image processing and analyzing. It contains image segmentation, registration and visualization. 3DMed is programed based on MITK with a friendly user interface. The multimodality image fusion and image processing are implemented by MITK and 3DMed.

Based on our previous work, the multimodality imaging software is designed to integrate MITK and 3DMed together. The image fusion and processing are performed by MITK. 3DMed is used as the user interface of our multimodality imaging software.

IV. Conclusions

We have reported the preliminary design of hybrid of MPI and optical multimodality imaging system. We can perform MPI and optical multimodality imaging sequentially with it. The hardware architecture, data acquisition flow and software framework are introduced. There are still lots of work to do before the real application of the system. Effective image registration and image fusion methods for different modalities have to be optimized. Currently our system acquires multimodality data sequentially, which is time-consuming. Further improvement will be addressed to acquire two or more modalities at one time.

ACKNOWLEDGEMENTS

This paper is supported by National Key Research and Development Program of China No. 2017YFA0205200, 2016YFC0103803, National Natural Science Foundation of China under Grant No. 81227901, 81527805, 81671851, 61231004, the International Innovation Team of CAS under Grant No. 20140491524, Beijing Municipal Science & Technology Commission No. Z161100002616022. : Supported by the Scientific Instrument Developing Project of the Chinese Academy of Sciences, Grant No. GJJSTD20170004.

REFERENCES

[1] W. Cai, X. Chen, "Multimodality molecular imaging of tumor angiogenesis," *Journal of Nuclear Medicine*, vol. 49, pp. 113S-128S, 2008.

[2] J. Tian, J. Bai, X. P. Yan, S. Bao, Y. Li, W. Liang, X. Yang, "Multimodality molecular imaging," *IEEE Engineering in Medicine and Biology Magazine*, vol. 27, no. 5, pp. 48-57, 2008.

[3] F. A. Jaffer, P. Libby, R. Weissleder, "Optical and multimodality molecular imaging insights into atherosclerosis," *Arteriosclerosis, thrombosis, and vascular biology*, vol. 29, no. 7, pp. 1017-1024, 2009.

[4] B. Gleich and J. Weizenecker. Tomographic imaging using the nonlinear response of magnetic particles. *Nature*, 435(7046):1217-1217, 2005. doi: 10.1038/nature03808.

[5] T. Knopp and T. M. Buzug. *Magnetic Particle Imaging: An Introduction to Imaging Principles and Scanner Instrumentation*. Springer, Berlin/Heidelberg, 2012. doi: 10.1007/978-3-642-04199-0.

[6] W. J. Mulder, A. W. Griffioen, G. J. Strijkers, D. P. Cormode, K. Nicolay, Z. A. Fayad, "Magnetic and fluorescent nanoparticles for multimodality imaging," *Nanomedicine*, vol. 2, no. 3, pp. 307-324, 2007.

[7] J. Culver, W. Akers, S. Achilefu, "Multimodality molecular imaging with combined optical and SPECT/PET modalities," *Journal of Nuclear Medicine*, vol. 49, no.2, pp. 169-172, 2008.

[8] H. Xing, W. Bu, S. Zhang, X. Zheng, M. Li, F. Chen, Q. He, L. Zhou, W. Peng, Y. Hua, J. Shi, "Multifunctional nanoprobes for upconversion fluorescence, MR and CT trimodal imaging," *Biomaterials*, vol. 33, no. 4, pp. 1079-1089,2012,

[9] D. Dong, J. Tian, Y. Dai, G. Yan, F. Yang, and P. Wu, "Unified reconstruction framework for multi-modal medical imaging," *Journal of X-Ray Science and Technology*, vol. 19, No. 1, pp. 111-126, 2011.

[10] J. Tian, J. Xue, Y. Dai, J. Chen and J. Zheng, "A novel software platform for medical image processing and analyzing," *IEEE Transactions on Information Technology in Biomedicine*, vol. 12, no. 6, pp. 800-812, 2008.

Analysis and Comparison of Magnetic Fields in MPI using Spherical Harmonic Expansions

Marija Boberg [a,b,*], Tobias Knopp [a,b], Martin Möddel [a,b]

[a] Section for Biomedical Imaging, University Medical Center Hamburg-Eppendorf, Hamburg, Germany
[b] Institute for Biomedical Imaging, Hamburg University of Technology, Hamburg, Germany
[*] Corresponding author, email: m.boberg@uke.de

I. Introduction

One of the fundamental building blocks of Magnetic Particle Imaging (MPI) scanner hardware are static and dynamic magnetic fields, as they generate and encode the MPI signal [1]. MPI scanners are characterized by the topology of their signal encoding field, which is either a field free point (FFP) or a field free line (FFL) [2].

Many reconstruction methods in MPI require some assumptions or knowledge about the magnetic fields. In x-space reconstruction the position of the field free point is required to grid the measured data to the spatial domain in one step of the reconstruction [3]. During the fast implicit multi-patch reconstruction, the center position of the different located FFP trajectories is required to avoid artifacts [4].

A concise way to represent magnetic fields within the scanner bore was proposed in [5]. There, the magnetic fields satisfy Laplace's equation $\Delta B_i = 0$ for $i = x, y, z$ and can be expanded into a basis of spherical harmonics around a central point. The coefficients of this expansion directly depend on the center position, such that the description of local magnetic fields with spherical harmonics is ambiguous.

In this work, we propose to remove this ambiguity by translating the center of the expansion into the FFP of a MPI system with focus fields switched off, leading to a unique representation of the magnetic fields. Furthermore, we propagate the errors of magnetic field measurements to remove non-significant coefficients, i.e. coefficients smaller than the propagated error, leading to a sparse representation of the fields. Moreover, we show how the expansion can be used to qualitatively and quantitatively analyze the local properties of a field, obtain the position of the FFP possibly shifted by focus fields, and compare different field configurations present in an FFP MPI system.

II. Material and Methods

The magnetic field inside a sphere $\mathcal{B}_r(q)$ can be represented by the series

$$B_i(a) = \sum_{l=0}^{\infty} \sum_{m=-l}^{l} \tilde{c}_{l,m}^i r^l Y_l^m \left(\frac{a}{r}\right), \quad i = x, y, z, \quad (1)$$

where $Y_l^m: \mathbb{S}^2 \to \mathbb{R}$ are the normalized real spherical harmonics on the unit sphere, $a \in \mathcal{B}_r(q) \subseteq \mathbb{R}^3$, $r = \|a\|_2$ and coefficients $\tilde{c}_{l,m} \in \mathbb{R}^3$. $\mathcal{B}_r(q)$ is a ball with radius r around the center q. $r^l Y_l^m \left(\frac{a}{r}\right)$ is in one to one correspondence to a polynomial in Cartesian coordinates.

To obtain this representation for a given field inside a sphere of radius R, the coefficients $\tilde{c}_{l,m}$ have to be computed from the inner product of B_i and Y_l^m. For quadrature we use t-designs as point set as it requires less nodes to achieve exact integration of the coefficients up to a given order L [6]. E.g. exact integration of the coefficients up to order $L = 4$ require an 8-design which consists of 36 points only. To account for the non-unit radius the norm r in equation (1) has to be normalized, e.g. by normalizing all coefficients via $\tilde{c}_{l,m}^i = \frac{c_{l,m}^i}{R^l}$.

The coefficients $c_{l,m}^x$, $c_{l,m}^y$, and $c_{l,m}^z$ describe the local magnetic field in x-, y-, and z-direction. The first coefficient $c_{0,0}^i$ describes the constant part of the field. If the magnetic field is expanded around an FFP this part vanishes. The coefficients for $l = 1$ represent the linear part of the field as the corresponding spherical harmonics are polynomials of degree 1. While $c_{1,-1}^i$ describes the linear part in y-direction, $c_{1,0}^i$ describes it in z-direction and $c_{1,1}^i$ in x-direction. Coefficients with $l > 1$ describe inhomogeneous and non-linear parts of the field. Fields in MPI are often designed homogeneous or linear, such that the coefficients drop off quickly for increasing l. Thus the spherical harmonic expansion (1) can be truncated at an index L without great loss of accuracy. A sparse field representation can be obtained by removing all coefficients smaller than their propagated error which stems from the field measurements.

The expansion is calculated around a specific point q, namely the center of the domain of the spherical harmonics. Calculating the spherical harmonic expansion around another point leads to different coefficients, which describe the same field. To get a unique representation, which is independent on the initial choice of the center position we propose to expand all fields of a MPI system around the initial position of the FFP. As the position of the FFP is not necessarily known in advance, the expansion around any other point may be obtained first and translated to the FFP later, as long as the FFP position lies inside the convergence radius R of the initial expansion. Finding the FFP position from the initial position is a simple root-finding problem. Using an adapted addition theorem of unnormalized complex solid harmonics the coefficients of a translated expansion can be directly obtained from the original ones [7].

These tools can also be combined to locally compare magnetic fields at different positions. Consider a field configuration, where the FFP is shifted away from its initial position, then we can shift the expansion into this new location and compare the local field around the shifted FFP with the local field around the initial FFP position on the basis of the two sets of coefficients as these contain information about the local fields.

We evaluated the proposed methods using a small experimental setup, i.e. an FFP field generator made of a coil pair with iron yoke, which can be individually driven by currents up to 14 A. Both coils are centered around the y-axis. All magnetic fields were measured at the same 8-design positions.

III. Results

The coefficients of the initial expansion of the magnetic field of the FFP field generator with a current of 14 A for each coil are shown in Fig. 1. Since the expansion was not centered around the FFP $c_{0,0}^i$ are not negligible. As it is described above the coefficients for $l = 1$ have a significant value for the corresponding directions. There is also visible that two coefficients $c_{1,0}^z$ and $c_{1,1}^x$ are the half of the third coefficient $c_{1,-1}^y$ and have the opposite sign as a direct consequence of Maxwell's equation $\nabla B = 0$.

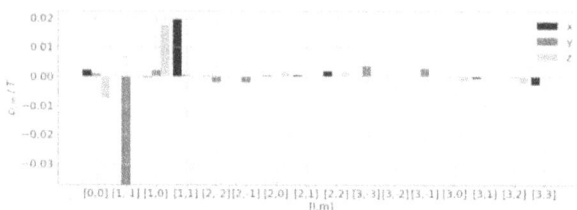

Figure 1: Plot of the coefficients of a spherical harmonic representation of the magnetic field in x- (black), y- (dark grey) and z-direction (light grey) without any translations.

Moreover, the coefficients for $l > 1$ decrease with increasing l. For $l > 3$ the coefficients are small compared to the error propagated from the field measurements. Thus the spherical harmonic expansion (1) can be truncated at an index $L = 3$ while maintaining the overall accuracy. If we compare the coefficients for $l > 1$ with those for $l = 1$ we conclude that the coils generate a good approximation of an ideal gradient field.

Fig. 2 shows all significant expansion coefficients in x-direction of two field configurations shifted into their respective FFP positions, with the generating coils driven by currents of 10 A (grey) and 14 A (black). A closer analysis reveals that the corresponding polynomial describing the field in x-direction is independent of y and z. The coefficients which correspond to quadratic or higher

order polynomials are small relatively to the coefficient $c_{1,1}^x$ corresponding to the linear part.

In comparison of the two expansions one observes that the distribution of the coefficients is the same. A quantitative analysis reveals that the reduction of the second current from 14 A to 10 A yields a reduction of the local field to 72% of its original value, which is approximately to the quotient of the currents of 10/14.

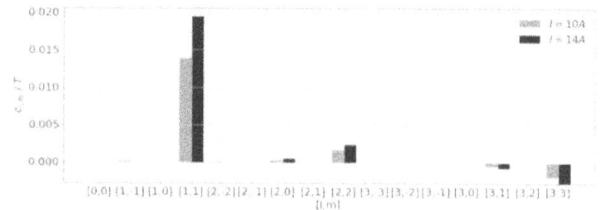

Figure 2: Plot of the coefficients of two spherical harmonic representation of the magnetic field in x-direction translated to the FFP (10 A grey and 14 A black). All coefficients smaller than the error estimation are set to zero.

IV. Discussion

We have shown that the coefficients of a spherical harmonic expansion provides a concise representation of the magnetic field. Translating the expansion to the FFP provides a unique representation independent of the initial position of the field measurements.

The expansion can be used to accurately locate the position of the field free point, which is especially important for the reconstruction of multi-patch imaging sequences [8]. Moreover, it can provide an accurate model to detect and incorporate deviation from ideal fields into a model driven reconstruction process.

The coefficients provide a direct access to the local properties of the field around the expansion point. As this point can be shifted they allow a qualitative and quantitative comparison of the same field at different points. Moreover, they allow a comparison of different magnetic fields at different points making them an ideal tool to describe and analyze magnetic fields in MPI.

ACKNOWLEDGEMENTS

The authors thankfully acknowledge the financial support by the German Research Foundation (DFG, grant number KN 1108/2-1) and the Federal Ministry of Education and Research (BMBF, grant number 05M16GKA).

REFERENCES

[1] J. Rahmer et al. Signal encoding in magnetic particle imaging. *BMC Med. Imaging*, 9, 4, 2009.

[2] T. Knopp et al. Magnetic particle imaging: from proof of principle to preclinical applications. *Phys. Med. Biol.*, 62, R124, 2017.

[3] P. W. Goodwill and S. M. Conolly. The X-space formulation of the magnetic particle imaging process: 1-D signal, resolution, bandwidth, SNR, SAR, and magnetostimulation. *IEEE Trans. Med. Imag.*, 29(11), 1851-9. 2010.

[4] P. Szwargulski et al. Fast Implicit Reconstruction of Focus Field Data in MPI. *IWMPI*, 2016.

[5] A. Weber. Imperfektionen bei Magnetic Particle Imaging. *Infinite Science Publishing*, 2017.

[6] C. H. L. Beentjes. Quadrature on a Spherical Surface. *Tech. Rep.*, University of Oxford, 2010.

[7] J. F. Rico et al. Translation of Real Solid Spherical Harmonics. *Int. J. Quantum Chem.*, 113(10), 1544-1548, 2013.

[8] T. Knopp et al. Joint reconstruction of non-overlapping magnetic particle imaging focus-field data. *Phys. Med. Biol.*, 60, L15, 2015.

Optimizing Transmit Coils for a Magnetic Particle Spectrometer

Xin Chen [a, *], Alexander Neumann [a], Thorsten M. Buzug [a]

[a] *Institute of Medical Engineering, University of Lübeck, Germany*
[*] *Corresponding author, email:{chen,buzug}@imt.uni-luebeck.de*

I. Introduction

In 2005 Bernhard Gleich and Jürgen Weizenecker introduced MPI as a novel imaging technology, it provides sub-millimeter spatial resolution and fast acquisition time for medical imaging [1, 2]. Three-dimensional real-time in-vivo experiments demonstrated a beating mouse heart with high temporal and spatial resolution, using a clinically approved tracer with tolerable concentration [3].

The three-dimensional Magnetic Particle Spectrometer (MPS) introduced in [4] can simulate the magnetic field inside an MPI imaging device and measure the response of the nanoparticles without moving the samples. Therefore, it can be used to estimate the characteristics of superparamagnetic iron oxide (SPIO) nanoparticles, as well as achieve the system matrix of imaging devices [5, 6].

The transmit coil setup used in this MPS is introduced in [4, 7]. However, the central solenoid coil was not optimized, and its size limits the further design of the receive coils as well as the implementation of a cooling system. Moreover, the previous coil setup was optimized by using a self-developed software. The geometrical size of the coils was changed manually to simulate the magnetic field. A coil with irregular shape is also not possible to be modeled in this software.

Therefore, a new optimization of the coil setup is desired. In this paper, different coils are compared with their power loss and homogeneity.

II. Material and Methods

The aim of this work is to optimize the geometrical size of the coils in order to reduce the total power loss of the coil setup, while ensuring the magnetic field at the center point reaches 20 mT.

As shown in Fig. 1, a solenoid coil in the center, which can generate a magnetic field in the X direction, is called X coil. Two pairs of solenoid coils in perpendicular directions Y and Z are called Y coils and Z coils.

Biot-Savart's law describes the magnetic field generated by an electric current

$$\mathbf{B}(r) = \frac{\mu_0}{4\pi} \int \frac{I \, dl \times r'}{|r'|^3}, \qquad (1)$$

where dl is the wire element in the direction of the current, r' is the displacement vector from the wire element l to the point r at which the field is being computed, μ_0 is the permeability of vacuum. I is the current. This equation is a line integral along the wire path in which the current flows.

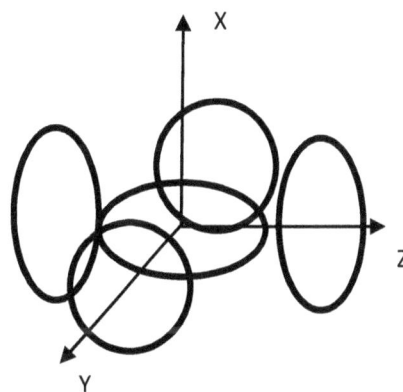

Figure 1: Transmit coil setup according to the coordinate system. Transmit coil in the X direction is a single solenoid coil, in Y or Z direction is a pair of identical solenoid coils.

Eq. (1) can be further simplified for a loop of circular wire or rectangular wire. For more complicated wire loop, numerical integration is used to calculate the magnetic field.

Except the regular circular and rectangular shape, other different shape of coils are also proposed to be compared, e.g. quasi-rectangular, quasi-circular and curved-rectangular coils (see Fig. 2). These kinds of shape ensure that the distance between coils can be further decreased without obstructing the access to the central chamber.

A solenoid coil can be approximately considered as a combination of different wire loops. Therefore, the accumulation of magnetic field generated by each wire loop is equal to the magnetic field generated by the corresponding solenoid coil.

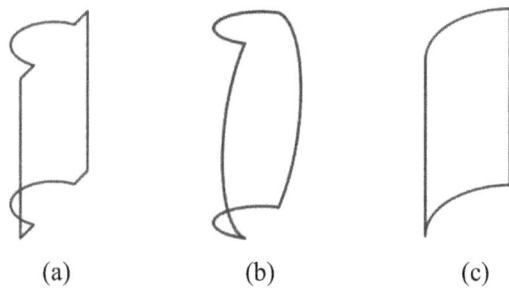

(a)   (b)   (c)

Figure 2: *Different shape of transmit coils. (a) Quasi-rectangular coil; (b) Quasi-circular coil; (c) Curved-rectangular coil.*

In MATLAB, an iterative program is written to compare the power loss of different coil setups. In the program, the radius of the X coil varies within a certain range, which will define the closest distance from the Y coils to the center point. The radius of the Y coil will as well limit the closest distance from the Z coils to the center point. And an iteration of all rational coil sizes will be implemented to calculate the power loss. The power loss of each coil in the coil setups will be summed up and compared.

III. Results

The wire used here is 1000×0.05 mm litz wire manufactured by Elektrisola, which has 2 mm diameter and $0.0092\ \Omega/m$ resistance.

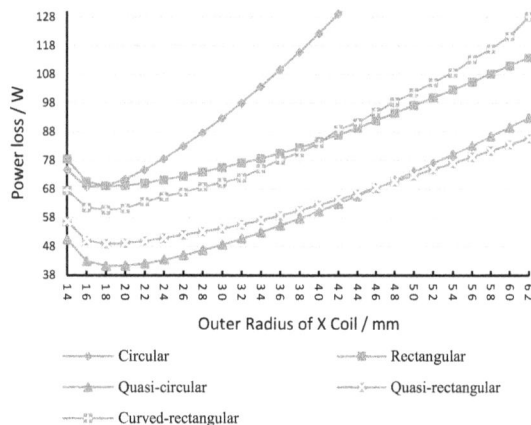

Figure 3: *Total power loss comparison between different coil setups.*

For the X coil, an inner chamber with 12 mm radius is reserved to place the sample vial and receive coils. As can be seen from Fig.3, quasi-rectangular coil setup has the lowest power loss of 41.26 W.

When set the X coil to be a circular solenoid coil with 20 mm outer radius and 18 mm length, the magnetic field along the axis of Y coils is calculated (see Fig. 4). The quasi-circular coil has a slightly worse homogeneity than the quasi-rectangular coils.

IV. Discussion

As in MPS, the sample is measured without moving it, the field homogeneity is not a restrictive factor in the design of transmit coil setup.

The quasi-rectangular coil has better field homogeneity but larger power loss. Moreover, during manufacturing, the sharp corners of the quasi-rectangular coil are more difficult to make than a circular coil. This imperfection will lead to an even larger power loss and worse homogeneity.

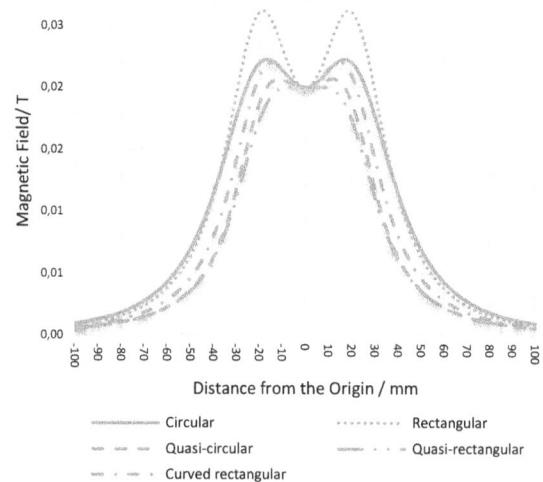

Figure 4: *The comparison of magnetic field along the axis of Y coils*

V. Conclusions

The quasi-circular coil setup is a better transmit coil design when optimizing the power loss. However, when optimizing the field homogeneity, the quasi-rectangular coil can be a better approach.

ACKNOWLEDGEMENTS

This work was supported by the Federal Ministry of Education and Research, Germany (BMBF) under grant 13GW0069A.

REFERENCES

[1] B. Gleich and J. Weizenecker. Tomographic imaging using the nonlinear response of magnetic particles. *Nature*, 435(7046):1214-1217, 2005. doi: 10.1038/nature03808.

[2] J. Weizenecker, J. Borgert and B. Gleich. A simulation study on the resolution and sensitivity of magnetic particle imaging. *Physics in Medicine and Biology*, 52(21):6363, 2007. doi: 10.1088/0031-9155/52/21/001.

[3] J. Weizenecker, B. Gleich, J. Rahmer, H. Dahnke and J. Borgert. Three-dimensional real-time in vivo magnetic particle imaging. *Physics in Medicine and Biology*, 54(5): L1, 2009. doi: 10.1088/0031-9155/54/5/L01.

[4] X. Chen, M. Graeser, A. Behrends, A. von Gladiss and T. M. Buzug. First measured result of the 3D Magnetic Particle Spectrometer, *In: International Workshop on Magnetic Particle Imaging*, 123, 2017.

[5] M. Grüttner, M. Graeser, S. Biederer, T. F. Sattel, H. Wojtczyk, W. Tenner, T. Knopp, B. Gleich, J. Borgert and T. M. Buzug. 1D-image reconstruction for magnetic particle imaging using a hybrid system function. *In Nuclear Science Symposium and Medical Imaging Conference (NSS/MIC)*, pages 2545-2548. IEEE, 2011. doi: 10.1109/NSSMIC.2011.6152687.

[6] A. von Gladiss, M. Graeser, P. Szwargulski, T. Knopp and T. M. Buzug. Hybrid System Calibration for Multidimensional Magnetic Particle Imaging. *Physics in Medicine and Biology*. 2016. doi: 10.1088/1361-6560/aa5340.

[7] X. Chen, A. Behrends, M. Graeser, A. Neumann and T. M. Buzug Optimizing the Coil Setup for a Three-Dimensional Magnetic Particle Spectrometer, *In: International Workshop on Magnetic Particle Imaging*, 59, 2016.

Design, Simulation and Construction of a Symmetrical Transmission Filter for an FFL-MPI

Huimin Wei [a,*], Jan Stelzner [a], Thorsten M. Buzug [a]

[a] Institute of Medical Engineering, Universität zu Lübeck, Ratzeburger Allee 160, Lübeck, 23562, Germany
[*] Corresponding author, email: wei@imt.uni-luebeck.de

I. Introduction

An external sinusoidal drive field is used in MPI to excite the superparamagnetic iron oxide nanoparticles (SPIONs) [1]. Due to the non-linear magnetization property of the SPIONs, the frequency spectrum of the induced magnetization contains not only the fundamental frequency of the drive field but also higher harmonics. The higher harmonics in the frequency domain can be used to reconstruct subsequently the spatial distribution of the nanoparticles. For the fact that the drive-field signal directly couples into the receive coils [2], previous filtering is necessary in an MPI system to keep a high spectral purity of the drive field signal.

In this work, a symmetrical band pass filter for a rabbit-sized FFL-scanner [3] is presented, which exclusively lets the desired excitation signal pass. Beneficial from its symmetry, the common-mode noise will be cancelled by measuring the difference at the output ports of the filter and hence has an advanced common-mode noise rejection.

II. Material and Methods

At first, a third order Chebyshev II band-pass filter is designed using a filter design software *FilterSolutions*. The symmetrical filter (Fig. 1) is a combination of two of this filter. One of the designed single-ended filter is mirrored vertically. The voltage source is connected between the two input ports. The load between the two output ports and the other ports are connected to the ground.

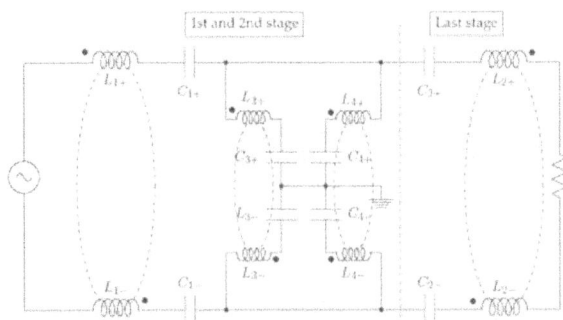

Figure 1: Design of the symmetrical transmission filter. The dashed ellipse indicates the winding cores of the coupled inductors.

The obtained filter shows horizontal symmetry and has a positive as well as a negative signal line. The common-mode noise on the filter is eliminated by taking the difference of the positive and negative signal line as the output signal. In this way, a balanced filter is obtained from two single-ended filters. The filter has a 25 kHz center frequency and a bandwidth of 5 kHz. The input impedance is 0.1 Ω to match the output impedance of the AC amplifier. The output impedance is 2 Ω to match the load impedance. The filter is designed to be capable to work with up to 100 V_{rms} voltage and 50 A current. The noise simulation is conducted using *LTspice*, random noise and 50 Hz frequency noise are introduced into the filter. The total harmonic distortion (THD) value of the voltage on the load is computed, which measures how much of the output signal is distortion caused by the harmonics, and is used to evaluate the effect of the noise on the signal. The toroidal air-core inductors are designed with an optimum cross-section shape that has maximum inductance for a given eddy-current and DC power loss per unit length of the wire [4]. CAD models of the toroidal cores are built according to the calculated cross-section shapes. The cores are hollow to reduce their weight and save material. They are divided into several segments to fit the size of the 3D printer. The segments are manufactured with 3D printing and assembled together to form the complete toroidal cores. Two inductors with same inductance are wound on one toroidal core to reduce the size. The inductance and resistance of each inductor are measured at different frequencies.

In order to protect the filter from external influences and couplings of the filter components, the filter is installed in two 9-mm-thick aluminum boxes. According to the thickness of the box wall and the skin depth of an interfering signal, the shielding box should be able to block the interfering signal with frequency above 82.25 Hz. The implemented filter is shown in Fig. 2.

III. Results

In simulation, where the components are considered ideal, the THD value of the symmetric filter stays zero when introducing common-mode noise. The verification of the noise property of the filter is not in the frame of this work. The measured self-resonant frequencies (SRF) of all inductors are above 3 MHz, therefore the inductors can work at 25 kHz frequency. The resistance increases with the frequency due to the influence of the skin effect. More parameters of the inductors are shown in Table 1.

The frequency response of the filter is measured by the *Keysight Technologies* E5061B LF-RF Network Analyzer. Baluns are used to provide an unbalanced to balanced circuit interface between the measurement ports and the filter and a 2 Ω resistor is connected in parallel between the two outputs of the filter to match the impedance.

The measured result of the network analyzer is shown in Fig. 3. The measurement of the transfer function verified 5 kHz for the pass bandwidth. At the passing frequency 25 kHz, the attenuation is -922.48 mdB, which is very low. The attenuation at frequencies between 50 kHz and 1 MHz are at least 50 dB. The attenuation of the first higher odd harmonic 75 kHz is 83.526 dB.

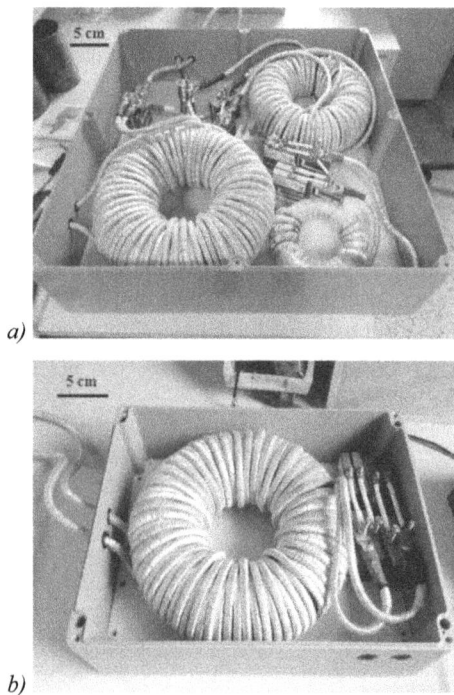

a)

b)

Figure 2: *The implemented filter with shielding boxes. a) The first and second stage. b) The last stage. The used litz wire contains 10000 strands with 63 μm diameter and is served with PEEK foil.*

Table 1: *Parameters of the inductors.*

Inductors	Inductance/μH	Outer Radius/m	Windings
L_1+L_1	61.47	0.1590	48
L_2+L_2	37.57	0.1390	48
L_3+L_3	2	0.0790	10
L_4+L_4	31.45	0.1340	48

IV. Discussion

The frequency response of the filter implies it is suitable to be used for the regarded FFL-scanner. The simulation results indicate that the symmetrical filter can eliminate the distortion of the signal and reduce disturbance caused by common mode noise. However, the implemented filter is

not perfectly symmetrical because the components of the positive and negative signal line are not exactly identical, which are produce through the manufacturing procedure. The measured common-mode rejection ratio (CMRR) at 25 kHz is 66.6 dB. Therefore, the performance of the filter with common-mode noise will be affected. Further test and measurement can be done to find out the practical capability of the filter to eliminate the common-mode noise. For this work, the filter only worked with small signals, the built-in AC source of the network analyzer has a maximum output power of 10 dBm. The filter can be tested with high voltage input signal to obtain its performance when carrying large current.

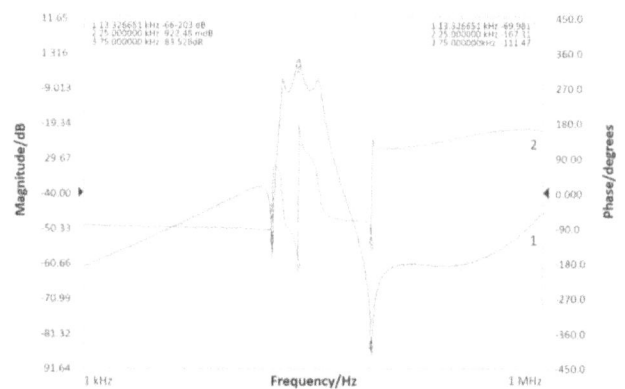

Figure 3: *The measured frequency response. 1. The magnitude response. 2. The phase response.*

V. Conclusions

Within the scope of this work, a symmetrical band-pass filter with a passing frequency of 25 kHz was designed and implemented. The next step in our development will include studies with noise and large-current measurement.

ACKNOWLEDGEMENTS

The authors would like to thank the German Federal Ministry of Education and Research (BMBF) in the framework Health Research (Gesundheitsforschung), contract number 13GW0230B, for financial support.

References

[1] B. Gleich and J. Weizenecker. Tomographic imaging using the nonlinear response of magnetic particles. *Nature*, 435(7046):1217-1217, 2005. doi: 10.1038/nature03808.

[2] M. Graeser, T. Knopp, M. Grüttner, T. F. Sattel, and T. M. Buzug. Analog receive signal processing for magnetic particle imaging. *Medical physics*, 40(4), 2013. doi:10.1118/1.4794482.

[3] G. Bringout, J. Stelzner, M. Ahlborg, A. Behrends, K. Bente, C. Debbeler, A. von Gladiß, K. Gräfe, M. Graeser, C. Kaethner, et al. Concept of a rabbit-sized ffl-scanner. In *Magnetic Particle Imaging (IWMPI), 2015 5th International Workshop on*, pages 1–1. IEEE, 2015. doi:10.1109/IWMPI.2015.7107032.

[4] P. Murgatroyd. Some optimum shapes for toroidal inductors. In *IEE Proceedings B (Electric Power Applications)*, 129:168–176, 1982. doi:10.1049/ip-b.1982.0023.

[5] T. M. Buzug, G. Bringout, M. Erbe, K. Gräfe, M. Graeser, M. Grüttner, A. Halkola, T. F. Sattel,W. Tenner, H.Wojtczyk, et al. Magnetic particle imaging: introduction to imaging and hardware realization. *Zeitschrift für Medizinische Physik*, 22(4):323–334, 2012. doi:10.1016/j.zemedi.2012.07.004.

Passive and Active Compensation of Drive Field Feed-Through for Multi-Frequency MPI

Dennis Pantke [a,*], Marcel Straub [a], Volkmar Schulz [a]

[a] *Department of Physics of Molecular Imaging, Institute for Experimental Molecular Imaging, RWTH Aachen University, Aachen, Germany*
[*] *Corresponding author, email: dennis.pantke@pmi.rwth-aachen.de*

I. Introduction

Conventional Magnetic Particle Imaging (MPI) devices quantitatively determine the spatial distribution of superparamagnetic iron oxide nanoparticles (SPIONs) by exploiting the characteristic nonlinear magnetization response to a changing magnetic field [1]. Although current scanners offer high temporal and spatial resolution, they are still limited in terms of sensitivity and their capability of measuring functional parameters as pH-value, temperature, binding status of the tracer or other biochemical parameters. While interest in using nanotechnology for cancer treatment is growing, continuous *in vivo* access to these parameters is highly desired, since it would allow the assessment of therapy progress and outcome. One promising approach to get information about functional parameters is particle excitation at multiple frequencies or at other than sinusoidal waveforms [2-4]. Current MPI systems use resonantly powered excitation fields to stimulate the SPIONs. Since the feed-through of the drive field is orders of magnitude higher than the particle signal, it is filtered by a narrow band-stop filter in conventional scanner designs. However, these approaches make the application of broadband excitation and different waveforms hardly possible.

Therefore, we propose a combined passive and active drive field feed-through compensation approach. By this, the whole dynamic range of the analog-to-digital converter shall be exploited. The compensation approach is intended to be used in a novel multi-frequency MPI device.

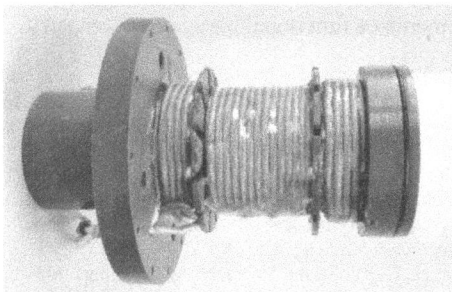

Figure 1: *Gradiometer coil design for Magnetic Particle Imaging at multiple frequencies.*

II. Material and Methods

Wideband passive compensation of the drive field feed-through was realized by inductive decoupling of separate transmit (TX) and receive (RX) solenoid coils in a gradiometer coil design (see Fig. 1). The TX/RX coils are designed for imaging applications. Their inner bore diameter is about 45 mm. Litz wire of 3 mm diameter was used. The TX coil was wound on top of the RX coil. Each coil has 19 windings (without second layer). The individual coils are subdivided in three sections. While the whole RX coil L_R and the central segment of the TX coil L_T are wound in one layer and one direction, the peripheral segments of the TX coil L_C are wound in two layers and the opposite direction. To find the winding number n of the second layer of L_C, a thin-wire approximation was used to compute the mutual inductance

$$M \propto \underbrace{\oint_{\partial A_T} \oint_{\partial A_R} \frac{dr_T \cdot dr_R}{\|dr_T - dr_R\|}}_{=: M_0} - \underbrace{\oint_{\partial A_C} \oint_{\partial A_R} \frac{dr_C \cdot dr_R}{\|dr_C - dr_R\|}}_{=: M_1} . \quad (1)$$

Fine tuning was achieved by connecting the coils to a network analyzer E5061B (Keysight Technologies, Inc., Santa Rosa/CA) and varying the second-layer winding number n. After tuning, the coils were fixed with epoxy.

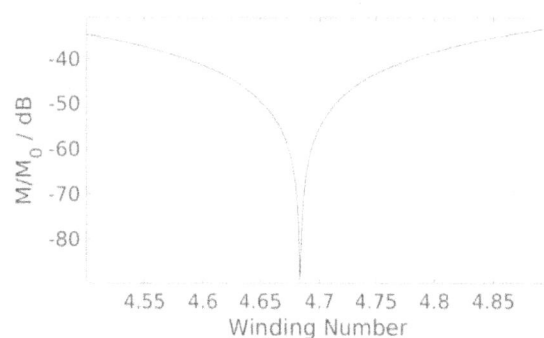

Figure 2: *Mutual inductance M divided by M_0 as a function of the winding number n of the second layer of L_C.*

The residual drive field feed-through is further attenuated actively by applying the inverse of the remaining feed-through signal via a transformer. Drive field and active compensation signals are generated by a remote controlled Keysight 33512B function generator. The drive field signal is amplified by an Omnitronic E-2000 MK2 power amplifier (Steincke Showtechnic GmbH, Waldbüttel-brunn/Germany). The residual feed-through is digitized by a PCIe-9852 analog-to-digital converter (Adlink Technology Inc., New Taipei City/Taiwan). A control circuit was implemented for proof-of-concept investigations, which allows to minimize the respective peak in the frequency spectrum that remains from the passive compensation stage.

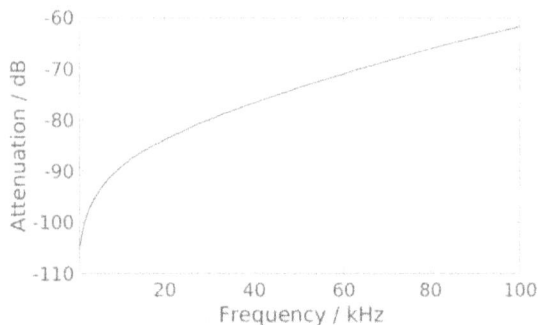

Figure 3: Broadband feed-through attenuation by passive decoupling determined with the Keysight E5061 network analyzer.

III. Results

The computed mutual inductance M divided by M_0 is depicted in Fig. 2. The result of the calculation set the starting condition for fine tuning. The frequency dependent drive field feed-through attenuation achieved by inductive decoupling can be seen in Fig. 3. At 20 kHz, an attenuation of -84 dB was reached. The frequency spectrum of the residual feed-through with and without applied active compensation for a drive field frequency of 20 kHz (max. active attenuation) is shown in Fig. 4. A further reduction of the residual feed-through by -42 dB was measured. Higher harmonics generated by the power electronics can be seen. The attenuation values of passive, active and combined passive and active compensation for a multitude of frequencies in the range of 5 kHz to 30 kHz are shown in table 1. The maximal, i.e. -126 dB, and minimal, i.e. -108 dB, attenuation were measured for 20 kHz and 30 kHz, respectively.

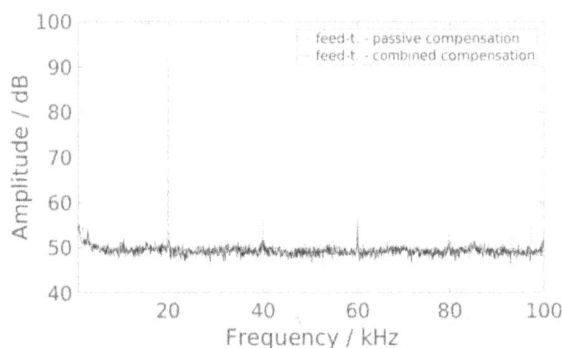

Figure 4: Averaged (40x) frequency spectra of the residual feed-through passively attenuated and with combined passive and active compensation exemplarily for 20 kHz.

Table 1: Feed-through attenuation reached by passive, active and combined passive and active compensation.

Frequency	Passive Compensation	Active Compensation	Combined
5 kHz	-94 dB	-19 dB	-113 dB
10 kHz	-90 dB	-32 dB	-122 dB
15 kHz	-86 dB	-38 dB	-124 dB
20 kHz	-84 dB	-42 dB	-126 dB
25 kHz	-82 dB	-33 dB	-115 dB
30 kHz	-80 dB	-28 dB	-108 dB

IV. Discussion

The results of the mutual inductance calculation showed a good agreement to the actual winding number with which maximum passive attenuation was reached. Only little fine tuning was necessary. A passive attenuation of up to -84 dB was measured (20 kHz). Tay et al. reached up to -67 dB (10 kHz) by inductive decoupling with their MPI spectrometer [4]. The frequency dependence of the decoupling curve results from the frequency dependent mutual induction of the coils. An additional attenuation of up to -42 dB was reached by active compensation at 20 kHz. The magnetic field strength and applicable frequency range is currently limited by the performance of the power amplifier. The output power determines the ratio between residual feed-through and noise level and thus, the amount of obtainable attenuation. A high power, broadband power amplifier, which performs well at a wide range of load impedances will enable a further increase of active attenuation at a greater bandwidth.

V. Conclusions

A combined passive and active compensation approach to attenuate the drive field feed-through was presented. This technique allows the use of multiple frequencies and other than sinusoidal waveforms for SPION excitations in MPI. Furthermore, it enables access to the first harmonic of the SPIONs response for conventional harmonic MPI. Passive compensation was realized by a gradiometer coil design. An attenuation of -84 dB could be shown for 20 kHz. The feasibility of active compensation was shown for frequencies between 5 and 30 kHz. The bandwidth and magnitude of active compensation was mainly limited by the power amplifier hardware. At 20 kHz the residual feed-through was further reduced by -42 dB. In total, a combined passive and active compensation of up to -126 dB (20 kHz) was shown, which enables imaging application. Thus, an initial step towards a multi-frequency MPI that allows measurements of functional parameters was performed.

REFERENCES

[1] T. Knopp and T. M. Buzug. *Magnetic Particle Imaging: An Introduction to Imaging Principles and Scanner Instrumentation.* Springer, Berlin/Heidelberg, 2012.

[2] C. Kuhlmann, A. P. Khandhar, R. M. Ferguson, S. Kemp, T. Wawrzik, M. Schilling, K. M. Krishnan und F. Ludwig, „Drive-Field Frequency Dependent MPI Performance of,“ *IEEE Transactions on Magnetics* 51, No. 2, 3-6, 2015.

[3] T. Viereck, C. Kuhlmann, S. Draack, M. Schilling und F. Ludwig, „Dual-frequency magnetic particle imaging of the Brownian particle contribution,“ *Journal of Magnetism and Magnetic Materials* 427, 156-161, 2016.

[4] Tay, Zhi Wei, et al. "A high-throughput, arbitrary-waveform, MPI spectrometer and relaxometer for comprehensive magnetic particle optimization and characterization." *Scientific reports* 6, 2016

A Hand-Held Single-Sided Explorer for Magnetic Particle Spectroscopy

Maximilian Gram[a], Cordula Grüttner[b], Alexander Kraupner[c], Karl-Heinz Hiller[d], Peter M. Jakob[a,d], Florian Fidler [d,*]

[a] Department of Experimental Physics 5, University of Würzburg, Würzburg, Germany
[b] micromod Partikeltechnologie GmbH, Rostock, Germany
[c] nanoPET Pharma GmbH, Berlin, Germany
[d] Magnetic Resonance and X-Ray Imaging MRB, Fraunhofer Institute for Integrated Circuits IIS, Würzburg, Germany
* Corresponding author, email: florian.fidler@iis.fraunhofer.de

I. Introduction

Small single-sided sensors allow the localization of tracer materials near the surface of an extended object. As an example, mammary carcinoma may be treated by the concept of sentinel lymph node identification [1]. In this work we describe such a sensor, comprising a cost-effective hand-held magnetic particle spectrometer (MPS) with extended capabilities in terms of a homogeneous excitation and readout field. With this sensor not only a localization of the tracer material is possible, it can also be used for characterization of the tracer material as well. This allows a wide range of applications from process control to medical applications.

II. Material and Methods

The detector consists of a single coil arrangement for excitation and signal detection. The signal acquisition is done as described in [2] by measuring the magnetic permeability of the probe volume. By means of this method, a single coil can be used for excitation and signal reception. Focus of this work was to develop a coil arrangement with a homogeneous field outside the surface. This results in both homogenous excitation and signal detection in the desired volume allowing to generate similar results to a regular MPS with a closed detection volume.

II.I. Development of the coil arrangement

The coil arrangement consists of three concentric stacked serial coils with individual diameter and number of turns allowing arbitrary current direction. The parameters have been iteratively optimized using FEMM 4.2 [3]. The desired field-of-view (fov) was a cylinder with a diameter of 20 mm and a height of 10 mm in front of the sensor.

The result is an arrangement of three serial coils with a maximum diameter of 46 mm. The central coil has a reverse direction. The sensor housing (Fig. 1) is manufactured with a 3D printer, the coils are wound up by hand according to the iteration result.

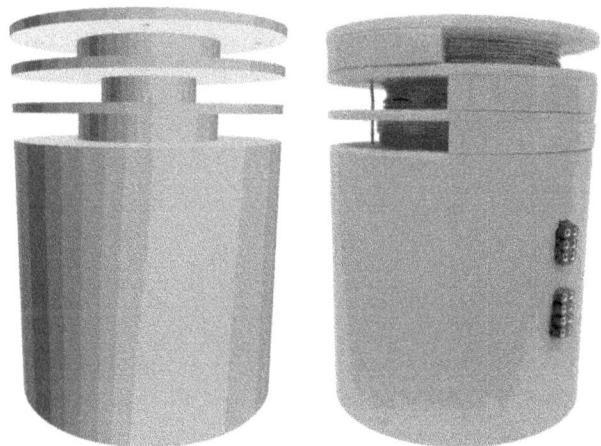

Figure 1: The CAD design of the sensor housing (left) and the built single-sided sensor (right) with cover partly removed.

II.II. Comparison with the simulation result

The alternating magnetic field is measured in the probe volume and compared with the simulation result. The normalized standard deviation in the fov deviates by 8.21% from the simulation result (Fig. 2). This is a sufficiently homogeneous field.

III. Results

For demonstration purposes, SPIONs with a volume of 1 ml are placed 1 mm above the surface in the sample volume. The generated alternating magnetic field was $B=(10.615 \pm 0.026)$ mT at a frequency of 18.424 kHz. The signal was acquired with a modified Drive^L (Pure Devices GmbH, Würzburg, Germany). Higher harmonics representing the particle properties, which are caused by the non-linear permeability of the sample volume, are measured in the recorded signal (Fig. 3).

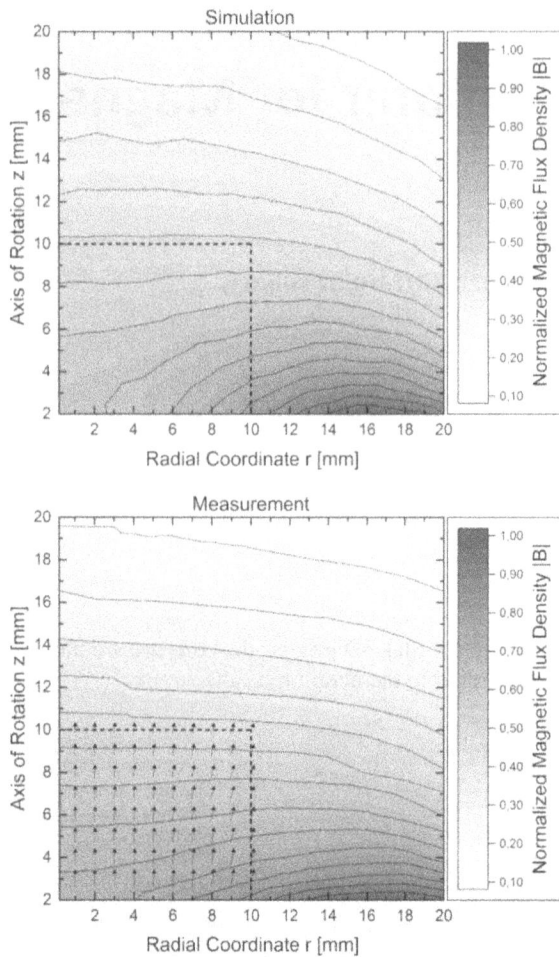

Figure 2: *Field map of simulation (top) and measurement (bottom). The fov is indicated by the rectangle, the magnetic field is indicated by vector arrows.*

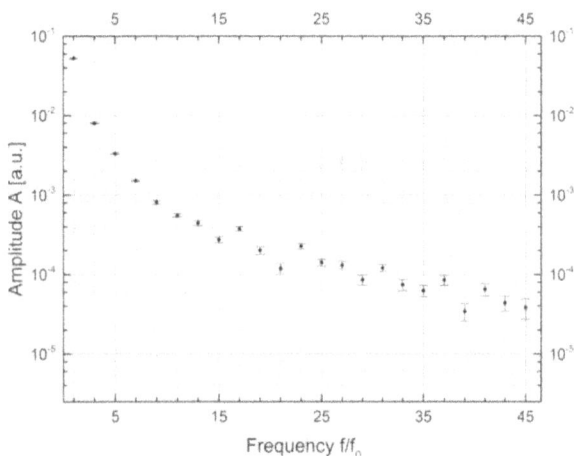

Figure 3: *Amplitude spectrum of odd harmonics of sample SPIONs at a frequency f_0=18.424 kHz.*

IV. Discussion

The developed single-sided sensor enables the detection and the characterization of SPIONs within the probe volume. The localization of the particles is given by the size of the sensor. Furthermore, since no averaging was applied, the sensor offers a high temporal resolution and can thus detect particles in nearly real time. For this purpose, the amplitudes of suitable harmonics are observed and recorded over time.

Additionally, the explorer is prepared for further optimization. Each coil can be modified in current and phase by adding lumped elements to the prepared connectors in the housing (Fig. 1) allowing modifying the field characteristic in the fov for the desired purpose.

V. Conclusions

The presented single-sided explorer allows a homogeneous excitation and signal detection similar to a regular MPS spectrometer of extended objects. This allows localization due to the small sensor size as well as particle characterization due to its relatively homogeneous excitation field and signal detection.

.ACKNOWLEDGEMENTS

This work was supported by the EU FP7 HEALTH program IDEA – "Identification, homing and monitoring of therapeutic cells for regenerative medicine – Identify, Enrich, Accelerate" under grant agreement no 279288.

REFERENCES

[1] D. Finas, K. Baumann, L. Sydow, K. Heinrich, K. Gräfe, A. Rody, K. Lüdtke-Buzug and T. Buzug. *Lymphatic Tissue and Superparamagnetic Nanoparticles - Magnetic Particle Imaging for Detection and Distribution in a Breast Cancer Model.* Biomedical Engineering / Biomedizinische Technik. 2013. 10.1515/bmt-2013-4262

[2] F. Fidler, K.-H. Hiller and P.M. Jakob. *Magnetic particle detection based on non-linear response to magnetic susceptibility changes.* IWMPI 2016

[3] D.C. Meeker. *FEMM 64-bit Executable.* Version 4.2 (12Jan2016 Build). http://www.femm.info/wiki/Download.

Complex Susceptibility Imaging of Magnetic Nanoparticles

Shiqiang Pi [a], Wenzhong Liu [a, b, *], Tao Jiang [a]

[a] *School of Automation, Huazhong University of Science and Technology, Wuhan 430074, China*
[b] *Key Laboratory of Image Processing and Intelligent Control, Huazhong University of Science and Technology, Wuhan 430074, China*
* *Corresponding author, email: lwz7410@hust.edu.cn*

I. Introduction

The tracer-based magnetic particle imaging (MPI), using the nonlinear magnetization response of magnetic nanoparticles (MNPs) under both gradient magnetic field and drive magnetic field, was first proposed by Gleich and Weizenecker [1]. Real-time and quantitative MPI with high image contrast and sensitivity has a great promising in biomedical applications, for instance, B. Zheng *et al.* performed *in vivo* experiments to monitor the transplantation, bio-distribution, and clearance of stem cells quantitatively [2].

Typically, the frequencies of drive magnetic fields used in MPI are over 10 kHz. However, due to the presence of magnetic relaxations, the magnetization response of the MNPs cannot instantaneously follow the applied ac magnetic field. The magnetization of the MNPs is accounted for by complex susceptibility [3], $\chi = \chi_0/(1 + i\omega\tau)$, where χ_0 is the equilibrium susceptibility which is proportional to the MNPs concentration, ω is the angular frequency of applied magnetic field, and τ is the effective relaxation time. Moreover, the complex susceptibility of MNP is strongly influenced by their surrounding microenvironment and applied magnetic fields that can provide significant implications for MNP-aided diagnosis and therapy.

Therefore, in this paper, we present an imaging method to map the spatial distribution of MNPs using the real part, imaginary part or magnitude of the MNP's complex susceptibility under gradient magnetic field, low-frequency drive magnetic field, and weak high-frequency magnetic field.

II. Material and Methods

II.I. Methods

Under a static and an ac magnetic fields $H(t) = H_{dc} + H_{ac}\cos(2\pi ft)$, the magnetization of the MNPs can be written as [4]

$$M\left(H(t)\right) = \phi m_s \left(\coth\left(\zeta_H\right) - 1/\zeta_H\right) \qquad (1)$$

where $\zeta_H = \mu_0 H(t)m_s/(kT)$, ϕ is particle concentration, $m_s = \pi M_s D^3/6$ is the saturation magnetic moment, M_s is the saturation magnetization, D is the diameter of the MNPs, k is the Boltzmann constant, and T is the absolute temperature. When the strength of the applied ac magnetic field H_{ac} is weak, the differential susceptibility of MNPs at static magnetic field H_{dc} can be then obtained from [5]:

$$\chi_d\left(H_{dc}\right) = \frac{\partial M}{\partial H}\bigg|_{H_{dc}} = \frac{\phi m_s^2}{kT} L'\left(\zeta_{dc}\right) \qquad (2)$$

where $\zeta_{dc} = \mu_0 H_{dc}m_s/(kT)$. Considering the magnetic relaxation of MNP, the differential complex susceptibility at static magnetic field strength H_{dc} is

$$\chi\left(H_{dc}\right) = \left(\frac{1}{1+\left(\omega\tau\right)^2} - i\frac{\omega\tau}{1+\left(\omega\tau\right)^2}\right)\chi_d\left(H_{dc}\right) \qquad (3)$$

The MNP with core size larger than 20 nm is dominated by Brownian relaxation. And the relaxation time of the components of magnetization parallel to external field is [6]

$$\tau = \frac{d\ln L\left(\xi_{dc}\right)}{d\ln \xi_{dc}}\tau_{B0} = \tau_{B0}\frac{\xi_{dc}}{L\left(\xi_{dc}\right)}L'\left(\xi_{dc}\right) \qquad (4)$$

where τ_{B0} is the relaxation time at a zero-dc magnetic field. For 1-D magnetic particle susceptibility imaging, the magnetic fields applied to the MNPs are $H(t) = Gx - H_{dc} + H_{ac}\cos(\omega t)$, the complex susceptibility of the MNPs can be calculated by

$$\chi'\left(x_p\right) = -\frac{1}{\kappa\omega H_{ac}}\frac{\omega}{\pi}\int_{-\pi/\omega}^{\pi/\omega} S\left(H_{dc},t\right)\cdot\sin\left(\omega t\right)dt \qquad (5)$$
$$= \chi\left(H_{dc}\right)\cos\left(\alpha\right)$$

$$\chi''\left(x_p\right) = \frac{1}{\kappa\omega H_{ac}}\frac{\omega}{\pi}\int_{-\pi/\omega}^{\pi/\omega} S\left(H_{dc},t\right)\cdot\cos\left(\omega t\right)dt \qquad (6)$$
$$= \chi\left(H_{dc}\right)\sin\left(\alpha\right)$$

where $S(H_{dc}, t)$ is the induced voltage of pick-up coil with sensitivity κ (herein we approximate κ as a constant in the FOV), α is the phase delay caused by the magnetic relaxations, and $x_p = H_{dc} / G$ is the zero static magnetic field point where the weak ac magnetic field is nonzero. The spatial differential susceptibilities can be then obtained by moving the zero static magnetic field point (by changing the value of H_{dc}). To improve the imaging speed, a low frequency drive magnetic field is used to replace the static magnetic field. The details of image reconstruction are described in our previous work [5].

II.II. Material

The 2-D imaging experiments were performed using our home-made imaging system [5].The commercial MNPs sample with a mean diameter of 25 nm (SHP-25, 5 mg-Fe/mL) purchased from Ocean Nanotech (San Diego, CA, USA) were used in the experiments. Moreover, the distilled water was used to dilute the MNPs solution.

III. Results

To compare the anti-noise ability, the simulation results of 1-D magnetic particle susceptibility imaging (MPSI) using the magnitude, real part and imaginary part of the complex susceptibility with different SNRs are shown in Figs. 1 and 2.

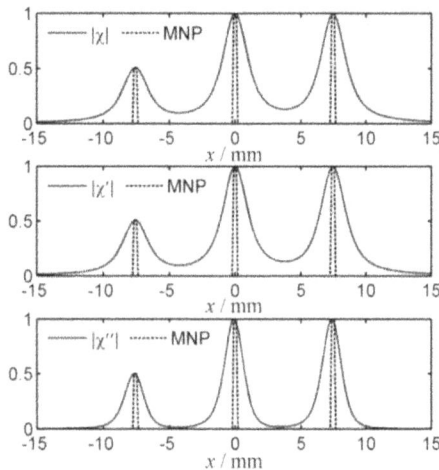

Figure 1: *Simulation of 1-D magnetic particle susceptibility imaging. $G = 2\ T/m/\mu_0$, $\tau_{B0} = 10^{-6}$ s, and SNR = 200 dB.*

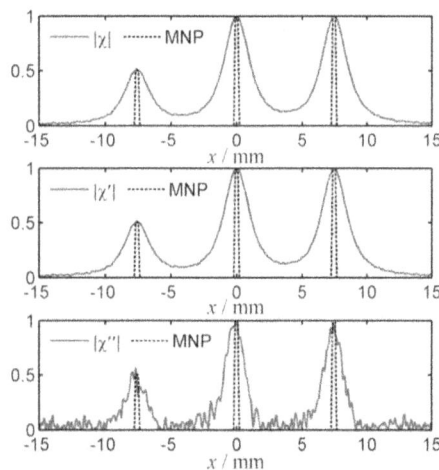

Figure 2: *Simulation of 1-D magnetic particle susceptibility imaging. $G = 2\ T/m/\mu_0$, $\tau_{B0} = 10^{-6}$ s, and SNR = 20 dB.*

Fig. 3 shows the images of single point tracer phantoms containing variant Fe quantities (500, 400, 300, 200, 100, 50, 25, and 12.5 μg). The 1st line shows the MNP solutions with different Fe concentrations. The 2nd ~ 4th lines show the images reconstructed using the magnitude, real part and imaginary part of ac susceptibility.

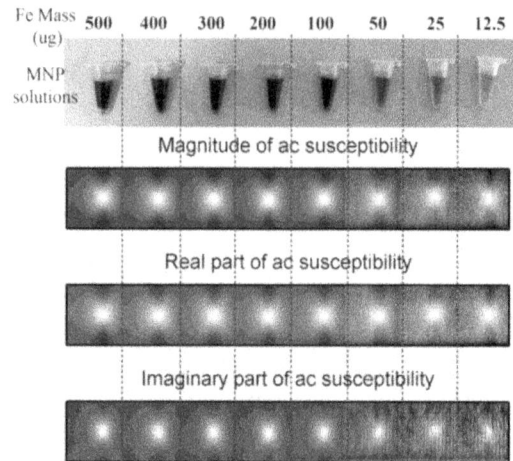

Figure 3: *Experimental results of 2-D magnetic particle susceptibility imaging.*

IV. Discussion

From both the simulation and the experimental results, we can find that the images reconstructed using imaginary part of ac susceptibility have higher spatial resolution but lower SNR. Moreover, sensitivity and linearity of MPSI are discussed in Ref. [5].

V. Conclusions

In conclusion, we achieve MPSI using the real part, imaginary part or magnitude of the MNP's complex ac susceptibility under gradient magnetic field, low-frequency drive magnetic field, and weak high-frequency magnetic field.

ACKNOWLEDGEMENTS

This work was supported by the National Natural Science Foundation of China under Grant number 61571199 and 61401168.

REFERENCES

[1] B. Gleich and J. Weizenecker. Tomographic imaging using the nonlinear response of magnetic particles. *Nature*, 435(7046):1217-1217, 2005. doi: 10.1038/nature03808.

[2] B. Zheng, M. P. von See, E. Yu, *et al.*, Quantitative magnetic particle imaging monitors the transplantation, biodistribution, and clearance of stem cells in vivo, *Theranostics,* vol. 6, pp. 291-301, 2016. doi: 10.7150/thno.13728.

[3] R. E. Rosensweig, Heating magnetic fluid with alternating magnetic field, J. Magn. Magn. Mater., vol. 252, pp. 370-374, 2002. doi: 10.1016/S0304-8853(02)00706-0.

[4] J. Rahmer, J. Weizenecker, B. Gleich, *et al.*, Signal encoding in magnetic particle imaging: properties of the system function,BMC Med. Imaging.vol. 9:4 2009. doi:10.1186/1471-2342-9-4.

[5] S. Pi, W. Liu, and T. Jiang, Real-time and quantitative isotropic spatial resolution susceptibility imaging for magnetic nanoparticles, *Meas. Sci. Technol.* 2017. https://doi.org/10.1088/1361-6501/aa9a55.

[6] Yu. L. Raikher, M.I. Shliomis, Relaxation phenomena in condensed matter. *Adv. Chem. Phys.*, 87 (1994), pp. 595-751 (Chapter 8).

Design of a Switched-Capacitor Array for High-Power Applications with Dense Coverage of Medium Frequency-Range

André Behrends [a,*], Thorsten M. Buzug [a], Alexander Neumann [a]

[a] Institute of Medical Engineering, University of Lübeck, Lübeck, Germany
* Corresponding author, email: {behrends,buzug}@imt.uni-luebeck.de

I. Introduction

I.I. Motivation

Magnetic hyperthermia has been studied for several years due to its possible uses in therapy such as cancer treatment [1] or targeted drug delivery [2]. The effectivity of the heating process depends on the used particles as well as the magnitude and frequency of the applied magnetic field [3]. Therefore, verification of the heating performance depending on these parameters is of high interest. It is possible to apply different field strengths [4, 5]. However, applying different frequencies is a challenging problem due to the necessary impedance matching. The only approach, known to the authors, is the measurement at widely spread discrete frequencies in the wanted frequency range. Numerical calculations indicate that optimal combinations of magnetic field strength, frequency and the size of the magnetic nanoparticles exist such that the increase of hysteresis loop area is maximal with respect to the applied magnetic field strength and frequency [6]. To find these combinations a dense coverage of the frequency-range is necessary.

I.II. Choice of Impedance Matching Type

The required field strengths to perform magnetic hyperthermia are up to $20\,\text{kA/m}$ ($25.08\,\text{mT}$), which makes an impedance matching of the magnetic field generator necessary. The topology of the impedance matching is shown in Fig. 1. The dc resistance is not shown in Fig. 1 but used in the calculations and the capacitors are assumed to be ideal. The typical frequency range for magnetic particle hyperthermia lies in the range $100\,\text{kHz} - 1\,\text{MHz}$. Unfortunately, most broadband impedance matching techniques, fail due to the combination of the broad frequency range and high power consumption of the system. Therefore, the approach proposed here is a capacitive impedance matching based on switched capacitors, which are selected such that the frequency range under examination can be matched in a dense manner.

II. Material and Methods

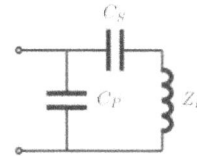

Figure 1: The matching capacitors C_P and C_S are used to transfer the power optimally from the power source to the field-generating coil Z_L. The dc resistance of the coil is not shown but used in the calculations and the capacitors are assumed ideal.

II.I. Dense Matching

The matching concept follows an approach of an earlier contribution [7], where it was exploited that every real impedance matching has a certain bandwidth, which can be termed a matching band (in [7] termed measurement ranges). If the matching frequencies are chosen in a way that the resulting matching bands overlap at appropriate values of load power, it is possible to have a sufficient matching for every frequency in the frequency range under consideration. This approach can be used to minimize the necessary number of matching frequencies.

II.II. Capacitor Selection

The first step in capacitor selection is to calculate the ideal values for the matching capacitors C_S and C_P for each targeted matching frequency, which can be done as discussed in [8]. The resulting ideal matching capacitances can be composed using capacitors following an E-series of preferred numbers. This ensures that the error produced by the approximation is below a maximum value, which is usually the fabrication error of the component. The choice of the specific E-series used, depends on the relative capacitance error, which is given by the designer of the system as well as the availability of suitable capacitors. The minimum and maximum values of the capacitors depend on the capacitance range the array is supposed to cover.

II.III. Array Synthesis

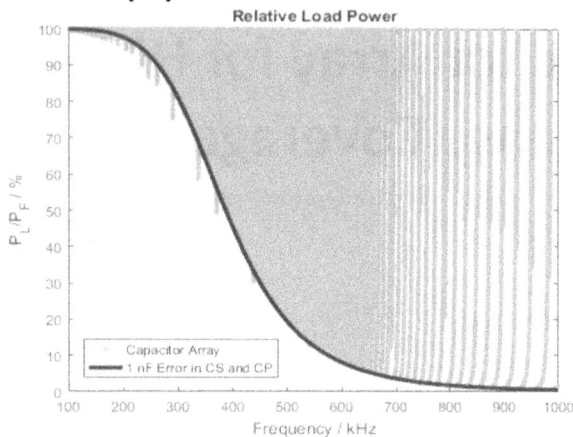

Figure 2: The relative load powers achieved for each matching frequency by the capacitor array are shown as light gray lines. Additionally, the dark curve shows the theoretical relative load power for ideal capacitance values provided with an absolute error of 1 nF in the series capacitor as well as the parallel capacitor of the impedance matching circuit.

For simplicity, the topology of the switched-capacitor array is restricted to parallel switched capacitors only. Therefore, the resulting capacitance can be easily calculated by the sum of single capacitances. However, each of the capacitors in the parallel strands has the value of an E-series capacitor mentioned in II.II and can be composed as a combination of parallel and series capacitors of the same capacitor model forming one *capacitor strand*, the capacitances resulting from this composition are therefore called *strand capacitances* C_{strand}. To determine the composition of each strand, one has to account for the current and voltage limits for each strand and the used capacitors, including a headroom for safety reasons. For further synthesis a catalogue of available capacitors has to be created, including the capacitances C_{comp}, the voltage limits u_{comp} and the current limits i_{comp} of the components. With the component properties and the calculated strand limits, n_p and n_s the minimum number of parallel and series capacitors for each capacitor strand can be calculated. However, due to this composition an effective capacitance C_{eff} forms. The array is finally synthesized by choosing the effective capacitances that are closest to the calculated strand capacitances and utilizes the least number of capacitors in a strand.

III. Results

The presented method has been applied for a system, which is supposed to work in the frequency range of 100 kHz – 1 MHz and utilizes a coil with an inductance of $L = 1.84\ \mu H$ and a dc resistance of $R_{DC} = 1.2\ m\Omega$. Both, the series as well as the parallel capacitor arrays, follow an E5-series ranging from 1 nF to 6.31 μF. The relative load power, defined as the load power P_L related to the forward power P_F of the amplifier, of the switched-capacitor impedance matching is chosen as a quality measure and is shown in Fig. 2. The maximum error is related to the choice of the lower bound of the E-series, which is 1 nF. The dark curve in Fig. 2 depicts the matching with ideal matching capacitances provided with a 1 nF error. A hull curve forms which covers the worst matched frequencies. To increase

the matching quality, the maximum allowable absolute error has to be discussed.

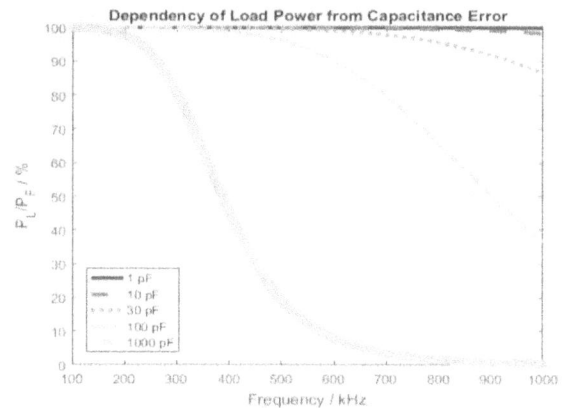

Figure 3 : The relative load power for ideal matching capacitances provided with 1 pF, 10 pF, 30 pF, 100 pF and 1 nF absolute error in the series capacitor as well as the parallel capacitor of the impedance matching are shown.

IV. Discussion

Fig. 3 shows multiple curves for the ideal values of the matching capacitors provided with 1 pF, 10 pF, 30 pF, 100 pF and 1 nF absolute error and their corresponding relative load powers. The curves indicate that an absolute error of 30 pF is acceptable. This can be achieved by either choosing a lower minimum capacitance of the E-series or by adding a motorized vacuum capacitor.

V. Conclusions

The proposed method has been validated computationally and gives a plausible solution. A discussion of possible matching improvements indicates that further components are necessary for good matching results. To ensure the suitability of this method a hardware implementation has to be realized and the results need to be compared to the calculated values.

ACKNOWLEDGEMENTS
We acknowledge the support of the Federal Ministry of Education and Research, Germany (BMBF) under the grant number 13GW0069A.

REFERENCES
[1]   Jordan A, Scholz R, Wust P, Fähling H, Felix R; J. Magn. Magn. Mater., 1999; 201:413-419.
[2]   Rose LC, Bear JC, Southern P, McNaughter PD, Piggott RB, Parkin IP, Qi S, Hills BP, Mayes AG; J. Mater. Chem. B 2016; 4:1704-1711.
[3]   Rosensweig RE; J. Magn. Magn. Mater. 2002; 252:370-374.
[4]   Hergt R, Andrä W, d'Ambly CG, Hilger I, Kaiser WA, Richter U, Schmidt HG.IEEE Trans. Magn. 1998; 34:3745-3754.
[5]   Garaio E, Collantes JM, Garcia JA, Plazaola F, Mornet S, Couillaud F, Sandre O. JMMM 2014; 368:432-437.
[6]   Carrey J, Mehdaoui B, Respaud M. J. Appl. Phys. 2011; 109:083921.
[7]   Behrends A, Graeser M, Buzug TM. Current Directions in Biomedical Engineering 2015; 1:249-253.
[8]   Kim J, Do-Hyeon K, Young-Jin P. IEEE Transactions on Industrial Electronics 2015; Vol. 62 No. 5:2807-2813.

Comparison of Extracellular and Intracellular Magnetic Hyperthermia Treatments Using Magnetic Particle Imaging

Kenya Murase*, Sayumi Kobayashi, Minori Tanoue, Yoshimi Inaoka, Akiko Ohki

Department of Medical Physics and Engineering, Graduate School of Medicine, Osaka University, Suita, Osaka, Japan
* Corresponding author, email: murase@sahs.med.osaka-u.ac.jp

I. Introduction

Magnetic hyperthermia treatment (MHT) is one of several hyperthermia treatments and utilizes the temperature rise of magnetic nanoparticles (MNPs) under an alternating magnetic field (AMF) [1]. MHT can selectively heat tumor cells without damaging normal tissues [1].

Recently, it has been reported that cell death by MNPs under AMF can occur without a noticeable global increase in temperature [2]. These results raised some debate in the literature, because it has been usually thought that it is necessary to achieve a homogeneous increase in temperature within the tumor for effective hyperthermia [2]. As a possible explanation for the above results, it has been hypothesized that even an increase in temperature localized in the vicinity of the MNPs could be enough to induce cell death without a significant global increase in temperature [2]. This study was undertaken to compare the therapeutic effect of extracellular MHT (Ex-MHT) and that of intracellular MHT (In-MHT) *in vivo* using tumor-bearing mice and to discuss the difference between them based on the temporal change of MNPs in the tumor measured using magnetic particle imaging (MPI) [3].

II. Material and Methods

II.I. Animal study

All animal studies were approved by the animal ethics committee at Osaka University School of Medicine. Seven-week-old male BALB/c mice weighing 24.3 ± 1.4 g (mean $\pm$ SD) were purchased. After one-week habituation to the rearing environment, 1×10^6 cells of colon-26 were implanted into the backs of the mice.

When the tumor volume reached approximately 100 mm³, the mice were divided into control (n=10), Ex-MHT (n=8), and In-MHT groups (n=7). In this study, we call the MHT performed immediately (15 min) and one day after the injection of MNPs "Ex-MHT" and "In-MHT", respectively. In the control group, MHT was not performed. The tumors in the Ex-MHT and In-MHT groups were directly injected with MNPs (Resovist®) (0.2 mL) with an iron concentration of 400 mM.

In the Ex-MHT group, MHT was started 15 min after the injection of MNPs and was performed by applying an AMF at a frequency of 600 kHz and a peak amplitude of 3.1 kA/m [1] for 20 min. During MHT, the temperatures of the tumor and rectum were measured in 3 mice using two fluorescence-type optical fiber thermometers. The MPI studies were performed using our MPI scanner [4] 13 min before MHT (2 min after the injection of MNPs), 22 min after MHT (37 min after the injection of MNPs), and 7 and 14 days after MHT. After the second MPI study (35 min after MHT), X-ray CT images were acquired using a 4-row multi-slice CT scanner with a tube voltage of 120 kV, a tube current of 210 mA, and a slice thickness of 0.5 mm. The X-ray CT images were also acquired 7 and 14 days after MHT. The MPI images were co-registered to the X-ray CT images for anatomical identification using the method reported in [1]. In the In-MHT group, MHT was performed one day after the injection of MNPs in the same manner as for the Ex-MHT group. The temperatures of the tumor and rectum were also measured during MHT in 4 mice. The MPI studies were performed 2 min after the injection of MNPs, 13 min before MHT, 22 min after MHT, and 7 and 14 days after MHT. The X-ray CT images were acquired 35 min, 7 days, and 14 days after MHT. After the MPI studies, we drew a region of interest (ROI) on the tumor in the MPI image and calculated the average MPI value within the ROI. In all groups, tumor volume was measured every day and the relative tumor volume growth (RTVG) was calculated [1].

II.II. Transmission electron microscopic study

For transmission electron microscopic (TEM) studies, tumor-bearing mice were sacrificed and the tumors were removed immediately (15 min) and one day after the injection of MNPs in the Ex-MHT (n=3) and In-MHT groups (n=4), respectively. The resected tumor tissues were fixed in 7.5% formaldehyde neutral buffered solution and TEM observation was performed under an electron microscope.

III. Results

The TEM studies showed that almost all the MNPs were aggregated in the extracellular space in the Ex-MHT group, whereas they were contained within the intracellular space in the In-MHT group. These results are consistent with the findings reported by Giustini et al. [5].

Fig. 1 shows the time courses of the temperature rise of the tumor, i.e., the temperature of the tumor minus that of the rectum, in the Ex-MHT (red circles, n=3) and In-MHT groups (blue circles, n=4). The temperature rise in the Ex-MHT group was significantly higher than that in the In-MHT group 30 s or more after the start of MHT.

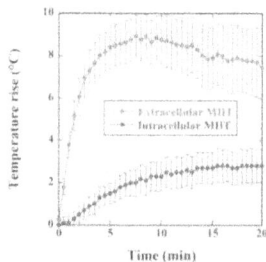

Figure 1: Time course of temperature rise.

Fig. 2 shows the temporal changes of the average MPI value within the ROI in the Ex-MHT (red bars, n=8) and In-MHT groups (blue bars, n=7). Note that the values immediately before MHT were normalized as unity. The normalized average MPI value in the In-MHT group was significantly higher than that in the Ex-MHT group immediately and 7 days after MHT.

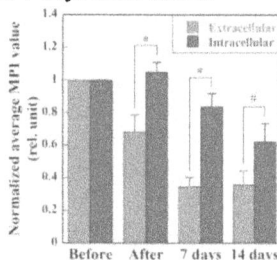

Figure 2: Comparison of normalized average MPI values.

Fig. 3 shows the time courses of the RTVG value in the Ex-MHT (red circles, n=8), In-MHT (blue circles, n=7), and control groups (black circles, n=10). The RTVG value in the Ex-MHT group was significantly lower than that in the control group 3 days or more after MHT. The RTVG value in the In-MHT group was significantly lower than that in the Ex-MHT group 3, 4, and 5 days after MHT.

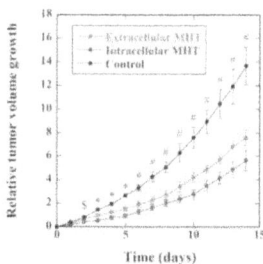

Figure 3: Time course of relative tumor volume growth.

IV. Discussion

Our results (Fig. 3) suggest that In-MHT is more cytotoxic than Ex-MHT in spite of the significantly lower temperature rise of the tumor (Fig. 1). Several hypotheses have been proposed to explain the cytotoxicity in the In-MHT. One of the leading hypotheses is based on recent experiments showing that the temperature rise is localized in the very close vicinity of the MNP surface. Riedinger et al. [2] experimentally demonstrated using a molecular temperature probe that the local temperature induced by AMF increased by several tens of degree at distances below 0.5 nm from the MNP surface and decayed exponentially with increasing distance. Furthermore, significant local-to-global temperature differences could be found at distances shorter than 3 nm [2]. This local heating could damage the surfaces of lysosomes where MNPs are stored and/or catalyze a chemical reaction in lysosomes such as the Fenton reaction. Our results suggest that the local temperature rise in cancer cells is more important rather than the global temperature rise for predicting the therapeutic effect of MHT and/or designing optimal treatment planning using MHT. In this respect, the present study offers important information regarding monitoring the temperature of the tumor during MHT.

As shown in Fig. 2, the normalized average MPI value in the In-MHT group was significantly higher than that in the Ex-MHT group immediately and 7 days after MHT. In addition, the temporal changes of the above parameter in the In-MHT group were smaller than those in the Ex-MHT group. As suggested by our TEM studies, this appears to be mainly due to the fact that once MNPs were internalized by tumor cells, their dispersion within the tumor and/or to the outside of the tumor is more likely to be reduced than that of the MNPs located outside the cells. This feature of the In-MHT would be useful especially when considering repeated applications of MHT.

V. Conclusions

Our results suggest that In-MHT is more cytotoxic than Ex-MHT in spite of the lower temperature rise of tumors, and that MPI is useful for evaluating the difference in temporal change of MNPs in the tumor between Ex-MHT and In-MHT.

ACKNOWLEDGEMENTS

This work was supported by JSPS KAKENHI Grant Numbers JP25282131 and JP15K12508.

REFERENCES

[1] K. Murase et al., Usefulness of magnetic particle imaging for predicting the therapeutic effect of magnetic hyperthermia, *Open J. Med. Imaging*, 5(2):85–99, 2015.

[2] A. Riedinger et al., Subnanometer local temperature probing and remotely controlled drug release based on azo-functionalized iron oxide nanoparticles, *Nano Lett*, 13: 2399-2406, 2013.

[3] B. Gleich and J. Weizenecker. Tomographic imaging using the nonlinear response of magnetic particles. *Nature*, 435(7046):1217-1217, 2005.

[4] K. Murase et al., Development of a System for Magnetic Particle Imaging Using Neodymium Magnets and Gradiometer. *Jpn J Appl Phys*, 53: 067001, 2014.

[5] A. J. Giustini et al. Magnetic nanoparticle biodistribution following intratumoral administration, *Nanotechnol*, 22: 345101, 2011.

Quantitative Assessment of Pulmonary Mucociliary Transport Using Magnetic Particle Imaging: Effect of Surface Potential of Magnetic Nanoparticles

Kohei Nishimoto, Satoshi Nagano, Kenya Murase*

Department of Medical Physics and Engineering, Graduate School of Medicine, Osaka University, Suita, Osaka, Japan
Corresponding author, email: murase@sahs.med.osaka-u.ac.jp

I. Introduction

Mucociliary transport (MCT) is an important defense mechanism for clearing the lung by removing inhaled aerocontaminants from airways [1]. The inhaled particles are trapped by mucus secreted from airway goblet cells and gland cells, and are transported from the peripheral lung via the airways and larynx into the gastrointestinal tract by ciliary beat [1].

Magnetically controlled drug delivery has been proposed, and is one of the most attractive therapeutic strategies for cancer and/or severe diseases, because this approach can enhance the efficacy of drugs and reduce the side effects [2]. When considering the application of magnetically controlled drug delivery to the lung, it is necessary to investigate the behavior of magnetic nanoparticles (MNPs) in the lung.

Magnetic particle imaging (MPI) is a new imaging method that was introduced in 2005 [3]. MPI utilizes the nonlinear response of MNPs to an alternating magnetic field, and can visualize the spatial distribution of MNPs in positive contrast and quantify the number of MNPs. It is expected that MPI can be used for long-term monitoring of MCT *in vivo*, because MPI uses insoluble MNPs as signal sources.

The purpose of this study was to develop a method for assessing the function of MCT using MPI and to investigate the effect of surface potential of MNPs on MCT.

II. Material and Methods

II.I. Magnetic nanoparticles

We used three kinds of MNPs with different surface potentials: carboxymethyl dextran magnetite (CMDM), alkalitreated dextran magnetite (ATDM), and trimethylammonium dextran magnetite (TMADM). Table 1 summarizes the mean diameters and zeta potentials of the three kinds of MNPs. The mean diameters of CMDM, ATDM, and TMADM were 50, 55, and 54 nm, respectively, whereas their zeta potentials were −24, −15, and +2 mV, respectively.

Table 1: Mean diameters and zeta potentials of three kinds of magnetic nanoparticles used in the present study (CMDM: carboxymethyl dextran magnetite, ATDM: alkalitreated dextran magnetite, and TMADM: trimethylammonium dextran magnetite).

	CMDM	ATDM	TMADM
Diameter (nm)	50	55	54
Zeta potential (mV)	−24	−15	+2

II.II. Animal study

All animal studies were approved by the animal ethics committee at Osaka University School of Medicine. Ten-week-old male ICR mice were divided into three groups (CMDM, ATDM, and TMADM). The mice in the CMDM (n=7), ATDM (n=6), and TMADM groups (n=7) were intratracheally administered with CMDM, ATDM, and TMADM, respectively, using a microsprayer [4]. The MPI studies were performed 30 min, 6 hours, 1 day, 3 days, and 7 days after the administration of the agents using our MPI scanner [5]. X-ray CT images were also acquired using a 4-row multi-slice CT scanner after the MPI studies and the MPI images were co-registered to the X-ray CT images for anatomical identification. After the MPI studies, we drew a region of interest (ROI) on the MPI image and calculated the average MPI value by taking the threshold value for extracting the lung as 30% of the maximum MPI value within the ROI (Fig. 1). We also calculated the retention fraction (RF) of the three kinds of MNPs in the lung by dividing the average MPI value by that in the first MPI study.

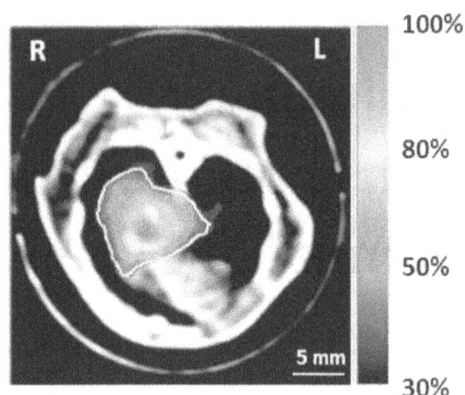

Figure 1: Example of the region of interest (ROI) drawn on an MPI image superimposed on an X-ray CT image.

III. Results

When using CMDM, the RF value in the lung (mean ± standard error) was 1.0, 0.82±0.03, 0.70±0.05, 0.44±0.04, and 0.32±0.05 at 30 min, 6 hours, 1 day, 3 days, and 7 days after the administration of CMDM, respectively. When using ATDM, the RF value was 1.0, 0.72±0.04, 0.55±0.04, 0.49±0.06, and 0.50±0.03 at 30 min, 6 hours, 1 day, 3 days, and 7 days after the administration of ATDM, respectively. When using TMADM, the RF value was 1.0, 0.92±0.07, 0.72±0.05, 0.67±0.05, and 0.67±0.05 at 30 min, 6 hours, 1 day, 3 days, and 7 days after the administration of TMADM, respectively. The RF value in the TMADM group was significantly ($p<0.05$) higher than that in the ATDM group at 6 hours and 7 days after the administration of the agents and tended to be higher than that in the ATDM group at 1 day ($p=0.077$) and 3 days ($p=0.053$). It was also significantly ($p<0.01$) higher than that in the CMDM group at 3 and 7 days. The RF value in the ATDM group was significantly ($p<0.05$) higher than that in the CMDM group at 7 days.

IV. Discussion

In the present study, we investigated the longitudinal change of the distribution of the MNPs given intratracheally into the lungs using MPI, and evaluated the effect of surface potential of MNPs on the MCT. We previously reported that there is an excellent linear correlation between the average MPI value and the iron concentration of Resovist® in phantom studies [6]. Based on these results, it appears that the change of the MPI value reflects that in the amount of MNPs per voxel and the change of the average MPI value reflects that in the amount of MNPs in the selected slice of the lung. Thus, our results suggest that MPI can evaluate the change of MNPs accumulated in the lung and that MPI is useful for visualizing the spatial distribution of MNPs and is applicable to quantitatively assessing the function of MCT.

We investigated the effect of the surface potential of MNPs on the MCT. For this purpose, we used three kinds of MNPs with different surface potentials, while we adjusted their diameters to be the same (approximately 50 nm) to minimize the size effect of MNPs (Table 1). As previously described, the MPI value tended to decrease with time in all groups, whereas the average MPI value in

the CMDM group did not show the rapid clearance during the first 6 hours. In contrast, the average MPI value in the TMADM group decreased slightly during the first 6 hours and remained almost constant up to 7 days. The RF value in the TMADM group was significantly higher ($p<0.05$) than that in the ATDM group at 6 hours and 7 days after the administration of the agents and tended to be higher than that in the ATDM group at 1 day ($p=0.077$) and 3 days ($p=0.053$). In addition, the RF value in the TMADM group was significantly higher ($p<0.05$) than that in the CMDM group at 3 and 7 days after the administration of the agents. Furthermore, the RF value in the ATDM group was significantly higher ($p<0.05$) than that in the CMDM group at 7 days. These results suggest that the difference in the clearance of MNPs observed in this study may be due to the difference in the surface potential of MNPs. Chen et al. reported that positively-charged nanoparticles (NPs) promoted to form the aggregation of mucin, thereby reducing the hydration and diffusivity of mucin [7]. In the present study, the retention of the positively-charged MNPs (ATDM) was higher than those of other negatively-charged MNPs. Thus, it appears that the higher retention of ATDM was mainly due to the reduction in the hydration and diffusivity of mucin, forming the MNPs-mucin gel complexes. In addition, Chen et al. also reported that negatively-charged (carboxyl-functional-ized) nanoparticles promote to disperse mucin gels by enhancing the network hydration [8]. Our results appear to support these reports. Thus, the observed differences in the retention among the MNPs with different surface potentials may be due to the fact that the surface potential of MNPs affects the formation of aggregated mucin and the hydration and dispersion of mucin.

V. Conclusions

Our results suggest that the surface potential of MNPs significantly affects MCT and that MPI is useful for quantitatively assessing the behavior of MNPs in the lung and factors affecting MCT.

ACKNOWLEDGEMENTS
This work was supported by JSPS KAKENHI Grant Numbers JP25282131 and JP15K12508.

REFERENCES
[1] M. B. Antunesa et al., Mucociliary clearance - a critical upper airway host defense mechanism and methods of assessment. *Current Opinion in Allergy and Clinical Immunology*, 7: 5–10, 2007.
[2] G. Mikhaylov et al., Ferri-liposomes as an MRI-visible drug-delivery system for targeting tumours and their microenvironment. *Nature Nanotechnol*, 6: 594-602, 2011.
[3] B. Gleich et al.. Tomographic imaging using the nonlinear response of magnetic particles. *Nature*, 435(7046):1217-1217, 2005.
[4] K. Nishimoto et al., Application of magnetic particle imaging using nebulized magnetic nanoparticles. *Open J Med Imaging*, 5: 49-55, 2015.
[5] K. Murase et al., Development of a system for magnetic particle imaging using neodymium magnets and gradiometer. *Jpn J Appl Phys*, 53: 067001, 2014.
[6] K. Murase et al., Usefulness of magnetic particle imaging for predicting the therapeutic effect of magnetic hyperthermia, *Open J Med Imaging*, 5(2):85–99, 2015.
[7] E. Chen et al., Functionalized positive nanoparticles reduce mucin swelling and dispersion, PLos One, 5: e15434, 2010.
[8] E. Chen et al., Functionalized carboxyl nanoparticles enhance mucus dispersion and hydration, *Scientific Reports*, 2: 211, 2012.

Session 11 - Talks

Applications III

Noninvasive Detection and Dynamic Quantification of Gastrointestinal Bleeding with Magnetic Particle Imaging

Elaine Y. Yu [a,+,*], Prashant Chandrasekharan [a,+], Ran Berzon [a], Zhi Wei Tay [a], Xinyi Y. Zhou [a],
Amit P. Khandhar [b], R. Matthew Ferguson [b], Scott J. Kemp [b], Bo Zheng [a], Patrick W. Goodwill [c],
Michael F. Wendland [a], Kannan M. Krishnan [b,d], Spencer Behr [e], Jonathan Carter [f],
Daniel W. Hensley [a], and Steven M. Conolly [a,g]

[a] Department of Bioengineering, University of California, Berkeley, California, USA
[b] Lodespin Labs, LLC., Seattle, Washington, USA
[c] Magnetic Insight, Inc., Alameda, California, USA
[d] Department of Material Science, University of Washington, Seattle, Washington, USA
[e] Department of Radiology and Biomedical Imaging, University of California San Francisco, California, USA
[f] University of California San Francisco Medical Center, California, USA
[g] Department of Electrical Engineering and Computer Sciences, University of California, Berkeley, California, USA

[+] These authors contributed equally to this work
[*] Corresponding author, email: elaineyu@berkeley.edu

I. Introduction

Gastrointestinal (GI) bleeding can occur spontaneously, after physical trauma or as a result of surgical complications, and are responsible for approximately 300,000 hospitalizations in the US [1]. Diagnostic techniques for GI bleeds rely on Nuclear Medicine (NM), CT Angiography (CTA) and MR Angiography (MRA). The NM technique to track red blood cells (RBCs) tagged with ^{99m}Tc is commonly the first test, because it is the most sensitive for detecting very slow bleeds. However, tradeoffs include radioactive dose to the patient, poor spatial resolution (~4 mm), bulky radio-pharmaceutical agent preparation and long scan times, which can delay surgical interventions. We present the use of Magnetic Particle Imaging (MPI) [2-5] to detect GI bleeding using long-circulating Superparamagnetic Iron Oxide nanoparticles (SPIO) as the vascular tracer agent. A mouse model of Familial Adenomatous Polyposis was used for this study, wherein polyps spontaneously develop with age, causing gastrointestinal bleeding.

II. Material and Methods

Five 12 week old C57BLK6/Apc$^{min/+}$ mice [6] with a genetic mutation in FAP (JAX® Laboratory) (Hct=0.21-0.30) [6] were used in this study. Three Wild-type C57BL/6 mice were used as control. SPIOs (LodeSpin-017, 5 mg Fe/kg in 100 μL) and heparin were injected through a lateral tail vein catheter for each animal. MPI was performed with a custom-built vertical bore field-free line (FFL) MPI scanner with a gradient strength of 6.3 T/m.

Twenty-one dynamic projection MPI scans were acquired with respiratory gating over 130 minutes. Region-Of-Interest based compartment fitting was performed after converting the MPI signal to iron concentration for flow quantification.

III. Results

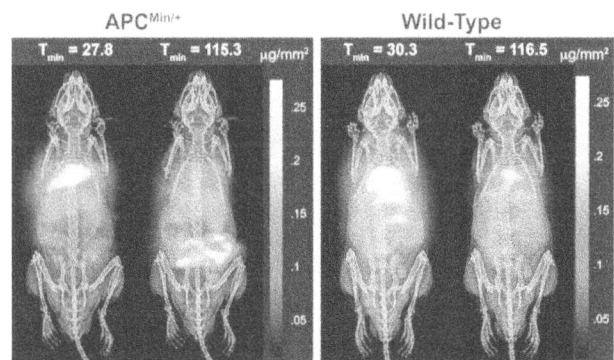

Figure 1 Representative MPI images with CT overlay of an Apc$^{Min/+}$ (left) and Wild-Type (right) mouse over time. MPI clearly captures dynamics of tracer extravasation into the gut in the Apc$^{Min/+}$ mouse, whereas no tracer extravasation into the gut is seen in the Wild-Type mouse.

2D MPI projection images of C57BLK6 and Apc$^{min/+}$ mice 30 min and 115 minutes post-SPIO injection are shown in Fig. 1. MPI signal was observed to accumulate in the gut lumen of the FAP model, whereas the wild type showed signal throughout the vascular compartment, typical of LS-017 (a blood pool tracer). In Fig. 2, the MPI image at the first time point was digitally subtracted from all images in time course with negative values set to zero to capture positive tracer accumulation. The GI bleed is visualized with extraordinary contrast in the Apc$^{min/+}$ mice, whereas minimal positive accumulation is observed in the control mice.

The tracer accumulation of the gut lumen of the Apc$^{Min/+}$ mice was linear with time with flow rates between $1-5$ µL/min. A representative two-compartment model fitting result is shown in Fig. 3.

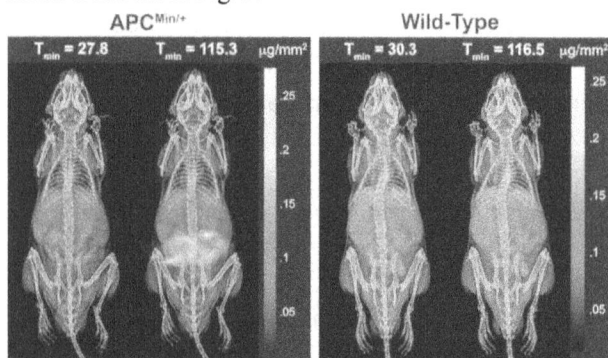

Figure 2 *Representative subtracted images of an Apc$^{Min/+}$ mouse (left) and a wild-type mouse over time. The GI bleed is visualized with extraordinary contrast in the Apc$^{Min/+}$ mouse, whereas for the Wild-Type mouse, the tracer was predominantly in the blood pool throughout the study and had no GI bleed, hence no subtracted signal was observed after subtraction.*

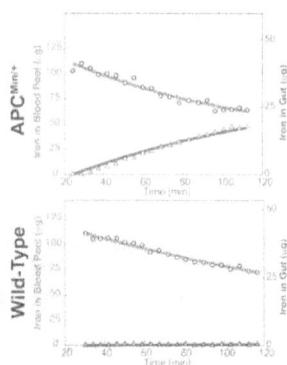

Figure 3 *Representative Non-linear least square fit results for Apc$^{Min/+}$ (top) mice and (d) wild-type mice. Axes: iron in blood on the left and iron in gut lumen on the right.*

IV. Discussion

Currently, ^{99m}Tc-labelled RBC is the most sensitive technique for detection of active bleeds over a long period of time [7]. In this work, we were able to detect GI bleeding using MPI at a sensitivity rivaling that of nuclear medicine techniques at clinically relevant doses, but by using a blood-pool, non-radioactive SPIO tracer [8]. Additional sensitivity improvement is possible through tracer and receive hardware optimization [9,10]. Since MPI is linearly quantitative throughout the body, we were able to quantify the bleed rate, and clearly visualize tracer dynamics over time. In addition, we have demonstrated that digital subtraction of baseline images from the rest of the images in the time course can dramatically improve image contrast.

V. Conclusions

In this work, we have demonstrated highly sensitive detection of GI bleeding in a murine model using MPI. Although there is still a long path to clinical translation for MPI tracers and imager, MPI is a clinically translatable imaging modality with superb contrast, sensitivity, linear quantitation and safety. We believe that in the future, MPI could complement the current clinical workflow for cases of occult or obscure GI bleeding. This may significantly improve the accuracy of diagnosis and ultimately reduce cost and improve outcome.

ACKNOWLEDGEMENTS

The authors would like to acknowledge funding support from NIH 5R01EB019458-03, NIH 5R24MH106053-03, UC Discovery Grant 29623, W. M. Keck Foundation Grant 009323, and NSF GRFP for this work. Additionally, work at Lodespin Labs and University of Washington was supported by NIH 1R41EB013520-01 and NIH 2R42EB013520-02A1.

REFERENCES

[1] B. S. M. Kim, B. T. Li, A. Engel, J. S. Samra, S. Clarke, I. D. Norton and A. E. Li, World Journal of Gastrointestinal Pathophysiology, vol. 5, pp. 467, 2014. doi: 10.4291/wjgp.v5.i4.467

[2] B. Gleich and J. Weizenecker. Tomographic imaging using the nonlinear response of magnetic particles. *Nature*, 435(7046):1217-1217, 2005. doi: 10.1038/nature03808

[3] T. Knopp and T. M. Buzug. *Magnetic Particle Imaging: An Introduction to Imaging Principles and Scanner Instrumentation.* Springer, Berlin/Heidelberg, 2012. doi: 10.1007/978-3-642-04199-0

[4] Goodwill, P. W. & Conolly, S. M. The X-space formulation of the magnetic particle imaging process: 1-D signal, resolution, bandwidth, SNR, SAR, and magnetostimulation. *IEEE Trans. Med. Imaging* 29, 1851–1859, 2010. doi: 10.1109/TMI.2010.2052284.

[5] Goodwill, P. W., Konkle, J. J., Zheng, B., Saritas, E. U. & Conolly, S. M. Projection x-space magnetic particle imaging. *IEEE Trans. Med. Imaging* 31, 1076–1085, 2012. doi: 10.1109/TMI.2012.2185247

[6] Wei, H., Shang, J., Keohane, C., Wang, M., Li, Q., Ni, W., O'Neill, K. & Chintala, M. A novel approach to assess the spontaneous gastrointestinal bleeding risk of antithrombotic agents using Apc(min/+) mice. *Thromb. Haemost.* 111, 1121–1132, 2014. doi: 10.1160/TH13-11-0926

[7] Graça, B. M., Freire, P. A., Brito, J. B., Ilharco, J. M., Carvalheiro, V. M. & Caseiro-Alves, F. Gastroenterologic and radiologic approach to obscure gastrointestinal bleeding: how, why, and when? *Radiographics* 30, 235–252, 2010. doi: 10.1148/rg.301095091

[8] Yu, E. Y., Chandrasekharan, P., Berzon, R., Tay, Z., Zhou, X. Y., Khandhar, A. P., Ferguson, R. M., Kemp, S. J., Zheng, B., Goodwill, P. W., Wendland, M. F., Krishnan, K. M., Behr, S., Carter, J., and Conolly, S. M. Magnetic Particle Imaging for Highly Sensitive, Quantitative, and Safe *in vivo* Gut Bleed Detection in a Murine Model. ACS Nano 2017. doi:10.1021/acsnano.7b04844

[9] Ferguson, R. M., Minard, K. R., Khandhar, A. P. & Krishnan, K. M. Optimizing magnetite nanoparticles for mass sensitivity in magnetic particle imaging. *Med. Phys.* 38, 1619–1626, 2011. doi: 10.1118/1.3554646

[10] Zheng, B., Goodwill, P. W., Dixit, N., Xiao, D., Zhang, W., Gunel, B., Lu, K., Scott, G. C. & Conolly, S. M. Optimal Broadband Noise Matching to Inductive Sensors: Application to Magnetic Particle Imaging. *IEEE Trans. Biomed. Circuits Syst.* (2017). doi: 10.1109/TBCAS.2017.2712566

Optimization of Tri-Modal Imaging Protocol for Comparison of Various SPIO Nanoparticles: Initial Approach Based on Subcutaneous Application in Mice

Pavla Francová [a,*], Kateřina Poláková [b], Aristides Bakandritsos [b], Kevin Jia-Jin Loo[c], Viktor Sýkora [a], Luděk Šefc [a]

[a] Center for Advanced Preclinical Imaging, 1st Medical Faculty, Charles University, Prague, Czech Republic
[b] Regional Centre of Advanced Technologies and Materials,Palacký University, Olomouc, Czech Republic
[c] Department of Biomathematics,Institute of Physiology, The Czech Academy of Sciences, Prague, Czech Republic
[*] Corresponding author, email: pavla.francova@lf1.cuni.cz

I. Introduction

Magnetic particle imaging (MPI) is a new functional imaging modality requiring co-registration with anatomical information for *in vivo* imaging. In this study, we propose using MPI in co-registration with magnetic resonance imaging (MRI) and computed tomography (CT). We developed and optimized a tri-modal MPI-MRI-CT imaging protocol to obtain datasets for 2D and 3D visualization of the MagAlg [1] SPIO nanoparticles in comparison with the MPI gold standard Resovist (ferucarbotran).

The goal of this study was to establish a workflow [2] between MPI, MRI and CT preclinical scanners for whole-body mouse *in vivo* examination to generate the first co-registered *in vivo* MPI-MRI-CT images, and finally to optimize *in vivo* comparison of the contrast agents.

II. Material and Methods

The prepared MagAlg SPIO nanoparticles were synthesized as condensed clustered colloids through a soft biomineralization process in the presence of a biopolymer alginate. The product was purified from by-products and fractionated. A detailed description of the synthesis and characterization of MagAlg SPIO nanoparticles can be found in previous work [1.3].

In vivo measurements were performed with the preclinical imaging systems MPI, 1 Tesla MRI ICON, and Albira CT (-PET/SPECT), all from Bruker BioSpin, Germany.

Prior to the animal imaging protocol, both variations of the MPI system functions - for samples and *in vivo* measurements - were performed for each kind of SPIO particle.

The tri-modal *in vivo* imaging protocol included pre-contrast and post-contrast measurements with MRI and CT scanners and post-contrast measurements on MPI on a group of healthy mice in anaesthesia (1.5-2% isoflurane) with total duration of 90 min. MRI and CT measurements were used for anatomical reference and validation of the subcutaneous locations of the applied superparamagnetic iron oxide (SPIO) particles. Position markers were placed on the dedicated multimodal bed (Bruker, Germany), and optimized for all modalities.

Obtained datasets were co-registered using P-MOD (PMOD Technologies, Germany) and MATLAB (MathWorks, USA) to obtain 2D and 3D visualizations of the contrast agents in the tissue.

III. Results

A workflow process for combined MPI-MRI-CT examination was established. Subcutaneous locations of SPIO particles (Resovist, MagAlg nanoparticles) were evaluated in both MPI and MRI modalities while neither one of used contrast agents is visible on CT.

The best fitting MPI evaluation parameters of both contrast agents were defined, and realized in-vitro MPI measurements were evaluated with both described set of parameters. Cross-reference of their results is taken as the main comparison parameter of the quality of the contrast agent in MPI.

In vivo MPI measurement were evaluated with the both sets of evaluation parameters, described on MPI sample measurements, and fused with MRI and CT datasets for 2D and 3D visualization. New contrast agent MagAlg proved to be feasible for MPI *in vivo* imaging when compared to Resovist.

IV. Discussion

Several challenges were observed during tri-modal imaging protocol implementation. Some of most important questions we focused on include:

The MPI system function's resolution versus duration; MPI measurement and evaluation of different parameter settings for widely applicable protocols useful for different contrast agents; location of position markers inside the FOV for multimodal *in vivo* measurements; and parameters for comparison of different contrast agents.

Choice of proper background modality for MPI – MRI or CT – always depends on the goals of chosen project. CT provides easy 3D visualization, short measurement time and no artefacts due to presence of SPIO particles as in MRI. MRI faces more challenged due to interactions of contrast media with the magnetic field but provides better resolution of the targeted tissue.

V. Conclusions

The acquisition of *in vivo* preclinical MPI-MRI-CT data is feasible and allows the combined analysis of MPI-MRI-CT information and comparison of both SPIO contrast agents.

Discussed MRI-MPI-CT protocol could be further used for other subcutaneous applications – like tumour imaging or (e.g. polymeric or gel-like) implant visualization.

ACKNOWLEDGEMENTS

This project was realized with the financial support of SVV 260371/2017, MEYS CR (LM2015062 Czech-BioImaging) and MŠMT NPU I LO1305.

REFERENCES

[1] G.Zoppellaro et.al. *Theranostics of Epitaxially Condensed Colloidal Nanocrystal Clusters, through a Soft Biomineralization Route.* Chemistry of Materials 2014; 26: 2062-2074. DOI: 10.1021/cm404053v

[2] M.G. Kaul, O. Weber, U. Heinen, A. Reitmeier, T. Mummert, C. Jung, N. Raabe, T. Knopp, H. Ittrich, G. Adam. *Combined Preclinical Magnetic Particle Imaging and Magnetic Resonance Imaging: Initial Results in Mice.* Fortschr Röntgenstr 2015; 187(05): 347-352. DOI: 10.1055/s-0034-1399344

[3] K.Tomankova et.al. *In vitro cytotoxicity analysis of doxorubicin-loaded/superparamagnetic iron oxide colloidal nanoassemblies on MCF7 and NIH3T3 cell lines.* Int J Nanomedicine 2015; 10: 949-961. DOI: 10.2147/IJN.S72590

First Temperature Measurements of Endovascular Stents in MPI

Franz Wegner [a,*], Thomas Friedrich [b], Nikolaos Panagiotopoulos [a], Sarah Valmaa [a], Jan P. Goltz [a], Florian M. Vogt [a], Martin A. Koch [b], Thorsten M. Buzug [b], Jörg Barkhausen [a], Julian Hägele [a,c]

[a] Department of Radiology and Nuclear Medicine, University Hospital Schleswig-Holstein, Lübeck, Germany
[b] Institute of Medical Engineering, University of Lübeck, Lübeck, Germany
[c] Zentrum für Radiologie und Nuklearmedizin, Korschenbroich, Germany
* Corresponding author, email: franz.wegner@uksh.de

I. Introduction

Stents are medical devices which are implanted into tubular structures (e.g. vessels, esophagus, bronchus) to keep passageways open. In clinical routine the implantation into vessels is visualized with x-ray based Digital Subtraction Angiography (DSA). With its high spatial and temporal resolution, the lack of ionizing radiation and kidney safe tracers MPI could be a valuable alternative for DSA for monitoring vascular interventions in the future.

In the therapy of arterial occlusive disease, there is an re-occlusion rate of up to 10% after dilation and stent implantation of stenosis and occlusions, even when very effective drug eluting stents are used [1]. Consequently, there is the need for a noninvasive imaging method to assess the patency of the stent after implantation. Imaging of stents with CT and MRI is limited by several artifacts which can artificially narrow the stent lumen on the images [2], [3]. It has to be evaluated, if MPI as a tracer based method can overcome these disadvantages and visualize the lumen of the stent to assess the patency reliable. In recent years there were several studies investigating the potential of MPI for vascular imaging and interventions [4]–[8], but none addressing MPI in the presence of endovascular stents. However, one study addressed heating of guidewires and catheters as a possible safety issue in MPI [9]. The purpose of this study was to evaluate the heating behavior of endovascular stents as a safety aspect for usage in MPI.

II. Material and Methods

Twenty-one commercially available endovascular stents of different sizes (diameter: 3, 3.5, 4, 5, 6, 7, 8, 10 mm, length: 11 – 99 mm) and materials (Stainless Steel, Nitinol=Nickel-Titanium, Platinum-Chromium, Cobalt-Chromium) were evaluated (Fig. 1). They were implanted into silicone tubes matching the stent diameter and placed into the center of the bore along the x-axis of a preclinical MPI-scanner (Bruker-Biospin, Ettlingen, Germany). The selection field gradient was 1.25 T/m in x- and y-direction and 2.5 T/m in z-direction. The excitation field strength was 12 mT in each direction. The excitation field frequencies were 24.5 kHz, 26.0 kHz, and 25.3 kHz in x-, y-, and z-direction, respectively. The duration of one excitation field cycle was 21.54 ms, amounting to a frequency of 46 images per second. Scans were performed with 20.000 repetitions (= total scan duration of 430.85 s). The hotspot of the stents was detected by thermography and the temperature change was measured with fiber optic-thermometers. One probe was directly placed at a stent strut at the hotspot of the stent with a balloon catheter. A second probe was placed at the bottom of the insert as a reference.

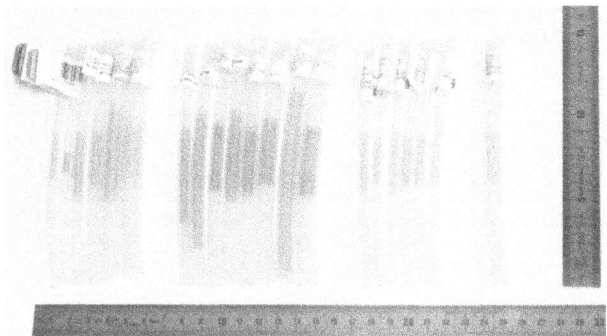

Figure 1: *Overview of the stents implanted in silicone tubes.*

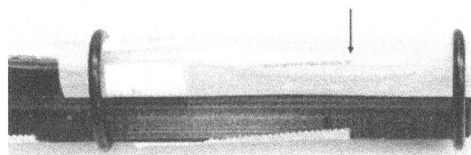

Figure 2: *The temperature probe is placed directly at a stent strut (pointer) with a balloon catheter at the hotspot of each stent.*

III. Results

An increase of temperature of 0.1 K (absolute accuracy of the temperature measurement) or more in relation to the reference temperature was defined as heating of the material. Nine stents showed no heating. Twelve stents showed heating of at least 0.1 K or more. Five stents showed heating of more than 3.0 K. The biggest temperature difference was 12.4 K (Table 1). The only significant predictor for the heating behavior of the stents was their diameter. Pearons's correlation coefficient depicted this dependency with a value r = 0.96. The length (r = 0.14) and the material had no measurable effect on the heating of the stents.

Table 1: *Detailed information of the stents: Stent Type, Material (316L=Stainless Steel, Nitinol, PtCr=Platinum-Chromium, CoCr=Cobald-Chromium), Diameter (Ø)/Length, measured temperature change (ΔT). Stents with a dual component stentdesign are marked with an asterisk (*).*

Stent Type	Material	Ø/Length (mm)	ΔT (K)
Biosensors, Biomatrix Neoflex	316 L	3/28	<0.1
Biosensors, Bio Freedom	316 L	3.5/11	<0.1
Boston Scientific, Taxus Liberté	316 L	4/38	0.2
Boston Scientific, Taxus Liberté	316 L	5/32	0.5
Boston Scientific, Express LD	316 L	7/57	5.6
Boston Scientific, Express LD	316 L	10/37	12.4
IDEV, Supera	Nitinol	4/40	1.0
IDEV, Supera	Nitinol	5/60	1.6
Gore, Tigris	Nitinol*	5/40	<0.1
IDEV, Supera	Nitinol	6/40	3.7
Gore, Tigris	Nitinol*	6/40	<0.1
Gore, Tigris	Nitinol*	7/40	0.1
Boston Scientific, Epic	Nitinol	7/99	3.3
Gore, Tigris	Nitinol*	8/40	<0.1
Boston Scientific, Promus Element	PtCr	3/32	<0.1
Boston Scientific, Promus Premier	PtCr	3/28	<0.1
Boston Scientific, Synergy	PtCr	3/38	<0.1
Boston Scientific, Promus Element	PtCr	4/28	<0.1
Boston Scientific, Promus Premier	PtCr	4/28	0.1
Boston Scientific, Rebel	PtCr	4/28	0.1
Boston Scientific, Carotid Wallstent	CoCr	7/30	3.6

IV. Discussion

This is the first study investigating the heating behavior of stents in MPI. The stent diameter was identified as the most influencing parameter concerning heating. This seems to be caused by orientation changes of the magnetic domains of the ferromagnetic stent material and eddy currents induced by the oscillating magnetic fields of the MPI scanner. This assumption was partially confirmed by a dual component stent design combining conductive and nonconductive material in the Tigris stents which prevented heating. All investigated stents were surrounded by air as an effective isolator and the magnetic fields were applied constantly for a duration of 431 seconds. Thus, this study is a worst case study. If the increase of temperature of stents with a larger diameter is still measureable under flow-conditions and thus relevant *in vivo* has to be further evaluated.

V. Conclusions

In principle, the safe use of endovascular stents in MPI concerning heating is possible as most of the stents showed no or mild increase of temperature. Commonly implanted coronary stents have diameters between 3 and 4 mm. Thus, especially cardiovascular imaging and coronary stent implantation with MPI seems to be safe.

REFERENCES

[1] J. W. Moses *et al.*, 'Sirolimus-eluting stents versus standard stents in patients with stenosis in a native coronary artery', *N. Engl. J. Med.*, vol. 349, no. 14, pp. 1315–1323, Oct. 2003. doi: 10.1056/NEJMoa035071.

[2] F. André *et al.*, 'In-vitro assessment of coronary artery stents in 256-multislice computed tomography angiography', *BMC Res. Notes*, vol. 7, no. 1, p. 38, 2014. doi: 10.1186/1756-0500-7-38.

[3] M. C. Burg *et al.*, 'MR Angiography of Peripheral Arterial Stents: In Vitro Evaluation of 22 Different Stent Types', *Radiol. Res. Pract.*, vol. 2011, 2011. doi: 10.1155/2011/478175.

[4] J. Salamon *et al.*, 'Magnetic Particle / Magnetic Resonance Imaging: In-Vitro MPI-Guided Real Time Catheter Tracking and 4D Angioplasty Using a Road Map and Blood Pool Tracer Approach', *PloS One*, vol. 11, no. 6, p. e0156899, 2016. doi: 10.1371/journal.pone.0156899.

[5] J. Haegele *et al.*, 'Magnetic particle imaging: visualization of instruments for cardiovascular intervention', *Radiology*, vol. 265, no. 3, pp. 933–938, Dec. 2012. doi: 10.1148/radiol.12120424.

[6] J. Haegele *et al.*, 'Magnetic Particle Imaging: A Resovist based Marking Technology for Guide Wires and Catheters for Vascular Interventions', *IEEE Trans. Med. Imaging*, Apr. 2016. doi: 10.1109/TMI.2016.2559538.

[7] J. Haegele *et al.*, 'Multi-color magnetic particle imaging for cardiovascular interventions', *Phys. Med. Biol.*, vol. 61, no. 16, pp. N415-426, Aug. 2016. doi: 10.1088/0031-9155/61/16/N415.

[8] J. Haegele *et al.*, 'Toward cardiovascular interventions guided by magnetic particle imaging: first instrument characterization', *Magn. Reson. Med.*, vol. 69, no. 6, pp. 1761–1767, Jun. 2013. doi: 10.1002/mrm.24421.

[9] R. L. Duschka *et al.*, 'Safety measurements for heating of instruments for cardiovascular interventions in magnetic particle imaging (MPI) - first experiences', *J. Healthc. Eng.*, vol. 5, no. 1, pp. 79–93, 2014. doi: 10.1260/2040-2295.5.1.79.

Exploiting Magnetic Relaxation in Magnetic Particle Imaging: First In Vivo Color MPI Results

Daniel Hensley [a,b*], **Zhi Wei Tay** [a], **Xinyi Y Zhou** [a], **Prashant Chandrasekharan** [a], **Bo Zheng** [a], **Patrick Goodwill** [b], **Steven Conolly** [a,c]

[a] *Department of Bioengineering, University of California, Berkeley, Berkeley, USA*
[b] *Magnetic Insight, Inc., Alameda, USA*
[c] *Department of Electrical Engineering and Computer Sciences, University of California, Berkeley, Berkeley, USA*
* *Corresponding author, email: dwhensley@berkeley.edu*

I. Introduction

Reporting physiologic contrast is of great interest to magnetic particle imaging (MPI) [1, 2], especially as the field explores new molecular imaging applications. One avenue to such contrast is through the rich dynamic magnetic physics (relaxation) of the tracers used in MPI [3]. Research has shown that magnetic relaxation can be used in sensing and imaging temperature [4], discriminating between different tracers [5,6], and quantifying micro-environmental conditions such as viscosity and pH [7]. A canonical way of reporting such information is via color images [5,6]. Here we show the first *in vivo* color MPI results.

II. Material and Methods

We have developed a custom colorizing algorithm depicted in Fig. 1. that aims to identify and disambiguate multiple tracers based on relaxation differences.

As shown in Fig. 1, we first take several consecutive MPI scans with different excitation amplitudes, reconstruct each with our standard x-space methods, and then produce our colorized image by solving a pixel-wise inverse problem in the reconstructed image domain. The forward model expresses a known or expected relaxation behavior across the excitation amplitude dimension, and in this work, contains information about how two tracer species behave differently, allowing us to implement a two-compartment fit. The forward model may be calibrated independently with known samples or per scan by including reference markers.

We first tested our approach with a calibration phantom: three vials containing 50 ul of 25 mg/ml tracer. One vial contains only Chemicell tracer (chemicell GmbH, Berlin, Germany), the other only nanomag MIP tracer (micromod Partikeltechnologie GmbH, Rostock, Germany), and the third contains a 50/50 mixture by volume.

We tested our approach *in vivo* by administering 0.229 mg of Chemicell tracer to a 0.2 kg female Fisher rat via tail vein injection followed by a second injection of 875,000 (0.08 mg Fe) macroaggregated albumin-tracer conjugates (MAA-perimag) derived from the Perimag (micromod Partikeltechnologie GmbH, Rostock, Germany) tracer as described in Zhou et al [8]. In this model, the Chemicell tracer immediately clears to the liver while the MAA-perimag initially gets stuck in the lungs before slowly clearing to the liver. In the initial period, we test our color algorithm's ability to disambiguate the liver and lungs that are tagged by the two different MPI tracers.

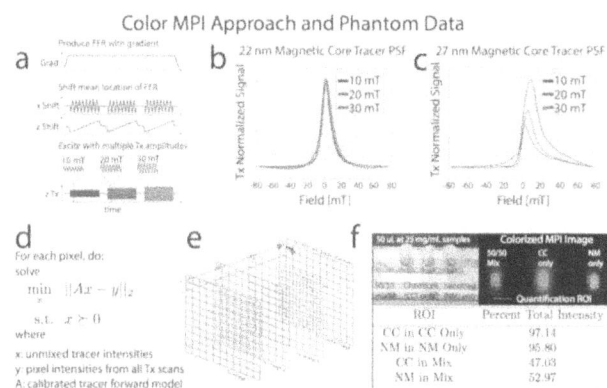

Figure 1: The x-space color MPI approach used in this work (a) Multiple x-space acquisitions are taken, each with a different excitation amplitude. (b,c) Tracers exhibit different relaxation-mediated changes to their PSF as a function of excitation amplitude per their relaxation properties. (d,e) We can use this as a basis to encode relaxation properties in MPI. Colorized images are produced by solving a pixel-wise inverse problem. (f) Initial vial phantom data and ROI quantification to test performance, especially unmixing of co-localized tracer.

Two reference markers (2 ul each) corresponding to the two tracers (Chemicell at 4.16 mg/mL and MAA-perimag at 0.67 mg/mL) were placed in the field of view (FOV) above the rat's chest. The rat was then scanned at four excitation amplitudes of 10, 15, 17.5, and 20 mT using our in house 7 T/m MPI field-free point (FFP) scanner [9] (4 x

3.75 x 10 cm FOV, approximately 10 min per scan, with respiratory gating). X-ray imaging was performed with a Kubtec Xpert 40. Our color algorithm was applied to the entire 3D data sets, providing 3D color MPI results.

III. Results

Fig. 1 (f) shows imaging results and ROI quantification of our color algorithm's performance when applied to the triple-vial phantom. Fig. 2 (a), shows MPI coronal slices from an *in vivo* experiment, including a standard x-space MPI image, separate MAA-perimag (Tracer 1) and Chemicell (Tracer 2) images provides by the color algorithm, and combined colorized images overlaid with an X-ray reference. Fig. 2 (b—e) show different slices of the 3D colorized data set, further demonstrating the ability of the algorithm to parse the lungs and liver, each tagged with a different tracer.

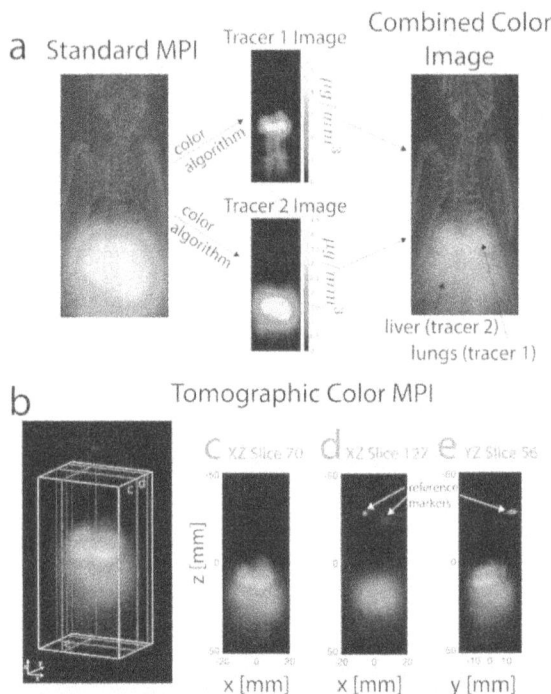

Figure 2: *In vivo color MPI results. (a) Coronal MPI image slice data from our standard x-space reconstruction and color algorithm. Separate MAA-perimag (Tracer 1) and Chemicell (Tracer 2) images are shown, disambiguating the lungs from the liver, along with a combined colorized image overlaid with a reference X-ray image. (b—e) Color MPI images from different slices show the fully 3D/tomographic application of the color algorithm and further demonstrate the separation of the lungs from the liver, which is not possible in the standard MPI images.*

IV. Discussion

The ROI quantification shown in Fig. 1 (f) indicates that our algorithm is able to identify and disambiguate co-localized tracers, and the data shown in Fig. 2 is the first demonstration of color MPI *in vivo*. We see that the color MPI algorithm successfully parses the MAA-perimag tracer in the lungs from the Chemicell tracer in the liver, converting a standard MPI image with no discernible distinction between the lungs and liver into a colorized image with clear distinction between these organs.

There are many ways to improve on the approach taken in this proof-of-concept work. For example, more sophisticated formulations that include other *a priori* information and global constraints would likely benefit the work described here. More generally, pushing the algorithm back to operate with time- or harmonic-domain data should provide better and more direct access to relaxation information. Leveraging different excitation techniques, such as recently described pulsed MPI methods [7], can fundamentally improve the quality and separability of relaxation information. This would greatly improve the posedness and possibilities associated with color algorithms. We also note that for some applications, directly reporting the continuous measure of relaxation, as opposed to carrying through a compartmental fit, will be more desirable.

V. Conclusions

We have reported the first proof-of-concept *in vivo* color MPI results. These data, together with the many other recent relaxation-based MPI demonstrations, are making clear that the rich relaxation physics of MPI tracers can enable new molecular imaging applications. More fully exploiting these physics will require improvements in multiple areas, such as tailored tracer design, how we encode relaxation information in MPI scans, and how we formulate reconstruction algorithms. In the long term, these color MPI methods may enable new applications such as monitoring of labeled cell metabolism, targeted binding contrast, and reporting local micro-environmental conditions in an imaging format.

ACKNOWLEDGEMENTS

We would like to acknowledge funding support from NIH 5R01EB019458-03, NIH 5R24MH106053-03, UC Discovery Grant 29623, W. M. Keck Foundation Grant 009323, and NSF GRFP.

REFERENCES

[1] B. Gleich and J. Weizenecker. Tomographic imaging using the nonlinear response of magnetic particles. *Nature*, 435(7046):1214-1217, 2005. doi: 10.1038/nature03808.

[2] P.W. Goodwill and S. M. Conolly. The X-space formulation of the magnetic particle imaging process: 1-D signal, resolution, bandwidth, SNR, SAR, and magnetostimulation. *IEEE transactions on medical imaging*, 29.11: 1851–1859, 2010.

[3] L. R. Croft, et al. Low drive field amplitude for improved image resolution in magnetic particle imaging. *Medical* physics, 43.1: 424–435, 2016.

[4] C. Stehning, B. Gleich, and J. Rahmer. Simultaneous magnetic particle imaging (MPI) and temperature mapping using multi-color MPI. *International Journal on Magnetic Particle Imaging* 2.2, 2016.

[5] J. Rahmer, A. Halkola, B. Gleich, I. Schmale, and J. Borgert. First experimental evidence of the feasibility of multi-color magnetic particle imaging. *Physics in medicine and biology*, 60(5), 1775, 2015.

[6] D. Hensley, P. Goodwill, L. Croft, and S. Conolly. Preliminary experimental x-space color MPI. *Magnetic particle imaging (IWMPI), 2015 5th international workshop on*, 2015.

[7] D. Hensley et al., Quantitative Magnetic Relaxation Mapping in Magnetic Particle Imaging using Pulsed Excitation Waveforms. *World Molecular Imaging Congress conference*, 2017.

[8] X.Y. Zhou, et al. First in vivo magnetic particle imaging of lung perfusion in rats. *Physics in Medicine and Biology*, 62(9), 3510, 2017.

[9] P. Goodwill, K. Lu, B. Zheng, and S. Conolly An x-space magnetic particle imaging scanner. *Review of Scientific Instruments*, 83(3), 033708, 2012.

Visualization of Spatial and Temporal Temperature Distributions in a Liver Tumor Ablation Model Using Magnetic Particle Imaging

Johannes Salamon [a,*], Jan Dieckhoff [a], Caroline Jung [a], Martin Möddel [b,c],
Michael Gerhard Kaul [a], Lukas Späth [a], Gerhard Adam [a], Tobias Knopp [a,b,c], Harald Ittrich [a]

[a]*Department of Diagnostic and Interventional Radiology and Nuclear Medicine, University Medical Center Hamburg-Eppendorf, Hamburg, Germany*
[b]*Section for Biomedical Imaging, University Medical Center Hamburg-Eppendorf, Hamburg, Germany*
[c]*Institute for Biomedical Imaging, Hamburg University of Technology (TUHH), Hamburg, Germany*
[*] *Corresponding author, email: j.salamon@uke.de*

I. Introduction

Thermal ablation especially of tumors, especially liver neoplasia has become an important minimal invasive treatment alternative to traditionally applied therapies, e. g., chemo-, radiation therapy or surgical resection, especially if surgery is associated with a higher risk of complications [1]. Ultrasound, computed tomography and MRI are clinically used for guidance of tumor ablations, but only MRI facilitates a simultaneous temperature measurement of the tumor and the surrounding tissue improving safety and success of the therapy [2].

The particles used as tracer in MPI are taken up by the mononuclear phagocytic system of the liver, enabling direct visualizations of healthy liver tissue [3]. Liver tumors like hepatocellular carcinomas or metastases with lacking accumulation of SPIONs [4] enable indirect tumor imaging [5]. Stehning, Gleich, and Rahmer estimated a temperature measurement precision of ± 0.5°C using a multi-color approach [6]. The main challenge of thermal tumor ablation represents the tradeoff between sufficient tumor heating in order to devitalize cancer cells and tolerable side effects to surrounding healthy tissue.

The purpose of this study was the evaluation of the feasibility of visualizing the temperature course during a thermal ablation in an *in vitro* liver tumor phantom using MPI and different iron oxide tracers.

II. Material and Methods

In vitro liver tissue phantoms with different iron oxide tracers (L93, Bayer-Schering; Perimag, Micromod Partikeltechnologie GmbH, Germany; Resovist, Bayer Schering Pharma AG, Germany; concentrations: 0.1-0.5 mg/ml) were generated in Eppendorf-Tubes using a 1:1 volume mixture of protein and water (Chicken White Protein, Sigma Aldrich) mimicking healthy liver tissue after the specific uptake of SPIONs with respect to the particle aggregation and mobility status [3]. The phantoms were heated by means of an inserted copper wire (1 mm diameter) and MPI-induced eddy currents. The heat-induced signal changes of the phantom were simultaneously imaged by MPI. In contrast to multi-color temperature MPI [6], image reconstruction was based on one room temperature calibration measurement utilizing corresponding reference samples. During thermal ablation, changes of the measured MPI particle distribution can be directly attributed to temperature changes, since the hepatic SPION distribution can be considered quasi-constant after the intravenous SPION injection and hepatic uptake process. As reference optical thermometer measurements (Optocon AG, Germany) were performed (Fig. 1a). As an *in vitro* liver tumor ablation model, tracer-free protein (pseudotumor) was embedded in protein (pseudo-liver tissue) mixed with L93 (CFe = 0.356 mg/ml). The pseudotumors were heated by means of an inserted copper wire with simultaneous detection of the MPI signal of the surrounding pseudo-liver tissue (Fig 2b). As reference IR camera measurements (Testo SE & Co., Germany) were performed. All experiments were carried out on a commercial MPI system (Philips/Bruker) with drive field amplitude and gradient strength set to 12 mT and 2 T m^{-1}, respectively resulting in an effective FOV of 24 × 24 × 12 mm^3. A 2D PDw TSE sequence was acquired as morphologic reference (Fig. 2b) using a preclinical 7T ClinScan MRI, Bruker, Germany).

III. Results

Heat-induced MPI signal increases could be detected with all tracers. L93 showed the highest temperature changes and therefore highest sensitivity (Fig. 1b).

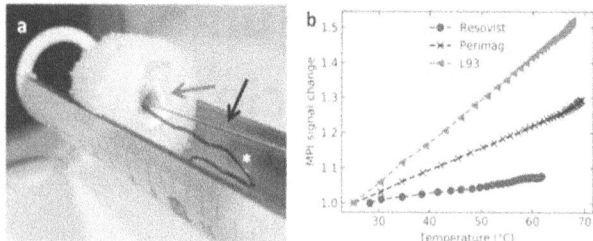

Figure 1: a) Photography of the experimental setup for evaluating the temperature sensitivity of the different tracers: The temperature probe (black arrow) was placed beside the copper wire (white asterix) within the liver tissue phantom inside an Eppendorf-tube (grey arrow). b) Correlation of MPI signal change and temperature change.

In the liver tumor ablation model, the ablation of the pseudo-liver tissue was visualized in 3D in real time by monitoring MPI signal changes of the surrounding liver tissue (Fig 2b) corresponding with IR camera temperature measurements (Fig 2a).

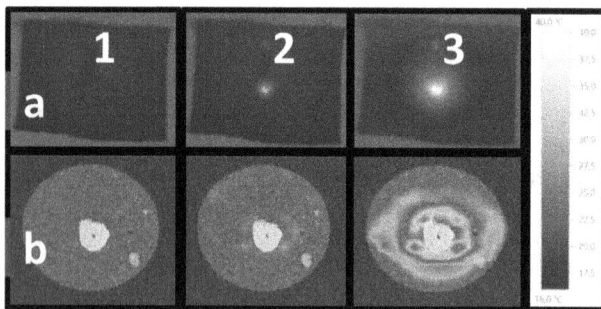

Figure 2: a) Thermographic captures with a range of 17 to 40 °C and b) corresponding visualization of the MPI signal change (MRI background with MPI overlay) at 0 s, 30 s and 210 s after start of heating.

IV. Discussion

While locally heating the phantoms to up to 40°C, temperature distribution could be imaged in real time. Signal changes in MPI showed a good correlation, so MPI-supported temperature monitoring of healthy tissue during thermal ablation is conceivable. The results need to be tested *ex vivo* in mouse liver tissue with induced tumors especially concerning the performance of different tracers in terms of spatial resolution and temperature sensitivity. For future *in vivo* studies available laser induced ablation platforms need to be tested for MPI compatibility in order to be able to perform imaging and heating independently. MPI data reconstruction was performed with only one calibration measurement (system matrix) minimizing the calibration effort in contrast to multi-color temperature MPI. In order to evaluate the full potential of MPI temperature measurements, the two calibration approaches need to be compared and a phantom allowing measurement of a system matrix at a constant temperature needs to be established.

V. Conclusions

MPI allows for spatial and temporal visualizing of temperature course and temperature distribution in a liver tumor ablation model. The sensitivity depends decisively on the used tracer. A temperature monitoring of healthy tissue for optimized MPI-guided tumor ablation in real time and 3D is feasible.

ACKNOWLEDGEMENTS

The authors acknowledge financial support by the Deutsche Forschungsgemeinschaft (DFG) under Sonder-forschungsbereich (SFB) 841 and tracer material support by Gunnar Schuetz (Bayer-Schering).

REFERENCES

[1] Ryan, Michael J. 2016. "Ablation Techniques for Primary and Metastatic Liver Tumors." *World Journal of Hepatology* 8 (3):191.

[2] Perälä, Jukka, Rauli Klemola, Raija Kallio, Chengli Li, Ilkka Vihriälä, Pasi I Salmela, Osmo Tervonen, and Roberto Blanco Sequeiros. 2014. "MRI-Guided Laser Ablation of Neuroendocrine Tumor Hepatic Metastases." *Acta Radiologica Short Reports*

[3] Dieckhoff, J, M G Kaul, T Mummert, C Jung, J Salamon, G Adam, T Knopp, F Ludwig, C Balceris, and H Ittrich. 2017. "*In Vivo* Liver Visualizations with Magnetic Particle Imaging Based on the Calibration Measurement Approach." *Physics in Medicine and Biology* 62 (9):3470–82

[4] Kawamori, Y, O Matsui, M Kadoya, J Yoshikawa, H Demachi, and T Takashima. 1992. "Differentiation of Hepatocellular Carcinomas from Hyperplastic Nodules Induced in Rat Liver with Ferrite-Enhanced MR Imaging." *Radiology* 183 (1):65–72.

[5] Dieckhoff, Jan, Michael G. Kaul, Tobias Mummert, Caroline Jung, Johannes Salamon, Gerhard Adam, Tobias Knopp, Dorothee Schwinge, and Harald Ittrich. 2017. "Magnetic Particle Imaging of Liver Tumors in Small Animal Models"

[6] Stehning, Christian, Bernhard Gleich, and Jürgen Rahmer. 2016. "Simultaneous Magnetic Particle Imaging (MPI) and Temperature Mapping Using Multi-Color MPI."

Session 12 - Diskussion

Survey on MPI Applications

An Eye on the Future of Magnetic Particle Imaging

During this session, the results of the questionnaire handed over at registration, will be presented. Following this short presentation, we will start an open panel discussion to find out what needs there are to shape the future of MPI.

The first objective is to identify and discuss potential high impact applications where MPI outperforms other methods by providing complementary information, better/faster diagnoses or therapies, or quantitative insights into technical or biological processes. For these applications, the next step will be to derive requirements in terms of tracer material, temporal and spatial resolution, system sensitivity and other requirements to make these applications come true in the near future.

As an MPI community, we have the opportunity to define and shape the future of magnetic particle imaging - together we are shaping the future of MPI.

Session 13 - Talks

Instrumentation IV

Parallel Magnetic Particle Imaging

Patrick Vogel [a,b,*], Thomas Kampf [a,c], Stefan Herz [b], Martin A. Rückert [a], Thorsten A. Bley [b], Volker C. Behr [a]

[a] Department of Experimental Physics 5 (Biophysics), University of Würzburg, 97074 Würzburg, Germany
[b] Department of Diagnostic and Interventional Radiology, University Hospital Würzburg, 97080 Würzburg, Germany
[c] Department of Diagnostic and Interventional Neuroradiology, University Hospital Würzburg, 97080 Würzburg, Germany
* Corresponding author, email: Patrick.Vogel@physik.uni-wuerzburg.de

I. Introduction

Since the first publication of Magnetic Particle Imaging (MPI) several hardware designs and scanner types have been presented [1]. In principle, a strong gradient (selection field) in the vicinity of a field free point (FFP) or field free line (FFL) is generated using permanent or electro magnets. Additional coils (drive coils) are used to move the FFP or FFL through the region of interest (ROI) along specific trajectories generating the MPI signal point-by-point or projection-wise. Due to the hardware design, in common MPI systems only one FFP or FFL can be used for imaging. This limits the possibility to scan a large FOV without increasing the acquisition time [2].

In a Traveling Wave MPI scanner (TWMPI) [3] a dynamic linear gradient array (dLGA) [4] is used for the generation of a sinusoidally shaped magnetic field (dynamic selection field). The zero-crossing points represent several FFPs traveling along the symmetry axis (z-direction) through the scanner. Additional saddle-coils are used to steer them on specific trajectories through the system to cover a full FOV. For a single receive coil design, the FOV is limited by the distance between two adjacent FFPs to ensure unambiguous encoding (Fig. 1 a).

In Fig. 1 (b) a simulation of the maximum of the magnetic field along the symmetry axis over a full period is shown indicating the area which could theoretically be used for imaging (l_{FOV2} vs. l_{FOV1}) [4].

In the following, the first concept of parallel imaging with a TWMPI scanner is presented, which offers scanning a larger FOV within the same time using multiple receive chains.

II. Material and Methods

To ensure a full encoding capability over the entire area, a number of receive coils have to be used to separate the signal from the same (or lower) number of FFPs. In Fig. 1 (c) a sketch of a TWMPI scanner using two receive chains for covering a larger FOV is shown.

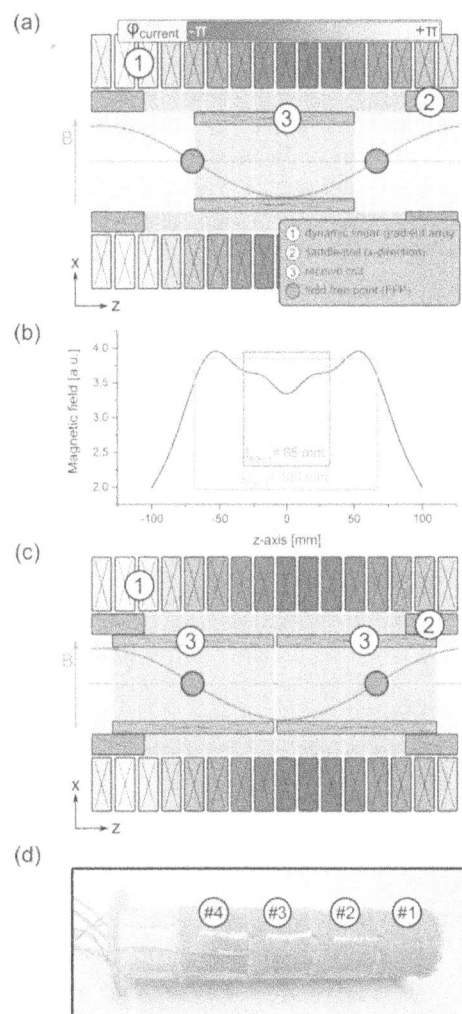

Figure 1: (a) Sketch of a 2D TWMPI system consisting of dLGA (1), saddle-coil (2) and receive coil (3). (b) The profile plot of the magnetic field along the symmetry axis shows the potentially operationable FOV. (c) With two receive chains a larger FOV can be encoded using two FFPs. (d) Photo of the new multi-channel receive coil.

Fig. 1 (d) shows a photo of the new multi-channel receive coil consisting of four separate elements aligned into z-direction [3]. This allows to investigate the behavior of different combinations of coils (here #1+#2 for channel-1 and #3+#4 for channel-2 and also #2+#3 for comparison) and their signal. Every element has a length of 30 mm and consists of 2×37 windings of litz wire (45×0.1, Rupalit Classic, Pack LitzWire, Germany).

III. Results

For imaging, the multi-channel receive coil was installed in a TWMPI scanner [3]. The signals of two receive channels (channel-1 with coils #1 and #2 in series and channel-2 with coils #3 and #4 in series) equipped with high- and low-pass filters as well as low-noise preamplifiers were acquired simultaneously. Both data streams were separately processed (receive chain correction and software-filtering) and reconstructed using an image-based reconstruction method [5]. For that, a model-based system matrix is calculated consisting of 10140×3799 entries sufficient to encode a FOV of 25×131 mm² with an isotropic resolution of 1 mm.

Furthermore, the signal of the coil combination #2+#3 is acquired for comparison in a separate experiment. As phantom a plastic-tube sample with an inner diameter of 0.86 mm filled with undiluted Resovist® (Bayer, Germany) is used.

In Fig. 2 the reconstructed images of the first parallel 2D MPI scan are shown. The following settings were used for the TWMPI experiments: frequencies for selection- and drive-field: f_z=723.57 Hz and f_x=18859.73 Hz generating a gradient of about G_z=2 T/m. The total acquisition time was 200 ms (10 averages).

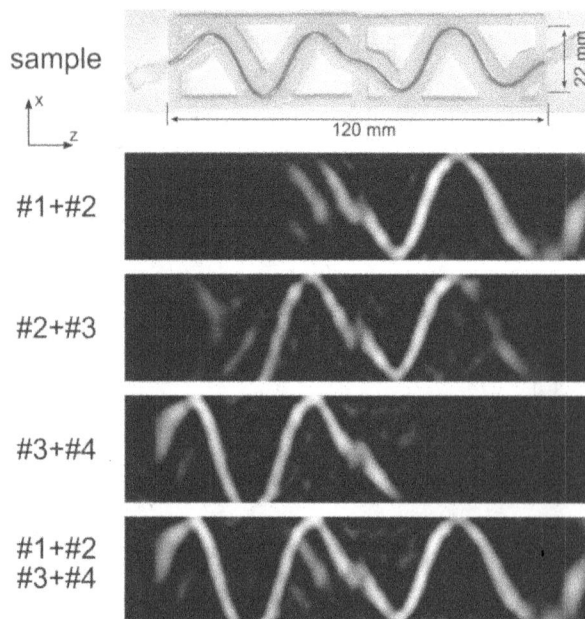

Figure 2: *Results of the first parallel TWMPI experiment: a sample filled with Resovist® (Bayer, Germany) is measured. The reconstructions of the receive coil combinations of #1+#2, #2+#3 and #3+#4 are shown as well as the overlay of #1+#2 and #3+#4.*

IV. Discussion

By using a Traveling Wave MPI approach it is possible to generate multiple FFPs traveling through the sample. Until now, the full potential of the TWMPI approach was not used (see Fig. (b)), which reduced the available FOV. With multiple receive coils, it is possible to enlarge the FOV without increasing the acquisition time. However, multiple receive coils require a multiple receive chains with optimally the same components properties (filter, LNAs, etc.). To amend minor variations, a more sophisticated calibration and correction algorithm has to be implemented in the postprocessing.

The electrical coupling between both receive chains can cause signal loss due to cross-talk between receivers. To minimize the electrical coupling an interleaved combination of the receive coils can be used: channel-1: #1-#3 and channel-2: #2-#4. For reconstructing the data several well-known algorithms can be borrowed from parallel magnetic resonance imaging (pMRI) such as PILS or SENSE [6, 7].

V. Conclusions

In this abstract the first result of a parallel MPI experiment is demonstrated. By using multiple receive coils it is possible to encode multiple FFPs traveling through an enlarged FOV at the same time. This increases the available FOV (here: 131 mm in length and 25 mm in diameter) without increasing the acquisition time.

REFERENCES

[1] T. Knopp, et al., Magnetic Particle Imaging: from proof of principle to preclinical applications, *Phys. Med. Biol.*, vol. 62(14), pp. R124-R178, 2017. DOI: 10.1088/1361-6560/aa6c99

[2] B. Gleich et al., Fast MPI demonstrator with enlarged field of view, Proc. ISMRM, vol. 18, pp.218, 2010.

[3] P. Vogel, et al., Traveling Wave Magnetic Particle Imaging, *IEEE TMI*, vol. 33(2), pp. 400-7, 2014. Doi:10.1109/TMI.2013.2285472.

[4] P. Vogel & P. Klauer, et al., Dynamic Linear Gradient Array for Traveling Wave Magnetic Particle Imaging, *IEEE Trans. Magn.*, (in press). Doi: 10.1109/TMAG.2017.2764440

[5] P. Vogel, et al., Flexible and Dynamic Patch Reconstruction for Traveling Wave MPI, *IJMPI*, vol. 2(2):1611001, 2017. Doi: 10.18416/ijmpi.2016.1611001

[6] M.A. Grisworld, et al., Partially parallel imaging with localized sensitivities (PILS), *MRM*, vol. 44, pp. 602-9, 2000. Doi: 10.1002/1522-2594(200010)44:4<602::AID-MRM14>3.0.CO;2-5

[7] K.P. Pruessmann, et al., SENSE: Sensitivity Encoding for Fast MRI, *MRM*, vol. 42, pp. 952-62, 1999. Doi: 10.1002/(SICI)1522-2594(199911)42:5<952::AID-MRM16>3.0.CO;2-S

An MPI-Compatible HIFU Transducer: Experimental Evaluation of Interferences.

Tim C. Kranemann[a,*], Thomas Ersepke[a], Jochen Franke[b] ,Thomas Friedrich[c], Alexander Neumann[c], Thorsten Buzug[c], Georg Schmitz[a]

[a] *Chair of Medical Engineering, Ruhr-Universität Bochum, Bochum, Germany*
[b] *Bruker BioSpin MRI GmbH, Ettlingen, Germany*
[c] *Institute of Medical Engineering, University of Lübeck, Lübeck, Germany*
[*] *Corresponding author, email: tim.kranemann@rub.de*

I. Introduction

The controlled application of heat to tumors is referred to as local hyperthermia in oncology. One clinically applied hyperthermia modality for various tumor entities is high intensity focused ultrasound (HIFU) [1]. The mechanical energy of an acoustic beam is precisely delivered to organs accessible by ultrasound (US). The acoustic energy is converted into heat in a small focal area, which leads to a rapid ablation. For an efficient and safe application, temperature monitoring of the tissue is necessary.

Monitoring of a HIFU treatment with US imaging is challenging [2]. Therefore, cost-intensive magnetic resonance imaging thermometry is the gold standard for HIFU monitoring to date [3]. The ability of magnetic particle imaging (MPI) to determine the nanoparticle tracer temperature has recently been demonstrated [4], [5]. Consequently, MPI has the potential to be used as an alternative hyperthermia monitoring device that delivers temperature maps sufficiently fast during rapid HIFU ablation. Further, MPI can be realized as a single-sided device, which would significantly reduce costs compared to a full MRI instrumentation.

During HIFU therapy, MPI is expected to deliver temperature maps in real-time that complement US-based therapy monitoring techniques. However, commercially available HIFU devices usually cannot operate inside MPI scanners. Due to the strong, alternating magnetic fields, eddy currents are induced in transducer components that can lead to a rapid destructive heating. To enable an MPI-HIFU combination, design guidelines for MPI compatible ultrasound hardware have already been proposed [6], [7].

To evaluate MPI as a HIFU monitoring modality, a first MPI adapted HIFU transducer is presented in this contribution. Its MPI compatibility is experimentally confirmed by infrared thermometry and measurements of electromagnetic interference. Thereof, the maximum possible acoustic intensity is deduced to determine if ablative acoustical intensities can be reached inside the MPI bore without overloading the MPI signal chain.

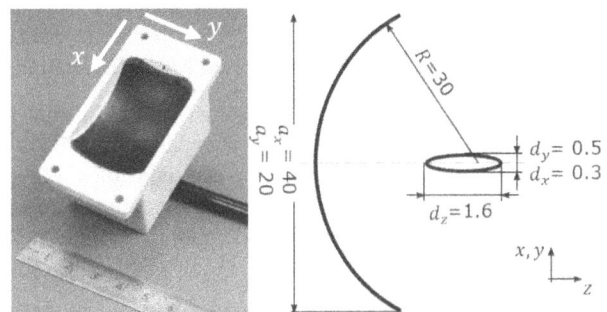

Figure 1: *Left: Transducer picture. Right: Schematic sketch of transducer and focus geometry and dimensions in units of mm.*

II. Material and Methods

The customized HIFU transducer (Imasonic, Voray sur l'Ognon, France) is a single element spherical transducer focused to a fixed target depth of 30 mm, see Fig. 1. The center frequency is $f_c = 3,5$ MHz but the excitation frequency can be adjusted (ca. 3 MHz – 4 MHz) to account for frequency dependent acoustic absorption phenomena. The device is designed to achieve an acoustic intensity of 5 kW/cm^2 at the focus.

To achieve MPI compatibility, the transducer electrode surfaces are patterned and any electrical shielding is removed to reduce eddy current heating by drive field coils at 25 kHz [6], [7]. Further, the electrode is divided up into five sub-electrodes to reduce the power per sub-electrode and thereby the cross-section of respective cables. To evaluate the effectiveness of these provisions, the transducer was placed inside the bore of a pre-clinical MPI scanner (MPI 25/20 FF, Bruker BioSpin MRI, Ettlingen, Germany) at a drive field strength of 12 mT/μ_0. Heating was monitored from outside the bore with a thermography camera (VarioCAM, InfraTec, Dresden, Germany).

To evaluate the electromagnetic interference in the MPI signal chain, at first an empty bore measurement was performed for comparison. Afterwards, the passive transducer was placed inside the bore and eventually connected to the US research platform (Vantage 256 HIFU,

Verasonics, Kirkland, WA) via five RG 58 C/U coaxial cables of 7 m length. For all these configurations, MPI spectra were recorded with the Bruker *Paravision* software. To evaluate the maximum power that can be transmitted to the transducer, the MPI signal chain was disconnected behind the MPI low noise amplifiers (LNA's). The transfer functions of the HIFU transducer to the LNA's were measured with a network analyzer (E5061B, Keysight Technologies, Santa Rosa, CA).

To characterize the generated sound field, US simulations with the k-wave toolbox [8] incorporating basic nonlinear ultrasound propagation were performed. The dimensions of the focal area and the average acoustic intensity therein were calculated.

III. Results

When the transducer was placed inside the scanner bore during imaging sequences, heating < 5K in steady state at an ambient temperature of 19 °C was observed. Thus, transducer operation is not limited by eddy current heating.

The empty bore spectra did not change when the transducer was placed inside the bore. However, overall spectral energy increased by 24 dB when the coaxial cables where connected and guided outside the shielding cabin. Hence, interferences were attributed to the degradation of the MPI shielding cabin.

The transfer functions between the transducer and the MPI LNA outputs are depicted in Fig 2. As the transmittance was −58 dB at the transducer center frequency, the maximum power is 58 dBm to avoid an LNA overload beyond 0 dBm. Since the transducer is designed for a maximum continuous power of +43 dBm, maximum acoustic power is not limited by MPI constraints.

Further spectra recorded with the Bruker *Paravision* Software revealed no significant rise in the noise level when the transducer was exemplarily driven with continuous wave excitation corresponding to 20 W active power. Simulations showed that with this electrical input power, an acoustic intensity of 5 kW/cm^2 is easily achieved in a focus with dimensions d according to Fig. 1.

IV. Discussion

The previously presented guidelines [6], [7] lead to an MPI compatible transducer. The acoustic power that can be transmitted inside the MPI is not limited by eddy current heating or interferences. Hence, acoustic intensities beyond those necessary for rapid ablation (2 kW/cm^2 [2]) are achieved without significantly influencing MPI signals. Contrary to prior assessment [7], this suggests that concurrent MPI reconstruction and HIFU therapy is feasible since the interferences are limited to the HIFU center frequency, thus, are above the frequency range relevant in MPI. For further investigations, the coaxial cables need to be guided through the shielding cabin via an electric filter to reduce the otherwise introduced noise. Nevertheless, since LNA's are not overdriven, it can be accounted for possible narrowband interferences by digital filtering during MPI reconstruction.

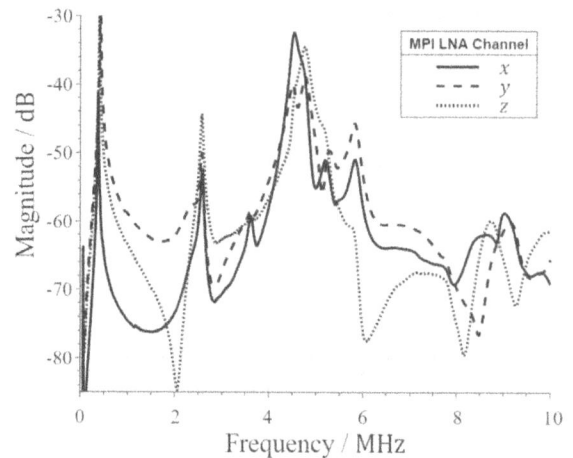

Figure 2: *Magnitude transmittance from the HIFU transducer to LNA output channels of the MPI scanner.*

V. Conclusions

With the insertion and operation of an ultrasound transducer inside the MPI scanner, the applicability of a HIFU and MPI combination has been confirmed. Accordingly, the presented HIFU transducer offers the opportunity to evaluate MPI as an alternative HIFU monitoring device.

ACKNOWLEDGEMENTS
This work was funded by the German Federal Ministry of Education and Research, contract number 13GW0069A-D (Project SAMBA-PATI).

REFERENCES
[1]   Focused Ultrasound Foundation, "Focused Ultrasound State of the Field," 2017.

[2]   E. S. Ebbini and G. Ter Haar, "Ultrasound-guided therapeutic focused ultrasound: Current status and future directions," *Int. J. Hyperth.*, vol. 2, 2015.

[3]   D. Schlesinger, S. Benedict, C. Diederich, *et al.* "MR-guided focused ultrasound surgery, present and future," *Med. Phys.*, vol. 40, no. 8, 2013.

[4]   E. W. Hansen, J. B. Weaver, and A. M. Rauwerdink, "Magnetic nanoparticle temperature estimation," *Med. Phys.*, vol. 36, 2009.

[5]   C. Stehning, B. Gleich, and J. Rahmer, "Simultaneous magnetic particle imaging (MPI) and temperature mapping using multi-color MPI," *Int. J. Magn. Part. Imaging*, vol. 2, no. 2 , 2016.

[6]   T. C. Kranemann, T. Ersepke, and G. Schmitz, "Design of a Magnetic Particle Imaging Compatible HIFU Transducer Array", presented at the IEEE Int. Ultrasonics Symp., 2016.

[7]   T. C. Kranemann, T. Ersepke, and G. Schmitz, "Towards the Integration of an MPI Compatible Ultrasound Transducer," *Int. J. Magn. Part. Imaging*, vol. 3, no. 1, 2017.

[8]   B. E. Treeby, J. Jaros, A. P. Rendell, and B. T. Cox, "Modeling nonlinear ultrasound propagation in heterogeneous media with power law absorption using a k-space pseudospectral method," *J. Acoust. Soc. Am.*, vol. 131, no. 6, 2012.

Permanent Magnet Selection Coils Design for Single-Sided Field-Free Line MPI

Grant Rudd [a], Alexey Tonyushkin [b,*]

[a] Engineering Department, University of Massachusetts Boston, Boston, MA, USA
[b] Physics Department, University of Massachusetts Boston, Boston, MA, USA
* Corresponding author, email: alexey.tonyushkin@umb.edu

I. Introduction

Over the last decade, Magnetic Particle Imaging (MPI) [1] evolved into a new imaging modality that holds promise for a variety of clinical applications [2]. One of the recent MPI developments is a single-sided MPI scanner based on a field-free point (FFP) [3]. In the single-sided scanner all the hardware is located on one side from the imaging volume, therefore it can alleviate spatial constraints particularly pertinent to imaging of large subjects. Although such scanner has a relatively shallow field of view, it could be a solution for a number of clinical applications [4].

Last year we presented a concept of a single-sided device based on a field-free line (FFL) with permanent magnet (PM) selection coils [5]. In this work, we show the actual design of the PM selection coils capable of producing strong field gradient at a height of 3 cm above the surface.

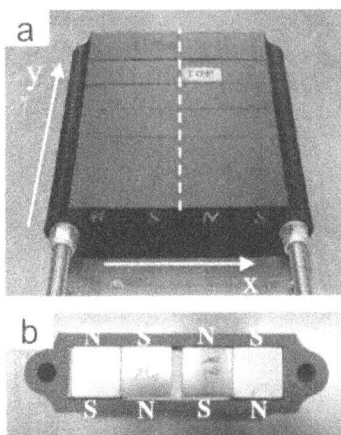

Figure 1: *Permanent magnet selection coils assembly. The assembly (a) consists of six identical elements (b) with four alternating pole magnets in each element. FFL is obtained above the surface in the isoplane (dashed line).*

II. Material and Methods

The parts of the PM coils' enclosure were prototyped on a 3D printer (*Markforged Mark* 2) out of carbon fiber reinforced nylon. The enclosure is assembled out of six identical elements (rows) with the total assembly size of 16.5 cm x 15.5 cm as shown in Fig. 1. Each row consists of four tightly packed 2.54 cm-cube NdFeB magnets with 0.5 cm spacer in the middle. The magnets in a row (x-axis) arranged with the alternating poles pointing at the surface of the coils that form the basis for the static selection field (Fig. 1b). The field gradient and the height of the FFL depend on the magnetizations and the magnets' separations. The magnetization in each column (y-axis) is defined by the remanence of the corresponding magnet's grade: N52 – the outer pair and N42 – the inner pair, with the magnetization ratio m=1.12.

To characterize the magnetic flux density **B** of the PM coils we carried out simulations and measurements using Wolfram *Mathematica* software and a gaussmeter (*Magsys*).

III. Results

The designed PM coils generate a FFL at the static height of z_0=2.9 ± 0.05 cm above the surface of the magnets that includes 0.635 cm thickness of the enclosure. The calculated and measured field gradients are G=3.25 T/m and G=2.91 T/m, respectively.

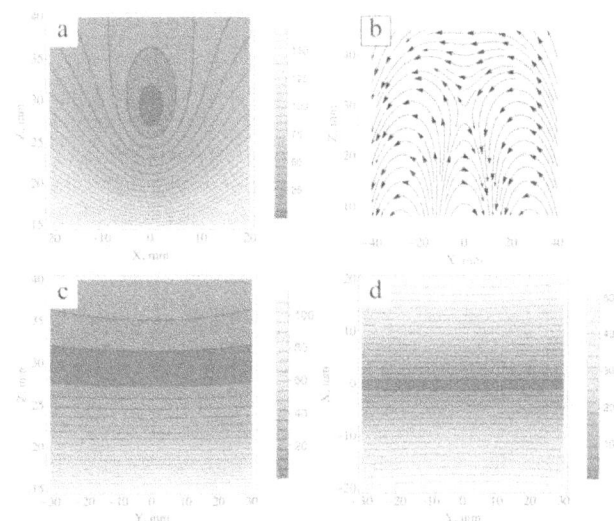

Figure 2: *Simulations of the PM coils: magnetic flux density contour plots (B/mT) in the xz-plane (a), the yz-plane (c), the yx-plane (d); vector plot of the B-field in the xz-plane (b).*

Fig. 2 shows simulations of the magnetic flux density **B** generated by the PM coils: the top row shows cross-section plots of the FFL in the *xz*-plane, the bottom row shows the curvature of the FFL in the *zy*- and *xy*-planes.

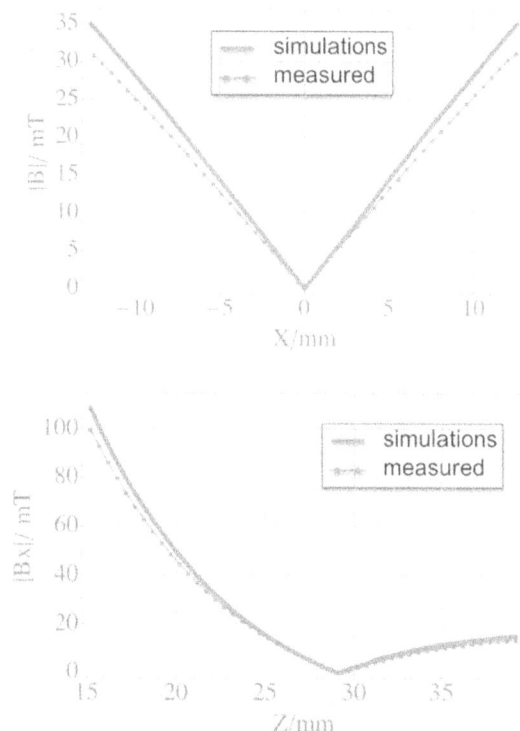

Figure 3: Simulations and measurements of the magnetic flux density from the PM coils, top: |B| along x-axis (z₀=29 mm), bottom: |Bₓ| along z-axis (x₀=0), where simulations – solid line, measurement – dot-solid line.

The simulated and measured magnetic flux densities generated by the PM coils along *x*- and *z*- axes are shown in Fig. 3. The measurement of the actual magnetic field shows good agreement with the simulations in the vicinity of the FFL, while the differences of ~10% at the edges of the depicted regions along *x*- and *z*- coordinates are attributed to the uncertainties in the specifications of PM magnetization.

IV. Discussion

The presented PM selection coils produce strong field gradient that is desired for an imaging with high spatial resolution. The calculated curvature of the FFL along *y*-axis is 320 μT/cm^2, which is sufficiently small to provide a few cm encoding region. Adding more elements to the assembly would further decrease the curvature. Depending on the application, the static height of the FFL, which defines the encoding slice, can be changed by modifying the design with various gaps between the pairs of magnets in each row or increasing the size of the magnets. For example, increasing the separation of the outer pairs by 2 cm would move the height up to 3.6 cm while decreasing the field gradient to 2.1 T/m.

The 3D operation can be achieved with the addition of AC electromagnets similarly as described in [6]. In such a hybrid design the PM coils would replace the top DC electromagnets, while the bottom row of the drive coils would provide translation of the FFL along *x*- and *z*- axes. For 2D imaging in the *xy*-plane only a single racetrack drive coil is needed that is placed along the isoaxis.

V. Conclusions

We designed permanent magnet selection coils for a single-sided FFL-based MPI scanner. The coils generate a static FFL at the height of 3 cm above the surface with the field gradient of *G*=3T/m. In combination with mechanical rotation and translation by the AC coils such a hybrid MPI device can provide a strong magnetic field gradient with a sufficient field of view at a reduced power consumption. The potential applications of a hybrid single-sided scanner may include human's interventional procedures.

ACKNOWLEDGEMENTS

We acknowledge support from University of Massachusetts President Office through OTCV Award.

REFERENCES

[1] B. Gleich and J. Weizenecker. Tomographic imaging using the nonlinear response of magnetic particles. *Nature*, 435(7046):1217-1217, 2005. doi:10.1038/nature03808.

[2] T. Knopp and T. M. Buzug. *Magnetic Particle Imaging: An Introduction to Imaging Principles and Scanner Instrumentation.* Springer, Berlin/Heidelberg, 2012. doi:10.1007/978-3-642-04199-0.

[3] T. F. Sattel, T. Knopp, S. Biederer, B. Gleich, J. Weizenecker, J. Borgert, and T. M. Buzug. Single-sided device for magnetic particle imaging. *J. Phys. D: Appl. Phys.*, 42(1):1–5, 2009. doi:10.1088/0022-3727/42/2/022001.

[4] C. Kaethner, M. Ahlborg, K. Gräfe, G. Bringout, T. F. Sattel, and T. M. Buzug. Asymmetric Scanner Design for Interventional Scenarios in Magnetic Particle Imaging. *IEEE Trans. Magn.*, 51(2):6501904, 2015. doi:10.1109/TMAG.2014.2337931.

[5] A. Tonyushkin. Single-sided hybrid selection coils for field-free line magnetic particle imaging. *Int. J. Magn. Particle Imag.*, 3(1): 1703009, 2017. doi:10.18416/ijmpi.2017.1703009.

[6] A. Tonyushkin. Single-sided field-free line generator magnet for multidimensional magnetic particle imaging, *IEEE Trans. Magn.*, 53(9):5300506, 2017. doi:10.1109/TMAG.2017.2718485.

First Phantom Measurements with a 3D Single-Sided MPI Scanner

Ksenija Gräfe [a,*], Anselm von Gladiss [a], Thorsten M. Buzug [a,*]

[a] Institute of Medical Engineering, University of Lübeck
* Corresponding author, email: {graefe,buzug}@imt.uni-luebeck.de

I. Introduction

Different coil topologies for single-sided magnetic particle imaging (MPI) concepts have been proposed over the last years [1, 2, 3]. First reconstruction result of a one-dimensional phantom, measured with a prototype of a single-sided MPI scanner has been presented already in 2009 [1]. In [2] a two-dimensional single-sided device and first reconstruction results have been published.

In this contribution, a three-dimensional single-sided MPI scanner and first reconstruction results of phantom measurements will be presented.

I.I. Single-Sided MPI Scanner

In comparison to other MPI scanner geometries [3] the single-sided concept has the advantage of an unconfined object size or patient access in a clinical scenario. Nevertheless, there is a limitation of the field of view (FOV) due to a penetration depth limitation of the spatial coding.

The coil geometry for a one-dimensional single-sided MPI scanner consists of two concentrically circular coils. Both coils feature a direct current (DC) that flow in opposite directions and generate the selection field, which contains the field free point (FFP). Additionally, there is an alternating current (AC) on the inner coil that moves the FFP on the middle axis of the device [1].

In order to enable the scanner for two-dimensional imaging a D-shaped coil pair has been added, which lies directly below the circular coils. An AC on this coil moves the FFP parallel to the scanner device. In combination with the AC on the inner coil the FFP is moved on a Lissajous trajectory [2].

I.II. Medical Application Scenario

One of many possible medical applications for a single-sided MPI scanner is the localization of the sentinel lymph nodes (SLN) in breast cancer treatment.

Today, blue dye injection or a radioactive tracer is used to label the SLN for subsequent dissection. Alternatively, biocompatible superparamagnetic nanoparticles could be injected as tracer material nearby the breast tumor and reach the SLN via the lymphatic system. Within the intervention, the tracer material inside the SLN could be detected with the single-sided MPI scanner and subsequently dissected. This way, radioactive tracer material could be omitted. Furthermore, this method would be much more precise than the SLN localization using blue dye or radioactive tracers. Therefore, the surgical procedure would be gentler and less invasive [4].

II. Material and Methods

In addition to the scanner setup presented in [2], another two D-shaped coil pairs are necessary to enable three-dimensional imaging with a single-sided scanner. One coil pair for the excitation part and one for the receive part. The additional D-shaped coil pairs are placed direct below the existing coils. This coil pairs are rotated by 90° with respect to the previous D-shaped coil pairs that enables two-dimensional lateral imaging. An AC on the excitation coil moves the FFP perpendicular to the existing excitation directions. In total, a three-dimensional Lissajous trajectory is generated. An overview of the coils is given in Tab. 1.

Table 1: *Overview of the different excitation coils.*

	coil	current	frequency	field
1	circular outer coil	56 A (DC)		selection field in combination with 2
2	circular inner coil	65 A (DC) 42 A (AC)	25.25 kHz	selection field in combination with 1 and drive field in x-direction
3	D-shaped coil pair	80 A (AC)	26.04 kHz	drive field in y-direction
4	D-shaped coil pair	80 A (AC)	26.88 kHz	drive field in z-direction

Fig. 1 (left) shows an exploded view of the three-dimensional scanner. A three-dimensional phantom (Fig. 2) has been measured and reconstructed. Each of the three dots inside the phantom is filled with 6.2 µl undiluted Resovist. The dots are located in the fifth and the eleventh z-plane.

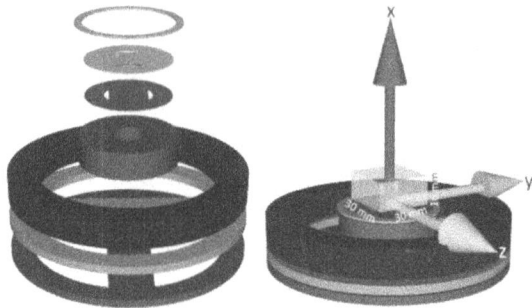

Figure 1: Exploded view of the single-sided scanner (left) and an illustration of the scanner with the FOV (right).

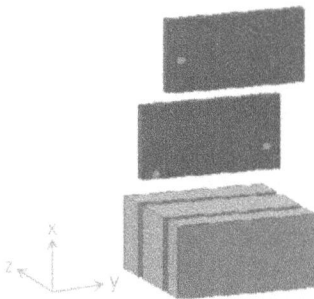

Figure 2: Schematic drawing of the phantom. The light dots on the dark squares indicate the particle samples.

Image reconstruction is performed by solving the linear system of equations

$$(\hat{S}^*W\hat{S} + \lambda I)c = \hat{S}^*W\hat{u} \tag{1}$$

with the unknown spatial particle concentration (c), the truncated system matrix ($\hat{S}$), the conjugate transpose of the truncated system matrix ($\hat{S}^*$), a weighting matrix (W), the regularization parameter (λ) in combination with the identity matrix (I) and the truncated measurement ($\hat{u}$). Equation (1) is solved by a modified iterative Kaczmarz algorithm [2].

The system matrix has been measured with a 2 x 2 x 2 mm³ particle sample of undiluted Resovist that has been moved in 8 x 15 x 15 steps of 2 mm over the FOV. The size of the FOV is 16 x 30 x 30 mm³ (Fig. 1, right).

III. Results

Fig. 3 shows the reconstruction result of the measured three-dimensional phantom (Fig. 2). Each rectangle represents one slice in z-direction. In slices three to six a signal of the dot in the fifth z-plane can be seen. A signal generated by the two dots in slice 11 can be seen from slice 13 to 16.

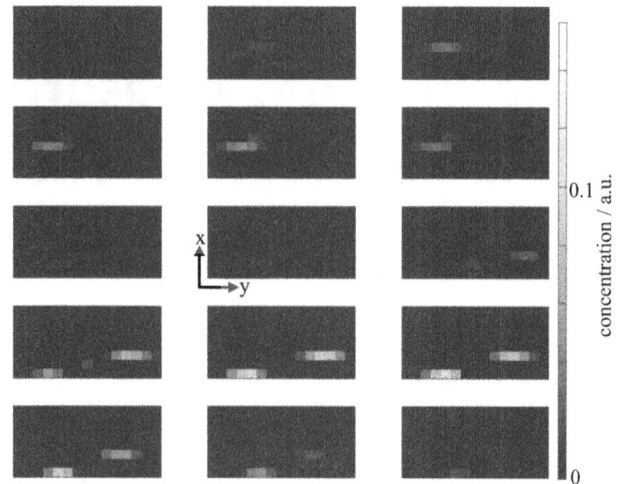

Figure 3: Reconstruction result of the phantom (Fig. 2) measurement. Each rectangle represents one slice in z-direction.

IV. Discussion

Three-dimensional imaging has been performed using a single-sided MPI scanner. The particle distribution inside a three-dimensional phantom has successfully been reconstructed.

The reconstruction result shows that the penetration depth of the FFP (in x-direction) is about 8 mm [2]. The spatial resolution in y- and z-direction is about 8 mm and the spatial resolution in x-direction is about 2 mm [2].

V. Conclusions

This contribution presents a first reconstruction result of a three-dimensional phantom measurement with a single-sided MPI scanner. Three-dimensional imaging is an important step towards clinical use, because neither the scanner nor the patient is required to move in order to image volumes.

Using the three-dimensional single-sided MPI scanner, an SLN may be localized in real-time, more precise than in the existing procedures and without harmful radiation.

ACKNOWLEDGEMENTS

The authors would like to thank the DFG (BU 1436/9-1) for the financial support.

REFERENCES

[1] T. F. Sattel, T. Knopp, S. Biederer, B. Gleich, J. Weizenecker, J. Borgert, and T. M. Buzug. Single-sided device for magnetic particle imaging, Journal of Physics D: Applied Physics, 42(2), pp. 1–5, 2009

[2] K. Gräfe, A. von Gladiss, G. Bringout, M. Ahlborg and T. M. Buzug. 2D Images Recorded With a Single-Sided Magnetic Particle Imaging Scanner, IEEE Transactions on Medical Imaging, 35(4), 1056-1065, 2016

[3] A. Tonyushkin. Single-Sided Field-Free Line Generator Magnet for Multi-Dimensional Magnetic Particle Imaging, IEEE Transactions on Magnetics, 53(9), 5300506, 2017

[4] D. Finas, K. Baumann, L. Sydow, K. Heinrich, A. Rody, K. Gräfe, T. M. Buzug and K. Lüdtke-Buzug, SPIO Detection and Distribution in Biological Tissue - A Murine MPI-SLNB Breast Cancer Model, IEEE Transactions on Magnetics, 51(2), 5400104, 2015

First Images from an Atomic-Magnetometry-Based 1D and (Hybrid) 2D MPI Scanner

Victor Lebedev[a,*], Simone Colombo [a], Simone Pengue [a], Zoran D. Grujić [a], Vladimir Dolgovskiy [a], Alexey Tonyushkin [b], Theo Scholtes [a], Antoine Weis [a]

[a] *Department of Physics, University of Fribourg, Fribourg, Switzerland*
[b] *Physics Department, University of Massachusetts Boston, Boston, USA*
* *Corresponding author, email: victor.lebedev@unifr.ch*

I. Introduction

We describe an atomic magnetometer-based Magnetic Particle Imaging (AM-MPI) scanner and present first 1D/2D images of magnetic nanoparticle (MNP) phantoms.

The AM-MPI differs essentially from both frequency and X-space MPI in the sense that it records directly a signal proportional to the magnetic susceptibility of the MNP sample in a frequency band from DC to a few kHz. Conventional MPI scanners rely on the Faraday induction law that requires RF frequencies and filtering of spectral harmonics in the MNP induction signal. Although posing constraints on scanner speed, our approach offers a way to avoid MPI biocompatibility issues, such as SAR limitations and PNS risk. Moreover, its operation at sub-kHz frequencies allows the deployment of MNPs with virtually any size, in any medium. In addition, the AM-MPI scanner can record magnetorelaxometry (MRX) maps using the same hardware and software.

Recently, we have addressed the prerequisites for realizing the receive part of an MPI scanner based on a robust atomic magnetometer [1-3]. Those prerequisites led us to develop a combination of a 1D magnetic scanner and a 1D mechanical sample motion unit. Inverse methods are applied to infer the magnitude and spatial distribution of the MNP sample from its (far-field) magnetic flux density $B(t)$ at the AM position.

II. Material and Methods

II.I. Coil system

The principle of the magnetic system of the AM-MPI scanner is described in a recent publication [3]. It consists of separately powered air-cooled offset (modulation) and gradient (selection) coils, produced by extended racetrack coils made from copper ribbon generating a (displaceable) field free line (FFL). Specifically designed passive compensation coils (Fig. 1) ensure that the flux density and its gradients are well below 1 μT and 100 nT/m, respectively, at the sensor position, while their own field is negligible at the sample position.

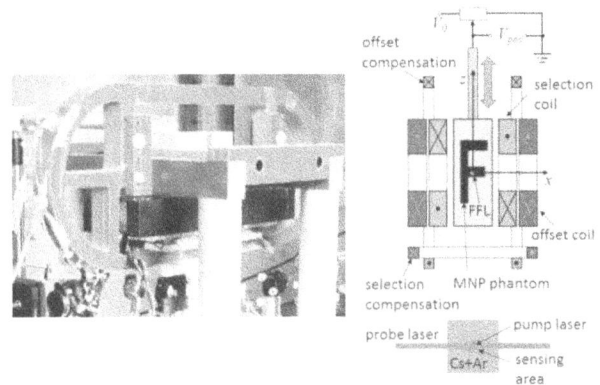

Figure 1: (color online) Left: Photograph of the magnetic system of the AM-MPI scanner. Right: transverse cross-section of the scanner

II.II. Atomic magnetometer

The experiments are performed in a walk-in double-walled cabin made each from 3 mm thick aluminum that suppresses magnetic power line interference. The deployed atomic magnetometer is a further development of the design presented in [3]. It has a $2 \times 2 \times 2$ mm^3 sensing volume defined by the intersection (at right angles) of a pump and a probe laser beam in a heated glass cell containing cesium and inert buffer gas. Magnetic resonance driven by a phase-locked feedback loop makes the system oscillate a frequency $v(t)$ that is proportional to the local flux density $|B(t)|$, yielding a few pT/Hz$^{1/2}$ sensitivity from DC to 3 kHz.

II.III. Magneto-mechanical scanner

Mechanical 1D scanning is realized by translational motion of the sample along z (Fig. 1) in a gradient up to 2 T/m. We supply a modulation current with small amplitude $I_{mod} \ll 1$ mT and frequency $f_{mod} = 121$ Hz to the offset coil. Lock-in demodulation of a voltage proportional to the magnetometer frequency $v(t)$ at f_{mod} then yields a signal S_{AM} that is proportional to the convolution of the MNP density distribution $\rho(x)$ with the derivative $L'(x)=dL(H)/dH(x)$ of the Langevin function (point spread function, PSF).

2D scanning is achieved by combining the mentioned mechanical scan along z with a 10 mT$_{pk}$ harmonic modulation of the offset field along x. The magnetic scan can yield a 20 mm field of view (FOV) along x, while the vertical motion covers 40 mm. The sample position is encoded by a voltage $V_{pos}(t)$ (Fig. 1) that is recorded, together with $I_{scan}(t)$ and $S_{AM}(t)$ by a 16-bit digital storage oscilloscope.

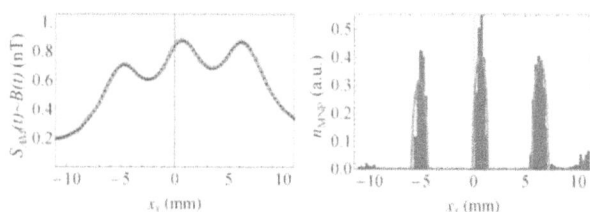

Figure 2: (color online) Left: Raw 1D mechanical AM-MPI image (dots) from three (1.5 mm diameter) tubes containing Resovist. Right: Reconstructed MNP distribution (blue histograms) with sub-mm resolution compared to anticipated distribution (solid magenta lines). The green (solid) line on the left graph is the forward-modeled signal from the inferred distributions on the right graph.

III. Results

Figure 2 shows an example of a 1D mechanical scan of a phantom consisting of 3 identical 1.5 mm diameter glass tubes filled with Resovist, and oriented parallel to the FFL. The extracted MNP distribution reflects well the tubes' cross section. We estimate the spatial resolution to be ~0.75 mm.

Figure 2 shows the first result of a hybrid 2D scanner. The raw 2D MPI image (center of Fig. 3) of an `F'-shaped phantom (Fig. 3, left) is obtained by representing $S_{AM}(I_{scan},V_{pos})$ after proper calibration of I_{scan} and V_{pos}. The blur reflects the finite width of the PSF $L'(x)$. Systematic effects from the offset coil's fringe field at the sensor position are suppressed by subtracting the background recorded separately with no inserted sample. We reconstruct the 2D MNP distribution (Fig. 3, right) by an offline deconvolution using the known PSF, thereby demonstrating 2×3 mm spatial resolution in the horizontal/vertical directions.

We observed comparable signals from structured phantoms filled with either Resovist (featuring a bimodal size distribution [2] with most particles larger than 20 nm) or Ferrotec EMG-700 (mostly containing 10 nm large particles). Both samples had similar iron content, yielding a sensitivity of 45 μg of iron per 25 mm^3 voxel.

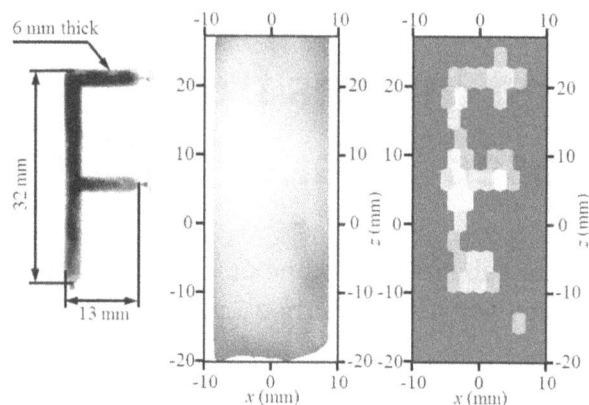

Figure 3: (color online) 2D AM-MPI scanner images: nanoparticle (Resovist, undiluted) phantom (left); recorded induction map (center); reconstructed nanoparticle distribution (right).

IV. Discussion

The demonstrated performance is limited by a trade-off between AM bandwidth and sensitivity. We currently investigate the so-called self-oscillating magnetometer mode of operation, which has the potential of substantially larger bandwidth without compromising the sensitivity. Image resolution can be further improved by forced coil cooling and a 3D FFL hybrid scanner using a rotating sample can be envisioned. The (currently off-line) image reconstruction is computationally not very demanding, and may then be feasible in real time.

V. Conclusions

We have demonstrated 1D/2D MPI imaging with an atomic magnetometer. The AM-MPI has a similar performance than the original MPI scanner [4], while operating at a much lower frequency and giving access to the sample's DC susceptibility.

ACKNOWLEDGEMENTS
Research supported by SNF Grant 200020_162988.

REFERENCES
[1] S. Colombo, V. Lebedev, Z. D. Grujić, V. Dolgovskiy, and A. Weis. MPS and ACS with an atomic magnetometer. *International Journal on Magnetic Particle Imaging*, 2 (1):1606002, 2016. doi: 10.18416/ijmpi.2016.1606002.
[2] S. Colombo, V. Lebedev, Z. D. Grujić, V. Dolgovskiy, and A. Weis. M(H) dependence and size distribution of SPIONs measured by atomic magnetometry. *International Journal on Magnetic Particle Imaging*, 2(1):1604001, 2016. Doi: 10.18416/ijmpi.2016.1604001.
[3] S. Colombo, V. Lebedev, A. Tonyushkin, Z. Grujić, V. Dolgovskiy, and A. Weis. Towards a mechanical mpi scanner based on atomic magnetometry, *International Journal on Magnetic Particle Imaging*, 3(1):1703006, 2017. doi: 10.18416/ijmpi.2017.1703006.
[4] B. Gleich and J. Weizenecker. Tomographic imaging using the nonlinear response of magnetic particles. *Nature*, 435:1214-1217, 2005. doi: 10.1038/nature03808.

A Magnetic Particle Detector for Margin Assessment in Breast-Conserving Surgery

Erica Mason [a,b,*], Clarissa Z. Cooley [b,c], Eli Mattingly [b], Jason Jensen [b], Priscilla Slanetz [d], Lawrence L. Wald [b,c]

[a] Harvard-MIT Health Sciences & Technology, Cambridge, MA, USA
[b] MGH/HST A.A. Martinos Center for Biomedical Imaging, Dept. of Radiology, Massachusetts General Hospital, Boston, MA, USA
[c] Harvard Medical School, Boston, MA, USA
[d] Beth Israel Deaconess Medical Center, Boston, MA, USA
* Corresponding author, email: ericamas@mit.edu

I. Introduction

I.I. Background & Motivation

Breast cancer is the most common cancer in women worldwide; an estimated 316,000 new cases of breast cancer will be diagnosed in 2017 in the US alone [1], [2]. Treatment options for early-stage, small breast tumors are: 1) mastectomy or 2) breast-conserving surgery (BCS, lumpectomy) combined with external radiotherapy. In the case of the breast-conserving approach, however, local tumor recurrence rates are high—23-38% of lumpectomies require reexcision and/or conversion to mastectomy [3], [4]. Recurrence occurs when the entire tumor is not removed—i.e. there are undetected positive margins. In recent years, methods for assessing surgical margins intraoperatively have been investigated, from the adoption of a clinical consensus on inked margins to the development of numerous intraoperative devices [3], [4].

While detection of magnetic particles has been considered for sentinel lymph node biopsy (SLNB) to discern whether breast tumors have metastasized [3], [5], it is also potentially valuable for margin assessment during BCS. To

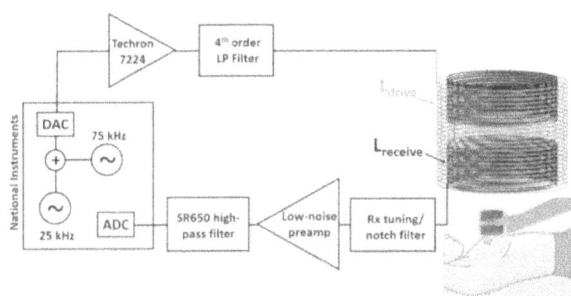

Figure 1: Schematic of MP detector system. Drive chain: NI-DAQ console produces a train of 25kHz sine waves lasting 12ms with adjustable 75kHz cancellation term; signal is amplified, low-pass filtered, and supplied to L_{drive}. Receive chain: Signal from $L_{receive}$ is tuned and notch filtered, amplified, high pass-filtered and sampled by ADC. Designed as handheld detector to be scanned over breast.
(Image of patient adapted from http://www.aafp.org/afp/2007/0601/afp 20070601p1660-f1.jpg)

this end, we propose applying the detection methods of Magnetic Particle Imaging (MPI) to develop a single-sided Magnetic Particle (MP) detector for intraoperative surgical margin assessment.

MPI is a tracer-based imaging modality developed over the past decade that identifies intravenously injected SuperParamagnetic Iron Oxide (SPIO) nanoparticles via their signature nonlinear magnetic response [6]. Through commonly observed passive mechanisms such as the Enhanced Permeability and Retention (EPR) effect, the precise mechanisms of which are still debated, the SPIO tracer will accumulate at tumor sites [7]–[9]. We propose a single-sided, handheld MP detector to detect passively accumulated SPIOs when scanned over tissue after intravenous injection. As the device is intended to be compact, hand-held, and used directly at the tumor location during surgery, spatial encoding is not considered for this application. The high sensitivity of MPI detection offers promise for detecting even slightly positive margins.

I.II. Detection Goals

Assessment of tumor margins via injected SPIOs relies on high-specificity accumulation of the SPIOs at the tumor site. Passive accumulation of coated nanoparticles ranges depending on particle size and coating, from 0.3-26% ID/g [10], [11].The approved human dose of Ferumoxytol is 5-7mg/kg Fe [12], [13]. Assuming a similar 5-7mg/kg dose in a 65kg patient (320-455mg total) and 1% ID/g tumor accumulation, a 1mm-diam. tumor would accumulate 1.7-2.4µg of SPIOs, solely via passive mechanisms. Additionally, active targeting methods, in which functional groups are conjugated to the SPIO coating, would allow for even higher-specificity SPIO accumulation [14], [15]. The work presented here aims initially to detect ~2µg SPIO, and to determine the maximal distance from the end of the detector at which this sample can be identified.

Current MPI systems have demonstrated detection limits down to 5ng Fe (in 2.14s) [16]. We have also developed an MP detector for functional detection in a rodent brain that is similar in technical concept and design to the breast detector, although is smaller and requires less current. It detects 45ng Fe with SNR of 5.4 [17]. By theoretical estimations, MPI has the potential to be sensitive to as little as 1pg Fe [18].

II. Material and Methods

II.I. MP Detector Design

The MP detector is a single-sided detector that does not utilize gradient fields to localize the MPI signal; its spatial localization capabilities are limited to those provided by the sensitive region beyond the detector's surface. The drive coil is a 3.5cm radius, 49 turn, 2-layer solenoid with inductance L = 140μH, wound with 20AWG Litz Wire (New England Wire, Lisbon, NH). It is driven with the NI USB-6363 DAQ (National Instruments, Austin, TX) console; the signal is amplified by an AE Techron (Elkhart, IN) 7224 power amplifier and filtered by a custom high-power low-pass filter. The coil produces 0.5mT at the surface per 1A current supplied (simulated). An adjustable control in the console allows for addition of a small amount of third-order harmonic to the drive field to cancel nonlinearities generated by the power amplifier. A gradiometer receive coil with two oppositely-wound coils (2cm long, 16 turn, 2.96cm radius, 1.1cm spacing) wound with 20 AWG Litz Wire is nested concentrically within the drive coil, providing first-order drive field cancellation. Unlike most MPI systems, we sample only the 3rd harmonic of the drive frequency. The gradiometer is tuned to the 3rd harmonic and notch-filtered to attenuate the drive frequency (59dB attenuation between f_3 and f_0). The received signal is fed into the Signal Recovery 5113

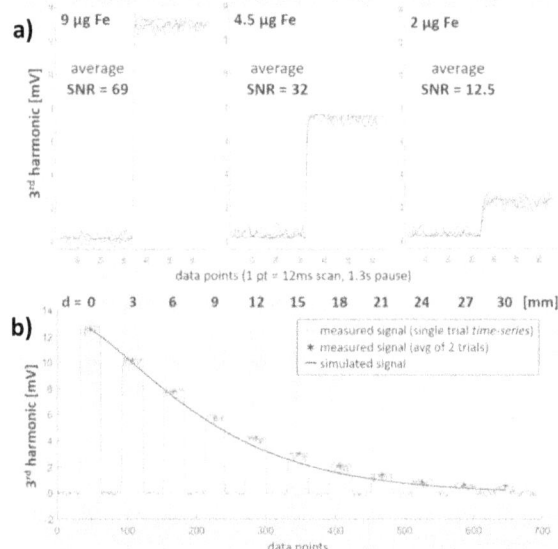

Figure 2: *a) Time-series voltage data for 9, 4.5 and 2μg VivoTrax SPIO samples moved from beyond detectable region (first ~30 data points) to d=0 (at the coil's surface, center of solenoid axis) (second ~30 data points). Each data point is accumulated over a 12ms pulse + 1.3s pause. Multiple runs are overlaid. b)Time-series voltage data of the 9μg Fe sample as it is moved to specified distances from surface (d=0,3,6,...,30mm). Sample is outside detectable region between measurements. A polynomial-fit baseline trend is removed to account for drift. Average measured signal and simulated signal (normalized) are plotted on top of time-series data.*

(Ametek Scientific Instruments, Berwyn, PA) low-noise preamplifier and then the SR650 (Stanford, CA) high-pass filter (cutoff at 40kHz) before console digitization. See Fig. 1 for system schematic.

II.II. Proof-of-Concept Experiments

The drive coil is supplied with a 30A, 25kHz signal to produce a 15mT sinusoidal magnetic field at the drive coil's surface. Samples of VivoTrax dextran coated SPIOs (Magnetic Insight, Alameda, USA) were diluted to concentrations of 0.5mg/ml, 0.25mg/ml, and 0.111mg/ml Fe and housed in 18μl bulbs (thus samples contain 9μg, 4.5μg, and 2μg Fe, respectively). The bulbs are placed in a holder that allows for adjustment of the distance of the sample from the end of the detector, and signal is acquired with 500kHz bandwidth in 12ms burst pulses, with a 1.3s pause between bursts to maintain a low duty cycle (1.22%). Acquired signal is amplified with a gain of 250. We also simulate the coils and MPI signal detection (using our in-house simulation tool implemented in MATLAB (Natick, MA)) for comparison to measurements.

III. Results

Fig. 2 shows time-series data of the received signal as the sample is moved to distances (d) from the surface of the MP detector. A phantom bulb containing 2μg Fe (the estimated passive SPIO uptake in a 1mm-diam. breast tumor) is detected with SNR=12.5 at the coil's surface. Simulated and measured signal show close agreement.

IV. Discussion

We present a custom-built MP detector for intraoperative assessment of tumor margins in breast-conserving surgery and demonstrate initial sensitivity measurements. Future work will investigate methods of noise reduction and additional system improvements to enhance sensitivity below 2μg Fe, as well as to detect SPIOs deeper within the breast tissue (further from the coil's surface).

ACKNOWLEDGEMENTS
Thank you to Suma Anand and Charlotte Sappo for work on the Tx filter. Funding: NIMH R24106053 and NSF GRFP 1122374.

REFERENCES
[1] Oeffinger *et al.*, *JAMA*, 2015.
[2] "How Common Is Breast Cancer?," *The American Cancer Society*. [Online]. Available: https://www.cancer.org/
[3] Thill and Baumann, "Breast Care," 2012.
[4] Morrow *et al.*, *JAMA Oncology*, 2017.
[5] Grafe *et al.*, *Magnetic Particle Imaging: A Novel SPIO Nanoparticle Imaging Technique*, 2015.
[6] Gleich and Weizenecker, *Nature*, 2005.
[7] Maeda *et al.*, *Adv. Drug Deliv. Rev.*, 2013.
[8] Grobmyer *et al.*, *Cancer Nanotechnol.: Methods & Protocols*, 2010.
[9] Heneweer *et al.*, *J. Nucl. Med.*, 2011.
[10] Perrault *et al.*, *Nano Lett.*, 2009.
[11] Lee *et al.*, *Nat. Med.*, 2007.
[12] Christen *et al.*, *Magn. Reson. Med.*, 2013.
[13] Qiu *et al.*, *Neuroimage*, 2012.
[14] Peng *et al.*, *Int. J. Nanomedicine*, 2008.
[15] Thorek *et al.*, *Ann. Biomed. Enginering*, 2006.
[16] M. Graeser *et al.*, *Sci. Rep.*, 2017.
[17] Cooley *et al.*, in *World Molecular Imaging Congress*, 2017.
[18] Gleich, *Principles and Applications of Magnetic Particle Imaging*. 2014.

Session 14 - Talks

Methods II

Metropolis Monte Carlo Simulations of Néel and Brownian Relaxation in Superparamagnetic Nanoparticles

Anton Lord, Marcel Straub, Volkmar Schulz*

Physics of Molecular Imaging, RWTH Aachen University Hospital, Aachen, Germany
* Corresponding author, email: volkmar.schulz@pmi.rwth-aachen.de

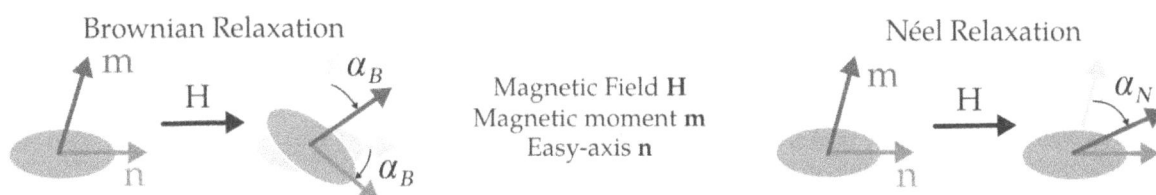

Figure 1: *The two processes governing the dynamic response of SPIONs. The Brownian rotation changes the Zeeman energy of the particle, while Néel changes both the Zeeman and the anisotropy energy.*

I. Introduction

The dynamic magnetic response of superparamagnetic iron oxide nanoparticles (SPIONs) is of great importance for modelling and optimizing magnetic particle imaging (MPI) experiments, and is governed by two mechanisms shown in Fig. 1. Brownian relaxation is when the particle itself rotates, with the magnetic moment remaining fixed relative to the crystal lattice. Conversely, for Néel relaxation, the internal magnetic moment rotates relative to the crystal lattice, keeping the particle fixed in laboratory frame. The two mechanisms may be described by two coupled stochastic differential equations (SDEs) [1], and numerical implementations have recently been investigated [1,2]. We present a Metropolis Monte Carlo (MMC) scheme, capable of simulating the single relaxation processes, and propose a way to couple them while being flexible in terms of parameter distributions and adding inter-particle effects such as dipole-dipole interactions.

II. Materials and Methods

We consider an ensemble of N SPIONs. Each SPION is characterized by a core volume V_C, a saturation magnetization M_S, an anisotropy constant K, anisotropy easy-axis direction n and a normalized magnetic moment m. According to the Stoner-Wohlfarth model, the energy of a particle placed in a magnetic field H is a combination of inner anisotropy and Zeeman energy [3]

$$E = E_A + E_Z = -KV_C(m \cdot n)^2 - M_S V_C(m \cdot H) \quad . \quad (1)$$

In the MMC algorithm, each particle is randomly perturbed, slightly changing the energy of the particle. The perturbations are small rotations of n and m (Brownian relaxation) or just m (Néel relaxation), as described in Fig. 1. The angles α_B and α_N are normally distributed $\alpha_{B,N} \sim N(0, \sigma_{B,N}^2)$ with a corresponding standard deviation $\sigma_{B,N}$. If the energy is lowered, i.e. $\Delta E < 0$, the perturbed state is always accepted as the new state of the particle. If the energy of the particle increases, i.e. $\Delta E > 0$, the so-called Heat Bath algorithm accepts the perturbed state only with a probability of $e^{-\Delta E/k_b T}$, k_B being Boltzmann's constant and T the environment temperature. Trying to change (but not necessarily changing) all of the particles in the system constitutes one Monte Carlo (MC) step, evolving the system in time. However, the physical time represented by an MC step depends on how big the perturbations are, i.e. the standard deviations. To avoid a tedious analysis of how this random process relates to physical time, both relaxation processes were simulated separately by solving the SDEs under simplified circumstances with their corresponding Fokker-Planck (FP) equations [4]. MMC simulations were then performed and fitted to the FP results, yielding two time constants characterizing the Néel and Brownian MC step size separately. Finally, a combined relaxation was simulated by intertwining small perturbations of each type during each MC step. A similar model for Néel relaxation have been solely investigated before [5], but to the best of our knowledge, a MMC model combining Brownian and Néel relaxation has not been presented so far.

To evaluate the relaxation, we simulated a static magnetic field of $12, 14, \ldots, 30$ mT that was instantaneously switched on, i.e. a step function. Corresponding experiments where performed with the MMC model as well as by solving the FP equations. An exponential decay law $M_Z(t) = M_0(1 - e^{-t/\tau_{B,N}})$ was fitted to the magnetization step responses from both models, yielding relaxation times $\tau_{B,N}$. 10 measurement points (per relaxation) were scaled by the same factor to minimize the total relative error between the relaxation times of the MMC model compared to the FP model. Assuming that the MC step is independent of magnetic field, this gives a MC step size dependent on the standard deviation $\sigma_{B,N}$, which was chosen sufficiently small, i.e. to see converging results.

The MMC model was realized as a system of 2940 particles modeled in 2D, i.e. $\mathbf{n}$ and $\mathbf{m}$ were only able to rotate around one axis.

III. Results

For a field strength of 22 mT, Fig. 2 shows the Brownian and Néel as well as the combined relaxation. In contrast to the single processes, an exponential decay law cannot be fitted to the combined relaxation, suggesting a need for a more complex description. To enable comparison with the single processes, a combined relaxation time τ_C was extracted as the point where the magnetization has reached 63 % of its saturated value.

Fig. 3 shows the relation between relaxation time and magnetic field strength for different relaxation types. We see that there is a slight discrepancy between the two models, but that the MMC model captures the main behaviour of the FP model, with the Néel relaxation spanning several orders of magnitude. For Brownian relaxation, the relative error between FP and MMC was on average 1.3 %, maximum 3.4 %, and for Néel on average 9.0 %, maximum 20.7 % for 30 mT. Comparing the combined relaxation to the often used effective relaxation time approximation $\tau_{Eff}^{-1} = \tau_B^{-1} + \tau_N^{-1}$, our results further support the notion of Deissler et al. [1] that this is a problematic description.

IV. Conclusions

We demonstrated a MMC model capable of replicating single Néel and Brownian relaxation in SPIONs. A proposed combined relaxation show disagreement between the often used effective relaxation time approximation and our MMC simulations of up to one order of magnitude. Together with a non-trivial relaxation behavior in time, this suggests that an effective relaxation time is an insufficient description of the process. In our opinion, realistic simulations of these processes are crucial to fully understanding and optimizing MPI experiments.

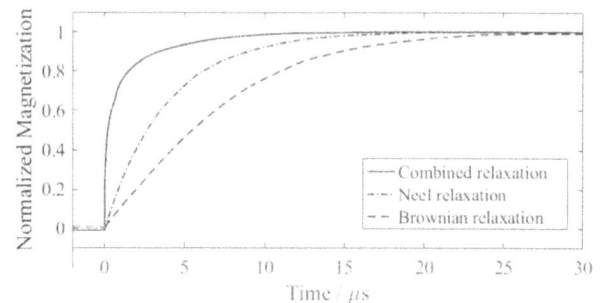

Figure 2: *MMC simulations of single and combined relaxation processes when instantly turning on a field of 22 mT at $t = 0$ ms. The single Néel and Brownian rotations are easily fitted to an exponential law, which is not the case with the combined relaxation.*

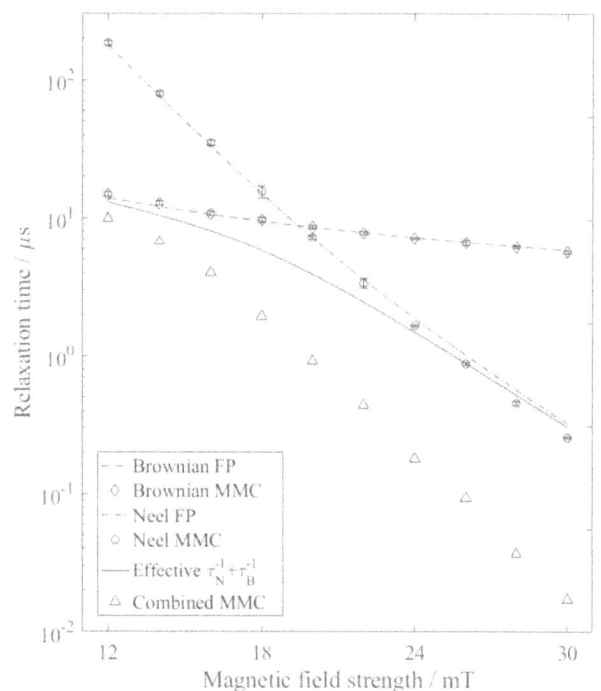

Figure 3: *Relaxation times for single and combined relaxation processes. Dashed lines are from Fokker-Planck simulations of each single process, the full line is the other two combined according to the effective relaxation constant approximation. Markers are from the MMC simulations for each single and combined relaxation. Error bars for the MMC single relaxations show the standard deviation of 5 repetitions. A clear discrepancy between the effective relaxation time and the MMC combined relaxation can be seen, differing with as much as one order of magnitude.*

REFERENCES

[1] M. Graeser, K. Bente, A. Neumann and T.M. Buzug. Trajectory dependent particle response for anisotropic mono domain particles in magnetic particle imaging. J. Phys. D, 49(4):045007, 2016. doi: 10.1088/0022-3727/49/4/045007

[2] D.B. Reeves and J.B. Weaver. Combined Néel and Brown rotational Langevin dynamics in magnetic particle imaging, sensing, and therapy. APL, 107(22):223106, 2015. doi: 10.1063/1.4936930.

[3] M.I. Shliomis and V.I. Stepanov. Theory of the Dynamic Susceptibility of Magnetic Fluids. *John Wiley & Sons, Inc.*, 1994. doi: 10.1002/9780470141465.ch1.

[4] R.J. Deissler, Y. Wu and M.A. Martens. Dependence of Brownian and Néel relaxation times on magnetic field strength. *Medical Physics*, 41(1):012301, 2014. doi: 10.1118/1.4837216.

[5] R. Tan, J. Carrey, M. Respaud. Magnetic hyperthermia properties of nanoparticles inside lysosomes using kinetic Monte Carlo simulations: Influence of key parameters and dipolar interactions, and evidence for strong spatial variation of heating power. *Phys. Rev. B*, 90(21):214421, 2014. doi: 10.1103/PhysRevB.90.214421

Relaxation Modeling and First Harmonic Recovery in Magnetic Particle Imaging

Ines Ayed [a,*], Marcel Straub [a], Volkmar Schulz [a]

[a] Physics of Molecular Imaging Systems, RWTH Aachen University Hospital, Aachen, Germany
[*] Ines Ayed, email: mpi@pmi.rwth-aachen.de

I. Introduction

Magnetic Particle imaging (MPI) is a novel functional imaging modality that offers a great potential in the field of tomographic imaging. It measures the spatial distribution of superparamagnetic iron oxide nanoparticles (SPIONs) by superimposing a static gradient field with homogeneous dynamic fields. The gradient field generates a field free point (FFP). Only those SPIONs in the vicinity of the FFP are affected by the dynamic fields. The dynamic fields, so called drive fields (DF), are used to change the magnetization of the SPIONs forth-and-backwards and to move the position of the FFP. The derived relation between time and position of the measured SPIONs is utilized by the *x-space* reconstruction [1].

In x-space MPI the magnetization of the SPIONs is usually modelled by the Langevin model, which assumes a thermodynamic equilibrium. For MPI, this does not hold because the frequency of the DFs is much higher than the relaxation times of the SPIONs. Hence, the reconstructed native image is blurred which is usually enhanced by deconvolution [2].

Since MPI does measure the SPIONs magnetization change while changing it, it is required to remove the excitation frequency, e.g. with a notch-filter, from the measured signal. In x-space MPI, the removal of the first harmonic causes intensity loss of the signal. Several groups are working on recovering this information loss. However, limitations are still reported: the relaxation's modeling lack of field-dependency [3], as well as the need for a-priori knowledge and the high computational complexity of the current first harmonic restoration technique [4].

This contribution addresses the modelling of the SPIONs' relaxation times and the loss of the first harmonic in magnetic particle spectroscopy (MPS). We present an experimental verification of the suggested methods.

II. Material and Methods

We model the non-equilibrium signal of the SPIONs by adopting the Debye theory of ferrofluids [5,6]. This allows the description of the relaxation blurring as a convolution of the magnetization with an exponentially decaying relaxation kernel k that is given by $k(t) = \tau^{-1} \cdot \exp(-t/\tau)$, for $t > 0$, where t is the time and τ is the relaxation time. Based on the x-space signal formulation

presented in [1] and the relaxation kernel $k(t)$, we derive the non-equilibrium signal equation

$$u^{ne}(t) = \sigma_r m \left[\rho(x) * \dot{L}\big(\beta G x_{FFP}(t)\big) * k(t) \right] \cdot \beta G \dot{x}_{FFP}(t)$$

with receive coil sensitivity σ_r, magnetic moment m of the particle, spatial tracer distribution $\rho(x)$, Langevin function L, a particle property (in m/A) β, gradient G, and FFP position $x_{FFP}(t)$. This fulfills the relation $u^{ne}(t) = u^e(t) * k(t)$, where $u^e(t)$ is the equilibrium x-space formulation from [1].

For a one-dimensional sinusoidal drive field, the FFP passes the same position twice during one period: in forward and backward direction. The voltage trace of the matching time ranges we call u_f^{ne} and u_r^{ne}, respectively. In frequency domain we can derive the relaxation time analytically as

$$\tau(x,f) = \frac{1}{j2\pi f} \cdot \frac{\big(U_f^{ne}(x,f)\big)^{\dagger} + U_r^{ne}(x,f)}{\big(U_f^{ne}(x,f)\big)^{\dagger} - U_r^{ne}(x,f)}$$

where $U_f^{ne}(x,f)$ and $U_r^{ne}(x,f)$ are the Fourier transformed of the time domain signals u_f^{ne} and u_r^{ne}.

The resulting τ is an effective relaxation time describing the observed blurring of an observed point spread function (PSF). For example, with a Wiener deconvolution it is now possible to restore the thermal-equilibrium signal and reconstruct an image without blurring degradation.

However, the removal of the first harmonic from the measured SIPON signal renders this deconvolution less robust. We recover the first harmonic by fitting the phenomenologically derived equations

$$y_{i,real} = \frac{1}{1+(\varphi x_i)^2}\left[r + x_i \varphi \left(a \exp\left(-bx_i^p\right) + c \right) \right]$$

$$y_{i,imag} = \frac{1}{1+(\varphi x_i)^2}\left[\left(a \exp\left(-bx_i^p\right) + c \right) - x_i \varphi\, r \right]$$

respectively to real and imaginary spectrum. Here, i denotes the index of the harmonic, $y_{i,real/imag}$ the value of the real and imaginary component of the signal, respectively, x_i is the frequency of the i-th harmonic, and $\varphi = 2\pi f_D \tau$ represents the phase lag caused by the relaxation time at an excitation frequency f_D. For the fit, the direct harmonics, starting with the third, of the spectrum with an SNR of above 4 are used.

The above described methods were verified with means of spectroscopy measurements using two different tracer samples: a sample from the commercial Perimag® (Micromod GmbH, Germany) series and an in-house sample called C2 (RWTH Aachen Medical Faculty, Germany). The measurements were conducted at a fixed excitation frequency of 24.25 kHz and different magnetic field values ranging from 10 $mT\mu_0^{-1}$ to 25 $mT\mu_0^{-1}$.

III. Results

The calculated relaxation times were found to decrease with increasing applied magnetic field for both used phantoms. The suggested spectral model for the first harmonic recovery enabled the restoration of the fundamental wave. The positivity of the MPS signal was restored as perceived in Fig. 1 for Perimag® at a drive field amplitude 25 $mT\mu_0^{-1}$. The intensity of the corrected signal increased by 50%.

Fig. 2 displays a comparison between the theoretical Langevin PSF, the measured PSF as well as the measured and corrected PSF. It is evident that the suggested method restores the Langevin PSF shape, which goes along with an enhanced magnetic resolution.

To quantify the resolution enhancement, we used the Houston resolution criterion that estimates a system's resolution with the FWHM of the PSF. The results are shown in Fig. 3. The resolution enhancement of C2 and Perimag® averaged out at 53.7% and 65.8%, respectively.

IV. Conclusions

In this contribution, we explored the tracer dynamics involved in MPI. The presented model is based on an extension of the Langevin theory with the Debye model for ferrofluids, whereas the latter was modified to phenomenologically account for the field-dependency of the relaxation times. The potential of the proposed method was demonstrated through experimental spectroscopic evaluation. The deconvolution by the relaxation times, leads to an enhanced FWHM. The recovery of the first harmonic rendered the positivity of the signal and enhanced its intensity.

REFERENCES

[1] Goodwill, P.; Conolly, S. (2010): *The X-Space Formulation of the Magnetic Particle Imaging Process: 1-D Signal, Resolution, Bandwidth, SNR, SAR, and Magnetostimulation.* In: IEEE transactions on medical imaging 29 (11), S. 1851-1559. doi: 10.1109/TMI.2010.2052284

[2] Goodwill, P.; Lu, K.; Zheng, B.; Conolly, S. (2012): *An x-space magnetic particle imaging scanner.* In: Review of Scientific Instruments 83 (3), S. 033708. doi: 10.1063/1.3694534

[3] Croft, L.; Goodwill, P.; Conolly, S. (2012): *Relaxation in x-space magnetic particle imaging.* In: IEEE transactions on medical imaging 31 (12), S. 2335-2342. doi: 10.1109/TMI.2012.2217979.

[4] Lu, K.; Goodwill, P.; Saritas, E.; Zheng, B.; Conolly, S. (2013): *Linearity and shift invariance for quantitative magnetic particle imaging.* In: IEEE transactions on medical imaging 32 (9), S. 1565-1575. doi: 10.1109/TMI.2013.2257177.

[5] Debye, P. (1929): *Polar Molecules.* The Chemical Catalog Company, Inc., New York, 1929.

[6] Goodwill, P.; Tamrazian, A.; Croft, L.; Lu, C.; Johnson, E.; Pidaparthi, R.; Ferguson, R.; Khandhar, A.; Krishnan, K.; Conolly, S. (2011):

Ferrohydrodynamic relaxometry for magnetic particle imaging. In: Applied Physics Letters 98, 262502. doi:10.1063/1.3604009

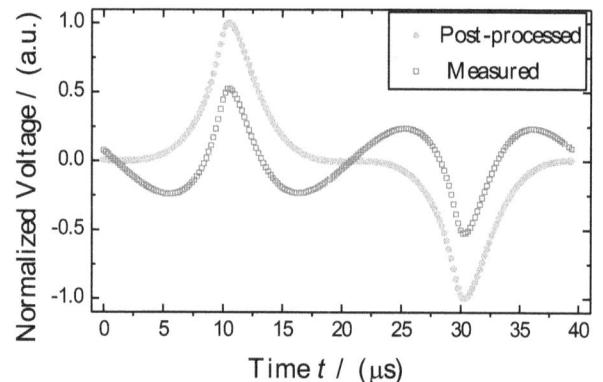

Figure 1: *Restoration of the first harmonic. Experimental MPS data of a Perimag® phantom at $H_D = 25$ $mT\mu_0^{-1}$ reconstructed without (□) and with (•) the proposed recovery method. The post-processed signal shows a higher intensity and a restored positivity i.e. a constancy around the zero-crossing area.*

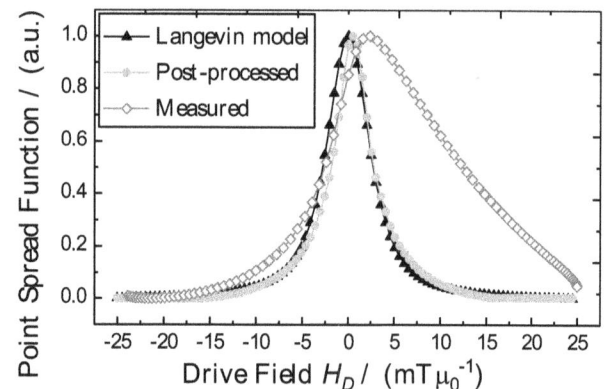

Figure 2: *PSF of Perimag® at $H_D = 25$ $mT\mu_0^{-1}$. Prior to the relaxation deconvolution (□), the PSF is broad and exhibits an asymmetric shape because of relaxation blur. The outcome of the relaxation deconvolution step (•) shows a good similarity to the theoretically expected Langevin PSF (▲). It is symmetric and as narrow as the theoretical PSF.*

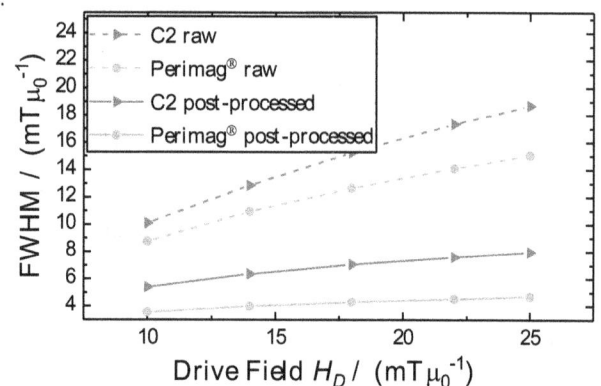

Figure 3: *Magnetic resolution (MR) of Perimag® and C2 at different drive field strength as well as with and without relaxation deconvolution. MR is defined as the FWHM of the PSFs. Experimental MR before and after relaxation deconvolution (dotted lines, solid lines) at several applied magnetic field values. A smaller FWHM value indicates a finer resolution.*

Stochastic Simulations of Magnetic Particles: Comparison of Different Methods

Alexander Neumann [a,*], Thorsten M. Buzug [a]

[a] Institute of Medical Engineering, Universität zu Lübeck, Lübeck, Germany
[*] Corresponding author, email: neumann@imt.uni-luebeck.de

I. Introduction

The behavior of magnetic (nano-)particles or structures are of interest for a broad range of applications ranging from information storage to medical applications. Micromagnetic simulation frameworks such as OOMMF [1], MicroMagnum [2], MuMax3 [3], VAMPIRE [4], FIDIMAG [5], etc. are commonly used to simulate the behavior of various magnetic materials or structures under different conditions. In general, those frameworks use a finite element approach to model the object of interest and solve the corresponding partial differential equation for each element. The equation used in the micromagnetic domain is the Landau-Lifschitz-Gilbert (LLG) equation or modified version of it including additional effects [1-5].

For medical applications, such as magnetic particle imaging (MPI) or magnetic particle hyperthermia, no general framework exist and the mentioned frameworks are not applicable because they do not include the possibility of the free mechanical rotation of the particles. Furthermore, those frameworks focus mainly on solving the ordinary differential equations (ODE) so that thermal effects are not properly taken into account. To include thermal effects the corresponding stochastic differential equations (SDE) and an appropriate solving method, such as the Euler-Maruyama method [6], have to be used. The mechanical (Brownian) rotation of the particles is given by the stochastic Euler equations of rotational motion and must be coupled to the stochastic LLG for a combined model (Yolk-Egg model as described in [7, 8]). This work compares the different published methods [9-11] solving the stochastic LLG and Euler equations, explains why the currently used methods in MPI [11-13] are not sufficient and introduces a general method that is fast and works for all possible cases without any additional limitations.

II. Material and Methods

In the following, the necessary equations to represent the motion of particles and magnetization are presented.

II.I. Landau-Lifschitz-Gilbert Equation

The Landau-Lifschitz-Gilbert equation describes the motion of the magnetization and is given by

$$\frac{\partial \vec{m}}{\partial t} = \underbrace{-\frac{\gamma}{1+\alpha^2} \vec{H}_{\text{eff}} \times \vec{m}}_{\vec{\omega}_{\text{L}}} + \underbrace{\frac{|\gamma|\alpha}{(1+\alpha^2)} \left(\vec{m} \times \vec{H}_{\text{eff}} \right) \times \vec{m}}_{\vec{\omega}_{\text{R}}}. \quad (1)$$

$\vec{m}$ is the unit magnetisation vector, α is the damping constant, γ is the (electron) gyromagnetic ratio and $\vec{H}_{\text{eff}}$ is the effective magnetic field given by (assuming uniaxial anisotropy) $\vec{H}_{\text{eff}} = 2K_{\text{u}}/M_{\text{S}} \left(\vec{m} \cdot \vec{n} \right) \vec{n} + \vec{H}_{\text{ext}} + \vec{H}_{\text{noise}}$. K_{u} is the anistropy constant, M_{S} is the saturation magnetization, $\vec{n}$ is the direction of the uniaxial anisotropy, $\vec{H}_{\text{ext}}$ is the external magnetic field and $\vec{H}_{\text{noise}}$ is a Gaussian white noise field.

II.II. Euler Equation

Euler's equations are used to describe the rotation of a rigid body. For particles in a viscose medium the equation is given by

$$I\frac{\partial \vec{\omega}_n}{\partial t} + \vec{\omega}_n \times I\vec{\omega}_n + 6\eta V_{\text{h}}(\vec{\omega}_n - \Omega) = \vec{\tau}_{\text{eff}}. \quad (2)$$

I is the inertia matrix, $\vec{\omega}_n$ is the angular velocity, η is the viscosity, Ω is the vorticity, V_{h} is the hydrodynamic volume and $\vec{\tau}_{\text{eff}} = 2K_{\text{u}}V_{\text{m}}(\vec{m} \cdot \vec{n})\vec{m} + \vec{\tau}_{\text{ext}} + \vec{\tau}_{\text{noise}}$ is the effective torque acting on the particle. (V_{m} is the magnetic volume of the particle). To simplifiy the equations it is assumed that I and Ω are (nearly) zero [7, 8] reducing the equation to $6\eta V_{\text{h}}\vec{\omega}_n = \vec{\tau}_{\text{eff}}$. To describe the orientation of a particle, a coordinate system associated with the particle must be defined. This defintion can either be done by using Euler angles or – in the case of uniaxial anisotropy – by only using the direction of the uniaxial axis $\vec{n}$ (as it is typically done in MPI [11-13]) which yields $\partial \vec{n}/\partial t = \vec{\omega}_n \times \vec{n}$.

II.III. Combined Equations

To combine equations (1) and (2) one has to use Newton's third law [7]. Since the magnetization can relax by a rotation of the particle, $\vec{\omega}_R$ in (1) must be replaced by the solution of

$$6\eta_m V_m(\vec{\omega}_R - \vec{\omega}_n) = M_S V_m(\vec{m} \times \vec{H}_{\text{eff}}) \quad (3)$$

where $\eta_m = M_S(1 + \alpha^2)/(6|\gamma|\alpha)$ is the magnetic viscosity. On the other hand, the relaxation of the magnetization creates an opposite force on the particle which alters equation (2) to

$$6\eta V_{\text{h}}\vec{\omega}_n + 6\eta_m V_m(\vec{\omega}_n - \vec{\omega}_R) = \vec{\tau}_{\text{eff}}. \quad (4)$$

II.IV. Stochastic Differential Equations

Equations (1) and (2) with the alterations (3) and (4) are SDEs, which cannot be solved with the methods of ODEs. One explicit solving method is the Euler-Maruyama scheme, which reads [6]

$$\vec{x}_{i+1} = \vec{x}_i + \left(\vec{a}(\vec{x}_i, t_i) + \vec{d}(\vec{x}_i, t_i) \right) \Delta t + b(\vec{x}_i, t_i) \Delta \vec{W}. \quad (5)$$

$\vec{x}_i$ ($\vec{x}_{i+1}$) is the current (next) state, $\vec{a}$ is the deterministic part, b is the stochastic matrix, $d_i = \frac{1}{2} b_{kj} \, \partial b_{ij}/\partial x_k$ is the drift correction, Δt is the time step and $\Delta \vec{W}$ is Gaussian white noise with zero mean and $\sqrt{\Delta t}$ width. $\vec{a}$, b and $\vec{d}$ are determined from the modified equations (1) and (2).

II.V. Implementation Details

Equations (1) and (2) have been implemented in Cartesian coordinates/uniaxial direction as well as spherical coordinates/Euler angles. The former is generally faster but limited to axial potentials whereas the latter is universal in usage but needs extra care due to numerical singularities at some angles. Furthermore, eq. (5) is not norm conserving in Cartesian coordinates making normalization of the unit vectors after each step necessary.

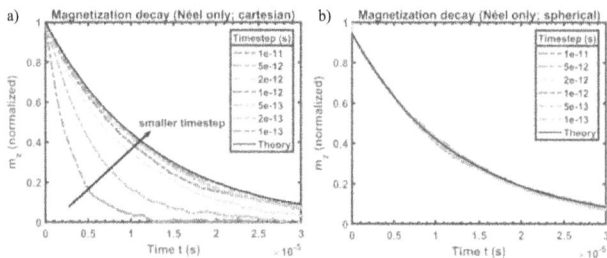

Figure 1: *Simulated magnetization decay of 10000 particles using Cartesian (a) and spherical coordinates (b). In (a) the simulation shows strong deviations from the theoretical behavior for larger time steps whereas in (b) the simulated and theoretical behavior are very similar even for bigger time steps. This indicates that spherical coordinates are better suited for obtaining the correct physical behavior.*

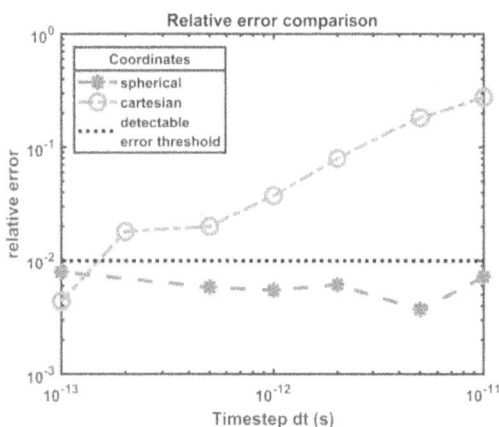

Figure 2: *Relative error extracted from Fig. 1 by calculating the sum of distances between simulation and theoretical behavior divided by the number of points (mean absolute error). The detectable error threshold is given by the inverse square root from the number of simulated particles. Using spherical coordinates gives an error below the detection threshold within the simulated range of time steps.*

III. Results and Discussion

To compare the different implementations, comparison tests have been performed. One of the test cases is the magnetization decay $M(t) = M_0 \exp(-t/\tau)$ of an aligned particle ensemble allowing only the motion of the magnetization with a first mean passage time τ of 12.4 µs [14]. Fig. 1 shows the results for Cartesian and spherical coordinates using different time steps Δt. For Cartesian coordinates a big difference between theoretical behavior and simulated behavior is observed whereas in spherical coordinates both agree very well and the error is below the detection threshold within the simulated range (Fig. 2). Additional results using the combined model will be presented.

V. Conclusions

From the performed studies it is evident that for simulations in Cartesian coordinates only very small time steps ($\ll 10$ ps) lead to the correct physical behavior. Although using spherical coordinates is about a factor of 2 to 4 slower per step, correct results even for bigger time steps makes it superior. The problem with using Cartesian coordinates is that eq. (5) is not norm conserving and normalization after each step is necessary. Without normalization, the simulations become unstable as shown in [15]. There are implicit methods like the midpoint scheme that are able to conserve the norm [9, 15] but due to the additional 100 to 10000 iterations needed for the implicit solver to converge those methods are too slow for practical usage. On a modern CPU (i7 7700K) the performed simulations using spherical coordinates run at approx. 250 ns/step. Without particle interactions, the simulations are parallelizable making it possible to simulate system matrices for MPI in adequate time by using an HPC cluster.

ACKNOWLEDGEMENTS

Funding by the Federal Ministry of Education and Research via the Project SAMBA-PATI (FKZ: 13GW0069A) is gratefully acknowledged.

REFERENCES

[1] M.J. Donahue & D.G. Porter. OOMMF User's Guide, Version 1.0, Interagency Report NISTIR 6376
[2] http://micromagnum.informatik.uni-hamburg.de/
[3] A. Vansteenkiste et al. AIP Advances 4, 107133 (2014)
[4] R. F. L. Evans et al. J. Phys.: Condens. Matter 26, 103202 (2014)
[5] David Cortés-Ortuño et al. (2016). Fidimag v2.0. Zenodo. http://doi.org/10.5281/zenodo.167858
[6] P. E. Kloeden & E. Platen. Numerical Solution of Stochastic Differential Equations, 2 ed. ,Springer (1995)
[7] M. I. Shliomis & V. I. Stepanov. Adv. Chem. Phys. Vol. 87, 1 (1994)
[8] W. T. Coffey & Y. P. Kalmykov. The Langevin Equation 3rd Ed. World Scientific (2012)
[9] M. d'Aquino et al. J. Appl. Phys. 99, 08B905 (2006).
[10] F. Roma et al. Phys. Rev. E. 90, 023203 (2014)
[11] J. Weizenecker et al. Phys. Med. Biol. 57, 7317-7327 (2012)
[12] M Graeser et al. J. Phys. D: Appl. Phys. 49, 045007 (2016)
[13] S. A. Shah et al. Phys. Rev. B 92, 094438 (2015)
[14] W. T. Coffey & Y. P. Kalmykov. J. Appl. Phys. 112, 121301 (2012)
[15] L. Banas et al. Stochastic Ferromagnetism. De Gruyter (2014)

Increasing the MPI Frame Rate by Excitation Signal Phase-Shifting and Receive-Signal Splitting

Anselm von Gladiss [a,*], Matthias Graeser [b,c], Thorsten M. Buzug [a]

[a] Institute of Medical Engineering, University of Lübeck, Lübeck, Germany
[b] Section for Biomedical Imaging, University Medical Center Hamburg-Eppendorf, Hamburg, Germany
[c] Institute for Biomedical Imaging, Hamburg University of Technology, Hamburg, Germany
* Corresponding author, email: {gladiss,buzug}@imt.uni-luebeck.de

I. Introduction

In Magnetic Particle Imaging (MPI), magnetic particles are excited by a sinusoidal magnetic field that drives the particles along their magnetisation curve towards saturation. A receive signal can be detected whose spectrum contains the excitation frequency and higher harmonics (see Fig. 2). Superposing a gradient field enables spatial encoding. The gradient field features a field free region, e.g. a field free point (FFP). Now, mainly the particles nearby the FFP contribute to the receive signal. The exciting magnetic field drives the FFP over the field of view (FOV) and therefore samples the FOV along a trajectory. In multidimensional imaging, different excitation fields of similar frequencies can be superposed from different spatial directions forming a Lissajous trajectory (see Fig. 1) [1].

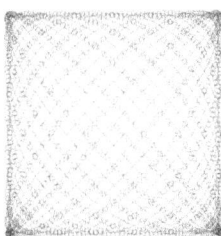

Sine wave Lissajous   Cosine wave Lissajous

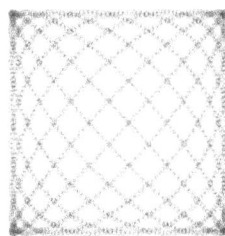

Figure 1: Lissajous trajectory in MPI using sine waves (left) and cosine waves (right). The first half (drawn line) and second half (dots) of the trajectory are shown separately. Using cosine waves, the sampling grid of the FOV is thinner and the first and second halves sample the same spatial positions.

As frequencies for the excitation field, frequencies nearby 25 kHz are common. Typical Lissajous trajectory periods are 0.65 ms and 21.54 ms for 2D and 3D imaging resulting in a possible frame rate per image of 1532 Hz and 46 Hz. With an imaging rate of 46 Hz per volume and a spatial resolution of about 1 mm, biological processes that have a velocity of about 0.025 m/s may be displayed as a movement from voxel to voxel following the Nyquist sampling theorem. The blood flow in human arteries that may have a velocity of 0.05 m/s could not be monitored exploiting the full spatial resolution of an MPI measurement. An increase in the frame rate by the factor of 2 could help for this. This work aims for increasing the frame rate for two-dimensional imaging by manipulating the phase of the excitation signal.

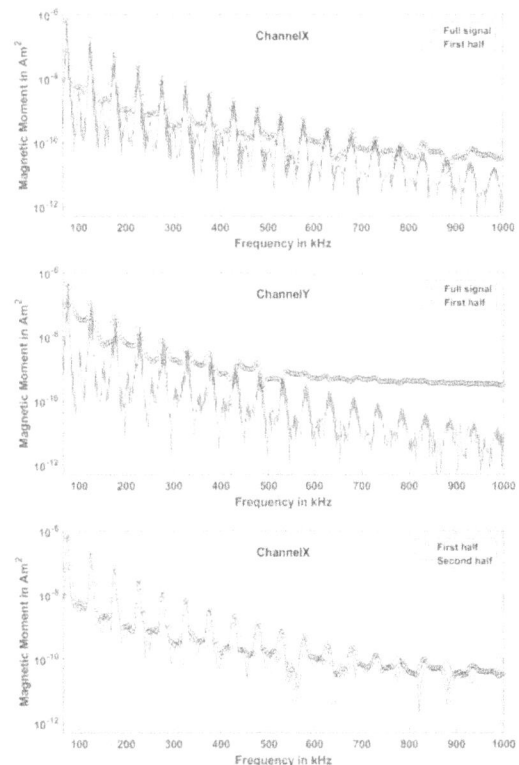

Figure 2: Amplitude spectra of measured signals. Top: Spectra of the entire receive signal and the first half of the x-channel. Middle: Same as top but of the y-channel. Bottom: Spectra of the first and second half receive signal of the x-channel.

II. Material and Methods

II.I. Splitting the Receive Signal

In order to increase the imaging rate of an MPI measurement, the phase of the magnetic excitation field is changed from sine to cosine excitation. Then, the Lissajous trajectory is symmetric at its temporal centre. This is due to the symmetric behaviour of cosine waves. The receive signal is split at its centre and the spectra of both halves are calculated (see Fig. 2 bottom). Then, the single spectra may be reconstructed separately resulting in two images per measurement frame. A corresponding system matrix needs to be acquired whose receive signal is split in half resulting in two system matrices for the two halves of the trajectory period.

II.II. Measurements and Reconstruction

The system matrices needed for reconstruction have been acquired with a multidimensional magnetic particle spectrometer [2, 3]. The single cube phantom measurements have been carried out using a commercially available MPI scanning device.

Image reconstruction has been performed using an unregularized Kaczmarz algorithm with 1 iteration when using the entire receive signal and 20 iterations when using only half of it [4]. Furthermore, the frequencies used for reconstruction have been selected based on their SNR using a threshold of 100 with a minimum frequency of 85 kHz and a maximum frequency of 1.25 MHz.

III. Results

A comparison of the amplitude spectra of an entire receive signal and halves of it are visualised in Fig. 2. The amplitudes of the half-signals match those of the entire signal at the harmonics and neighbouring frequencies up to about 800 kHz and 550 kHz at the x-channel and y-channel, respectively. Both the spectra of the half-signals match at the harmonics up to about 750 kHz.

Fig. 3 shows the reconstruction results of the single cube measurements. In all the reconstructed images the phantom has been reconstructed to a similar spatial position. However, reconstruction artefacts as background noise and fringing of the phantom can be observed when reconstructing with only half the receive signal.

IV. Discussion

The amplitude spectra in Fig. 2 show a mismatch of harmonics at higher frequencies and intermediate frequencies between the entire receive signal and the half-signals. An analysis of the time signal shows that the split receive signal is not fully periodically, which may be caused by a shift of the excitation signal. In Fourier domain artefacts arise that may induce reconstruction artefacts as in Fig. 3 (c) and (d) including a varying spatial position.

The spectral resolution is decreased when using a split receive signal. This may decrease the spatial resolution for multidimensional MPI as mixing frequencies are not resolved.

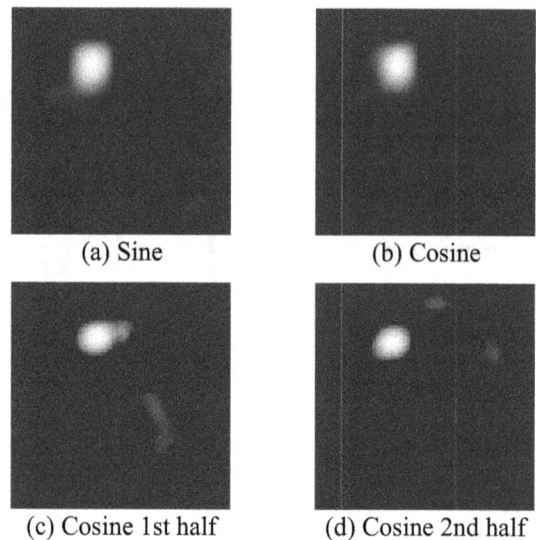

(a) Sine   (b) Cosine

(c) Cosine 1st half   (d) Cosine 2nd half

Figure 3: *Reconstruction results of a single cube phantom measurement using the entire receive signal performing (a) sine and (b) cosine excitation and (c, d) using the halves of the receive signal using cosine excitation.*

V. Conclusions

It has been shown that the receive signal of an MPI measurement can be split in order to increase the imaging rate of an MPI scanner when exciting with cosine waves. Image reconstruction can be performed successfully using only half of the receive signal. Additional symmetries of the excitation trajectory might be found that increase the imaging rate even more.

It needs to be analysed if the spatial resolution of an MPI measurement remains constant when applying cosine excitation as then only half of the FOV is sampled (see Fig. 1). If so, the spatial resolution should be constant when using only half of the receive signal as the spatial sampling does not change. However, the impact of mixing frequencies on the spatial resolution needs to be investigated.

In this work, increasing the imaging rate has been performed with a two dimensional dataset. Applying the same method on three dimensional data will exploit the full use for clinical practice. Then, a higher imaging rate of three dimensional volumes might enable the monitoring of fast biological processes as the blood flow in human arteries at full spatial resolution.

ACKNOWLEDGEMENTS

The authors thankfully acknowledge the financial support by the German Research Foundation (DFG, grant number BU 1436/10-1) and the Federal Ministry of Education and Research (BMBF, grant number 13GW0069A).

REFERENCES

[1] B. Gleich and J. Weizenecker. *Nature*, 2005.
    doi: 10.1038/nature03808.
[2] A. von Gladiss, M. Graeser, et al. *PMB*, 2017.
    doi: 10.1088/1361-6560/aa5340.
[3] M. Graeser, A. von Gladiss, et al. *PMB*, 2017.
    doi: 10.1088/1361-6560/aa5bcd.
[4] T. Knopp, J. Rahmer, et al. *PMB*, 2010.
    doi: 10.1088/0031-9155/55/6/003.

Stenosis Analysis by Synergizing MPI and Intravascular OCT

Florian Griese [a,b,*], **Sarah Latus** [c], **Matthias Gräser**[a,b], **Martin Möddel**[a,b], **Matthias Schlüter**[c], **Christoph Otte**[c], **Thore Saathoff**[c], **Alexander Schlaefer**[c] **and Tobias Knopp**[a]

[a] *Section for Biomedical Imaging, University Medical Center Hamburg Eppendorf, Hamburg, Germany*
[b] *Institute for Biomedical Imaging, Hamburg University of Technology, Hamburg, Germany*
[c] *Institute of Medical Technology, Hamburg University of Technology, Hamburg, Germany*
[*] *Corresponding author, email: f.griese@uke.de*

I. Introduction

Magnetic Particle Imaging (MPI) proved to resolve super-paramagnetic iron oxide particles (SPIO) with high temporal resolution, full 3D spatial resolution and high sensitivity [1]. With these characteristics, MPI was successfully used for interventional application labeling medical instruments such as catheters and guide wires [2-4]. Simple navigation experiments with coated instruments were demonstrated at high temporal resolution. In [5] Salamon et al. cleared an artificial stenosis with a coated balloon catheter and used Resovist as a tracer to verify the clearance of the stenosis. Further, multi-color MPI was used to differentiate between two different types of tracer material, one coated to the catheter and the other used as blood pool tracer [6]. Recently, MPI proved to be a suitable imaging modality to quantify vascular stenosis and to determine the degree of stenosis [7]. However, as analyzed by Vaalma et al. [7] the degree of stenosis could be determined quite well although the spatial resolution still lacks behind digital subtraction angiography (DSA) providing sub-millimeter resolution [8]. In comparison with DSA, low gradient MPI has only a resolution of a few millimeters. To overcome this limitation, we combine MPI with intravascular OCT (IVOCT). IVOCT provides micrometer scale axial resolution while acquiring A-scans with a high temporal resolution. The penetration depth is only a few millimeter, but IVOCT is able to asses vascular walls and distinguish between healthy tissue and different plaque stages and formation [9]. IVOCT benefits from an additional imaging modality to determine the catheter's position in order to reconstruct morphologically correct 3D volume images. DSA provides only 2D projection information [10] while MPI has full 3D spatial information. MPI is non-ionizing and allows a longer imaging time by using tracers that stay in the blood pool over several hours. The low spatial resolution of low gradient MPI can be mitigated with a sub-voxel approach presented in [11] allowing for position estimation in the sub-millimeter range. The combination of MPI and IVOCT uses the strengths of both modalities (no radiation, high spatial resolution, high temporal resolution) and compensates for the individual weaknesses of each modality. In this work, we analyze a steady stenosis phantom to show the potential of combining MPI with IVOCT.

II. Material and Methods

MPI measurements are performed with a preclinical MPI scanner (Philips/Bruker) with sinusoidal excitation fields. Perimag (micromod) with an iron concentration of 10 mmol/l is used as MPI tracer. The estimated 3D positions of the IVOCT catheter head is retrieved from the static 3D MPI tomogram by calculating the center of mass slice-wise within the yz-plain as in [11]. The IVOCT measurements are done with the catheter Dragonfly Duo Kit (St. Jude Medical) in combination with a commercial OCT acquisition device (Thorlabs, Telesto I). The OCT device offers an A-scan rate of 91 kHz and a customized catheter driver is able to rotate the catheter with a velocity of 1000 rpm. The pullback of the catheter is performed with a pullback velocity of 0.75 mm/s over a distance of 25 mm. A constant refractive index of water 1.33 is assumed for the A-scan resulting in a pixel spacing of 4.5 μm/px.

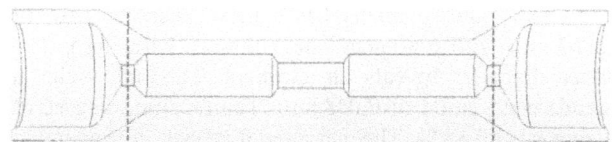

Figure 1: *CAD drawing of the stenosis phantom with outer diameter of 2.5 mm and inner diameter of 1.5 mm. The dashed lines mark the two constrictions that are used as landmarks for co-registration of MPI and IVOCT.*

IVOCT and MPI measurements are performed with a stenosis phantom shown in Fig. 1. It has a length of 20 mm, an outer diameter of 2.5 mm and an inner diameter of 1.5 mm resulting in a degree of stenosis of 64% calculated as in [7]. At first, the stenosis phantom is filled with Perimag and a static 3D MPI volume is acquired. Afterwards, the IVOCT catheter is moved inside the stenosis phantom and the OCT data is acquired while the catheter rotates and is slowly pulled back.

III. Results

In Fig. 2 the native volumetric IVOCT reconstruction is shown and it becomes visible that the shape is twisted and contains rotational artifacts due to missing position information.

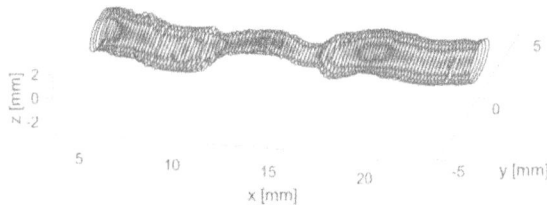

Figure 2: Native volumetric IVOCT reconstruction without the catheters position information.

The volumetric IVOCT reconstruction using the estimated catheter position determined slice-wise from the MPI volume image can be seen in Fig. 3. The IVOCT MPI reconstruction shows no artifacts and its shape and dimensions agree very nicely with the ground truth from the CAD drawings.

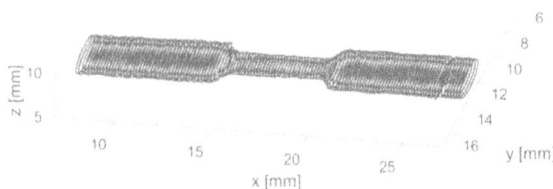

Figure 3: Volumetric IVOCT reconstruction with position information.

The mean outer diameter has a mean absolute error of 0.063 mm with a standard deviation of 0.026 mm. The inner diameter reveals an error of 0.093 mm with a standard deviation of 0.048 mm. The resulting degree of stenosis is 69.84 %. The measured diameters for inner and outer diameters are shown in Fig. 4.

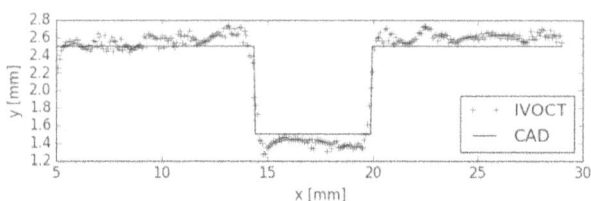

Figure 4: Diameter of volumetric IVOCT reconstruction with position information.

IV. Discussion

The presented method combining IVOCT and MPI shows a high precision in determining the diameters of the stenosis. The slice-wise center of mass approach using MPI volume images provides accurate enough 3D coordinates to reconstruct the volumetric IVOCT image. However, it could be further improved by using a MPI marker attached to the catheters head that could be tracked during pullback. With this improvement, a non-linear pullback behavior caused by elastic catheter material could be compensated. A similar artifact is the non-linear rotational velocity caused by friction inside the catheter that still needs to be addressed. Despite that, the results have clearly demonstrated that the combination of both imaging modalities yields accurate reconstructed 3D OCT volumes.

V. Conclusions

This study underlines the beneficial combination of MPI and IVOCT synergizing high temporal and high spatial resolution, non-ionization, artifact reduction and full 3D characteristics of both imaging modalities. For further investigations, the combination of IVOCT and MPI has to be become truly bimodal and MPI has to provide the actual trajectory of the catheter head. By realizing these steps, the synergy of IVOCT and MPI becomes a promising technique for intravascular applications.

ACKNOWLEDGEMENTS

The authors thankfully acknowledge financial support by the German Research Foundation (DFG, grant number KN 1108/2-1).

REFERENCES

[1] B. Gleich and J. Weizenecker. Tomographic imaging using the nonlinear response of magnetic particles. *Nature*, 435(7046):1217-1217, 2005. doi: 10.1038/nature03808.

[2] J. Haegele, J. Rahmer, B. Gleich, et al. Magnetic particle imaging: visualization of instruments for cardiovascular intervention. *Radiology* 265(3), 933–938 (2012).

[3] J. Haegele, S. Biederer, H. Wojtczyk, et al. Toward cardiovascular interventions guided by magnetic particle imaging: First instrument characterization. *Magnetic Resonance in Medicine* 69(6), 1761–1767 (2013).

[4] Panagiotopoulos, S. Cremers, et al. Magnetic particle imaging: A resovist based marking technology for guide wires and catheters for vascular interventions. IEEE Transactions on Medical Imaging, 35(10), 2312–2318 (2016).

[5] J. Salamon, M. Hofmann, C. Jung, et al. Magnetic particle/magnetic resonance imaging: in-vitro mpi-guided real time catheter tracking and 4d angioplasty using a road map and blood pool tracer approach. *PloS one* 11(6), e0156899 (2016).

[6] J. Haegele, S. Vaalma, N. Panagiotopoulos, et al. Multi-color magnetic particle imaging for cardio-vascular interventions. *Physics in Medicine and Biology* 61(16), N415 (2016).

[7] S. Vaalma, J. Rahmer, N. Panagiotopoulos, et al. Magnetic particle imaging (mpi): Experimental quantification of vascular stenosis using stationary stenosis phantoms. *PloS one* 12, 1–22 (2017).

[8] W. R. Brody. Digital subtraction angiography. *IEEE Transactions on Nuclear Science*, 29(3):1176–1180, 1982.

[9] Huang D, Swanson EA, Lin CP, et al. Optical Coherence Tomography. *Science (New York, NY)*. 1991;254(5035):1178-1181.

[10] De Cock, S. Tu, G. J. Ughi, et al. Development of 3d ivoct imaging and co-registration of ivoctand angiography in the catheterization laboratory. Current Cardiovascular Imaging Reports 7, 9290 (2014).

[11] F. Griese, T. Knopp, R. Werner, et al. Submillimeter-Accurate Marker Localization within Low Gradient Magnetic Particle Imaging Tomograms. *International Journal on Magnetic Particle Imaging* 3(1) (2017).

Author Index

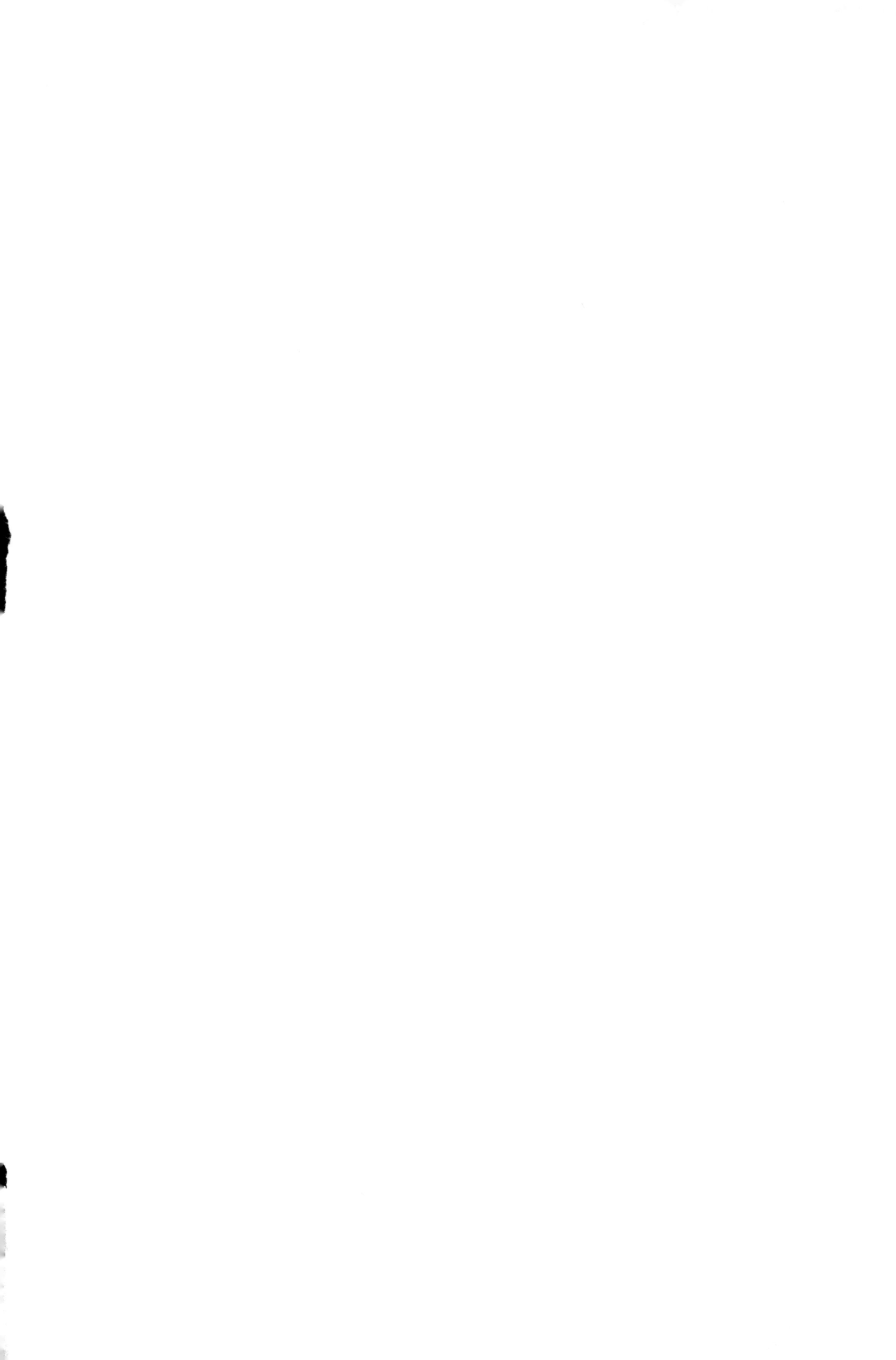